TREATING COMPLEX TRAUMATIC STRESS DISORDERS IN CHILDREN AND ADOLESCENTS

Treating Complex Traumatic Stress Disorders in Children and Adolescents

Scientific Foundations and Therapeutic Models

Edited by
JULIAN D. FORD
CHRISTINE A. COURTOIS

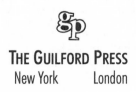

THE GUILFORD PRESS
New York   London

*To all victims and survivors of complex trauma
in childhood and adolescence:
Support is available and healing is possible.*

© 2013 The Guilford Press
A Division of Guilford Publications, Inc.
370 Seventh Avenue, Suite 1200, New York, NY 10001
www.guilford.com

Paperback edition 2016

Printed in the United States of America

This book is printed on acid-free paper.

Last digit is print number: 9 8 7 6 5 4 3

The authors have checked with sources believed to be reliable in her efforts to provide
information that is complete and generally in accord with the standards of practice
that are accepted at the time of publication. However, in view of the possibility of
human error or changes in behavioral, mental health, or medical sciences, neither the
author, nor the editors and publisher, nor any other party who has been involved in
the preparation or publication of this work warrants that the information contained
herein is in every respect accurate or complete, and they are not responsible for any
errors or omissions or the results obtained from the use of such information. Readers
are encouraged to confirm the information contained in this book with other sources.

Library of Congress Cataloging-in-Publication Data

Treating complex traumatic stress disorders in children and adolescents : scientific
foundations and therapeutic models / edited by Julian D. Ford, Christine A. Courtois.
    pages cm
  Includes bibliographical references and index.
  ISBN 978-1-4625-0949-2 (hardcover : alk. paper)
  ISBN 978-1-4625-2461-7 (paperback : alk. paper)
  1. Psychic trauma in children—Treatment.   2. Psychic trauma in adolescence—
Treatment.   3. Child psychotherapy.   I. Ford, Julian D.   II. Courtois, Christine A.
  RJ506.P66T743 2013
  616.85′2100835—dc23   2013002334

About the Editors

Julian D. Ford, PhD, ABPP, a clinical psychologist, is Professor of Psychiatry, Psychology, and Law at the University of Connecticut, where he is also Director of the Center for Trauma Recovery and Juvenile Justice. He has served on the Steering Committee of the National Child Traumatic Stress Network, as Associate Editor of the *Journal of Trauma and Dissociation* and the *European Journal of Psychotraumatology,* as Co-Chair of the Presidential Task Force on Child Trauma for Division 56 (Trauma Psychology) of the American Psychological Association (APA), and as a board member and Vice President of the International Society for Traumatic Stress Studies (ISTSS). With Christine A. Courtois, Dr. Ford is a recipient of the Print Media Award from the International Society for the Study of Trauma and Dissociation (ISSTD) for their coedited volume on treating complex traumatic stress disorders in adults; he has also published several other books on trauma-related topics. Dr. Ford developed and conducts research on the Trauma Affect Regulation: Guide for Education and Therapy (TARGET) psychosocial intervention for adolescents, adults, and families.

Christine A. Courtois, PhD, ABPP, a counseling psychologist in private practice in Washington, DC, is National Clinical Training Director of Elements Behavioral Health; cofounder and past Clinical and Training Director of The CENTER: Posttraumatic Disorders Program, in Washington, DC; chair of APA's Guideline Development Panel for Posttraumatic Stress Disorder; past president of APA Division 56; and past founding Associate Editor of the Division's journal, *Psychological Trauma: Theory, Research, Practice, and Policy.* She is a recipient of the Outstanding Contributions to Professional Practice Award from APA Division 56, the APA Award for Distinguished Professional Contributions to Applied Psychology as a Professional Practice, the Lifetime Achievement Award from ISSTD, and the Sarah Haley Award for Clinical Excellence from ISTSS, among other honors. She has published numerous books (four of them coedited or coauthored with Dr. Ford), book chapters, and articles on trauma-related topics.

Contributors

Pamela C. Alexander, PhD, JBS International, North Bethesda, Maryland

Lisa Amaya-Jackson, MD, MPH, UCLA–Duke National Center for Child Traumatic Stress, Center for Child and Family Health, Duke Evidence-based Practice Implementation Center, Duke University Medical Center, Durham, North Carolina

Rebecca Babcock, MA, Department of Psychology, University of Denver, Denver, Colorado

Margaret E. Blaustein, PhD, The Trauma Center at Justice Resource Institute, Brookline, Massachusetts

Sandra L. Bloom, MD, School of Public Health, Drexel University, Philadelphia, Pennsylvania; Sanctuary Institute, Andrus Center, Yonkers, New York

Robyn Bluhm, PhD, Department of Philosophy and Religious Studies, Old Dominion University, Norfolk, Virginia

John Briere, PhD, Department of Psychiatry and Behavioral Sciences, Keck School of Medicine, University of Southern California, Los Angeles, California

Adam D. Brown, PsyD, Department of Child and Adolescent Psychiatry, NYU School of Medicine/Child Study Center, New York, New York

Judith A. Cohen, MD, Department of Psychiatry, Allegheny General Hospital, Pittsburgh, Pennsylvania

Christine A. Courtois, PhD, Courtois & Associates, PC, Washington, DC

Anne P. DePrince, PhD, Department of Psychology, University of Denver, Denver, Colorado

Ruth R. DeRosa, PhD, Cognitive Behavioral Associates, Great Neck, New York

Christine L. Dobson, PhD, The ChildTrauma Academy, Houston, Texas

B. Heidi Ellis, PhD, Department of Psychiatry, Boston Children's Hospital, Boston, Massachusetts

Kenneth E. Fletcher, PhD, Behavioral Science Research Core, University of Massachusetts Medical School, Worcester, Massachusetts

Julian D. Ford, PhD, Department of Psychiatry, University of Connecticut School of Medicine, Farmington, Connecticut

Paul A. Frewen, PhD, Departments of Psychiatry and Psychology, University of Western Ontario, London, Ontario, Canada

Jennifer J. Freyd, PhD, Department of Psychology, University of Oregon, Eugene, Oregon

Damion Grasso, PhD, Department of Psychiatry, University of Connecticut School of Medicine, Farmington, Connecticut

Carolyn Greene, PhD, Department of Psychiatry, University of Connecticut School of Medicine, Farmington, Connecticut

Mandy Habib, PsyD, Department of Psychiatry, North Shore University Hospital, Manhasset, New York

Laura A. Kaehler, MS, Department of Psychology, University of Oregon, Eugene, Oregon

Richard Kagan, PhD, HEROES Project and Psychological Services, Parsons Child and Family Center, Albany, New York

Amy Klatzkin, MA, private practice, San Francisco, California

Matthew Kliethermes, PhD, Children's Advocacy Services of Greater St. Louis, Department of Psychology, University of Missouri–St. Louis, St. Louis, Missouri

Ruth A. Lanius, MD, PhD, Departments of Psychiatry and Neuroscience, University of Western Ontario, London, Ontario, Canada

Cheryl Lanktree, PhD, private practice and professional training, Santa Monica, California; Department of Psychiatry and Behavioral Sciences, Keck School of Medicine, University of Southern California, Los Angeles, California

Christopher M. Layne, PhD, UCLA–National Center for Child Traumatic Stress, Los Angeles, California

Alicia F. Lieberman, PhD, UCSF Child Trauma Research Program, Division of Infant, Child, and Adolescent Psychiatry, San Francisco General Hospital, San Francisco, California

Anthony P. Mannarino, PhD, Department of Psychiatry, Allegheny General Hospital, Pittsburgh, Pennsylvania

Kathleen Nader, PhD, private practice, Cedar Park, Texas

Carryl P. Navalta, PhD, Mental Health Counseling and Behavioral Medicine Program, Boston University School of Medicine, Boston, Massachusetts

Amanda Nisewaner, MSW, Lincoln Child Center, Oakland, California

Bruce D. Perry, MD, PhD, The ChildTrauma Academy, Houston, Texas; Department of Psychiatry and Behavioral Sciences, Feinberg School of Medicine, Northwestern University, Chicago, Illinois; The Berry Street Childhood Institute, Melbourne, Australia

Jill H. Rathus, PhD, Department of Psychology, Long Island University, C. W. Post Campus, Brookville, New York

Glenn N. Saxe, MD, Department of Child and Adolescent Psychiatry, NYU School of Medicine/Child Study Center, New York, New York

Allan N. Schore, PhD, Department of Psychiatry and Biobehavioral Sciences, UCLA David Geffen School of Medicine, Northridge, California

Francine Shapiro, PhD, Mental Research Institute, Palo Alto, California

Joyanna Silberg, PhD, Sheppard Pratt Health System, Baltimore, Maryland

Susan Timmer, PhD, Mental Health Services and Clinical Research, CAARE Diagnostic and Treatment Center, Department of Pediatrics, UC Davis Children's Hospital, Sacramento, California

Anthony J. Urquiza, PhD, Mental Health Services and Clinical Research, CAARE Diagnostic and Treatment Center, Department of Pediatrics, UC Davis Children's Hospital, Sacramento, California

Patricia Van Horn, PhD, UCSF Child Trauma Research Program, Division of Infant, Child, and Adolescent Psychiatry, San Francisco General Hospital, San Francisco, California

Rachel Wamser Nanney, MA, Children's Advocacy Services of Greater St. Louis, Department of Psychology, University of Missouri–St. Louis, St. Louis, Missouri

Debra Wesselmann, MS, The Attachment and Trauma Center of Nebraska, Omaha, Nebraska

Sandra Wieland, PhD, private practice, Victoria, British Columbia, Canada

Preface

Treating children and adolescents with complex trauma histories and complex traumatic stress disorders provides countless challenges and opportunities for therapists and researchers. These children often come into treatment with many diagnoses, medications, and unsuccessful past treatments and placements, as well as with what may seem to be intractable emotional and behavioral problems. A complex trauma perspective can provide the clinician with an invaluable unifying framework for understanding these children, as well as for doing case conceptualization, assessment, and treatment in the midst of the chaos and turmoil of their lives. The aim of this book is to provide clinicians with this unifying perspective and with a comprehensive and up-to-date guide to the treatments available for children and adolescents with complex traumatic stress disorders.

Remarkable progress has taken place in recent years in the identification of complex trauma early in life and in the development, evaluation, and dissemination of treatments to help children and adolescents recover from its various aftereffects. These therapeutic interventions for children and adolescents with complex trauma histories are crucially important because they have the potential to prevent or attenuate trauma-related changes that otherwise may lead to a lifetime of recurrent developmental interruptions and challenges, as well as trauma-related reactions, symptoms, and impairments.

In this book, as in its predecessor, *Treating Complex Traumatic Stress Disorders: An Evidence-Based Guide* (Courtois & Ford, 2009; focused on the treatment of adults), we address the challenges facing clinicians when they treat young survivors of complex forms of psychological trauma. The book begins with a seven-chapter overview of recent advances in the science of early childhood brain development, attachment bonding, development of the self, emotion regulation, and the translation of these into clinical practice. The 11 chapters that follow describe cutting-edge therapeutic models that span the theoretical spectrum, each with a case vignette to which the model is applied. This book is intended primarily for clinicians within the mental health and behavioral health professions who evaluate and treat traumatized children and adolescents and their families, and for clinical researchers and graduate-level trainees in those professions (e.g., psychology, psychiatry, counseling, social work, marriage and family therapy, addiction treatment, employee assistance program staff). It informs allied professionals who work directly with trauma survivors, or consult with and refer to mental health colleagues who treat trauma survivors—such as medical and nursing practitioners, attorneys and judges, educators, personal coaches, child protective services workers, family or parent advocacy or support services providers, or police and other forensic and juvenile justice personnel. This book could be used as either a primary or secondary text in psychology, psychiatry, social work, marriage and family therapy, or counseling training programs.

We define complex psychological trauma as experiences that (1) are interpersonal and often involve betrayal; (2) are repetitive or prolonged; (3) involve direct harm through various forms of abuse (psychological/emotional, physical, and sexual), neglect, or abandonment by persons who are responsible for the care, protection, or guidance of others, especially youngsters and offspring (such as parents, family caregivers, teachers, coaches, or religious advisors), or traumatic losses in those relationships; and (4) occur at developmentally vulnerable times in life, such as early childhood, or undermine important developmental attainments at any point in the lifespan. Potential examples of complex trauma include identity- or gender-based victimization, ongoing domestic or sexual violence, historical trauma, torture, mass political violence, kidnapping and human trafficking, physical and homeland displacement and becoming a refugee, or genocide.

Whether freestanding or building on previous traumatization, such experiences tend to compromise or derail a child's primary relationships and ability to trust, connect to, and be intimate with others. Severe and pervasive complex traumatic stress disorders can develop as a result of this fundamental threat or harm at any point across the lifespan, but especially when it involves a child or adolescent's bodily or personal integrity or the security and stability of primary relationships. Problems associated with complex traumatic stress disorders include dissociation, emotional dysregulation, impulsivity and associated high-risk behaviors, aggression toward self and others, addictions and compulsions, pervasive states of anxiety, and hopelessness, isolation, and profound alienation. They extend well beyond the classic symptoms of posttraumatic stress disorder (PTSD) and are difficult to diagnose accurately and treat effectively. This book's primary aim is to provide practicing therapists with an overview of these disorders and the variability of their symptoms and clinical presentations, a thorough and practical overview of the biological and psychosocial foundations of effective treatment, and an introduction to contemporary evidence-based treatment approaches that can immediately inform their clinical work with complexly traumatized children and adolescents.

Unique features of this book include its comprehensive overview of a variety of state-of-the-art and evidence-based treatments for children and adolescents with complex traumatic stress disorders. It also offers a complete and authoritative summary of the neurobiological, attachment, and developmental substrates and emotional, behavioral, and relational features of children's and adolescents' complex traumatic stress disorders beyond those captured by the classic diagnosis of PTSD. In this volume we present a detailed review of assessment strategies and instruments for both trauma exposure and the range of self-regulation problems experienced by children and adolescents with complex traumatic stress disorders. Clinical vignettes enable readers to experience and understand moment-to-moment interactions and the course of sophisticated treatments for children and adolescents with these disorders.

In this book you will also find a careful consideration of how a complex trauma perspective helps clinicians engage otherwise unreachable children and adolescents who are mistrustful of and often resistant and hostile toward authority figures, including counselors and psychotherapists. These clients are emotionally, behaviorally, interpersonally, and somatically dysregulated. Clinicians struggle to help them gain control over the accompanying emotional firestorms, out-of-control behavior, alienation from others, and sense of being permanently damaged in order to enable them to heal their profound psychological and interpersonal wounds. The chapters addressing these particularly difficult challenges also offer support and empathy for therapists facing the frustrations and challenges of treating these children and adolescents.

Several key themes run through all of the chapters in this book. The core foundation for treating children with complex trauma histories is an understanding of the source and nature of their symptoms and impairment. First, exposure to complex traumatic stressors in early life has a biological impact that can fundamentally alter the structure and functioning of areas in the brain that are essential to a child's development of nonverbal/implicit and emotional forms of intelligence and an integrated and positive sense of self (see Chapters 1 and 2). Second, when the shock and threat of traumatic stressors are compounded by the obviation, disruption, or loss of fundamental attachment bonds, brain development is particularly vulnerable to impairment (see Chapters 1 and 2), jeopardizing the development of a sense of self (see Chapter 3). The associated capacity to trust and engage in healthy relationships (see Chapters 3 and 4) often is profoundly impaired as well.

Third, children and adolescents who have experienced complex trauma from an early age may require qualitatively different approaches to treatment than even the most severely traumatized child who has not had to survive multiple forms of victimization (see Chapter 5). These children often have been labeled as unable to benefit from treatment, while simultaneously being overmedicated or treated with methods that require a degree of self-regulation that complex trauma has prevented them from developing (see Chapters 1–3). It is essential that therapy not inadvertently contribute to the sense of betrayal and hopelessness that these children have experienced (see Chapter 4). In order to avoid the pitfall of continued "failures" in treatment, clinicians must be able to bring to the treatment of complexly traumatized children a combination of "clinical creativity, guided by sound clinical theory, evidence-based assessment, wise clinical judgment, and an evolving evidence base" (see Chapter 6, p. 112). The remainder of the book provides clinicians with several templates for effective treatment of children and adolescents who are complex trauma survivors.

We begin the treatment section of the book by considering how assessment can cover not just PTSD and other familiar Axis I symptoms of psychiatric disorders but also the child's strengths and problems in several domains of self-regulation—including physiological, affective, cognitive, behavioral, relational, and identity (see Chapter 7). We turn next to approaches to treatment that draw on scientific and clinical innovations in the traumatic stress field. We provided an overview of this empirically based approach to treating children and adolescents with complex traumatic stress disorders in a chapter (Ford & Cloitre, 2009) in our previous edited book (Courtois & Ford, 2009). Chapter 8 (on integrated treatment of complex trauma) begins with a thorough overview of the impressive and growing range of treatment options and suggestions for customizing them to the needs of the client and family.

Treatment of children who have complex trauma histories and correspondingly complex problems with self-regulation typically must address not just one but several of the fundamental types of posttraumatic dysregulation. Dissociation is a particularly challenging manifestation of trauma-related impaired self-regulation that requires a sophisticated understanding of fragmented self-states and their manifestation in the developing child (see Chapter 9). At the other end of the spectrum, children and adolescents with complex trauma histories often emotionally shut down and "act out" in an attempt to avoid painful trauma reminders. Treatment must enable these children to safely create a narrative of their traumatic experiences that they can emotionally face and process—no small feat when their trauma-related dysregulation is so complex and extended that identifying and organizing memories of past traumatic experiences is a substantial clinical challenge (see Chapters 10 and 11). These children, and particularly adolescents, exhibit severe emotional and behavioral dysregulation for which they need practical self-regulation skills and finely attuned guidance (see Chapters

12–14). Often, the families, communities, and therapeutic programs and providers caring for these children and youth need a framework to guide them in creating systems of care that intentionally support self-regulation (see Chapters 14, 15, 17, and 18) across several generations (see Chapter 16), and ultimately that become a sanctuary from trauma (see Chapter 15).

Creating such a system of care is a tall order, indeed, but one that is within the grasp of any provider or program willing to become "complex trauma informed."

It is to that goal, and to the clinicians who are willing to take on the daunting challenges that are involved in providing psychotherapy to children with complex traumatic stress disorders, that this book is dedicated.

Acknowledgments

The editors gratefully acknowledge the courage and resilience of the girls and boys and young women and men whom they've had the privilege of working with and learning from in therapy, as well as the compassion and strength of their caregivers and families. The capacity of these youth and families to recover from complex trauma has been an inspiration that has sustained us in this challenging work. We also want to sincerely thank each author who contributed to this book—they are our irreplaceable colleagues, role models, and friends. And we are appreciative of the wisdom and support we've received from many other esteemed professional colleagues, including coleaders and team members in the Center for Trauma Recovery and Juvenile Justice and the Complex Trauma Treatment Network; the larger National Child Traumatic Stress Network of the Substance Abuse and Mental Health Services Administration and SAMHSA's Trauma-Informed Care Initiative (J.F.); our colleagues in the International Society for Traumatic Stress Studies (with special thanks to the members of the Complex Trauma Task Force); Division 56 of the American Psychological Association and its journal *Psychological Trauma*; and the International Society for the Study of Trauma and Dissociation and its *Journal of Trauma and Dissociation*. Dr. Ford also thanks his colleagues in Connecticut's Child Health and Development Institute and Judicial Branch Court Support Services Division, and in the Child Division and the larger Department of Psychiatry and School of Medicine at the University of Connecticut. Dr. Courtois thanks members of her personal and professional support system for their ongoing tolerance and encouragement and for their reminders to take breaks and have some fun in the midst of it all. This book would not be possible without the mentoring and support that they've provided to us and through their tireless efforts on behalf of children and families.

We want to specially acknowledge Guilford Senior Editor Jim Nageotte and Editorial Assistant Jane Keislar, who provided us with the benefit of their invaluable experience, expertise, and perseverance. We also owe a debt that can never be fully repaid to each of our spouses, Judy and Tom, for their love, brilliant insights, and patience above and beyond the call.

References

Courtois, C. A., & Ford, J. D. (Eds.). (2009). *Treating complex traumatic stress disorders: An evidence-based guide*. New York: Guilford Press.

Ford, J. D., & Cloitre, M. (2009). Best practices in psychotherapy for children and adolescents. In C. A. Courtois & J. D. Ford (Eds.), *Treating complex traumatic stress disorders: An evidence-based guide* (pp. 59–81). New York: Guilford Press.

Contents

II. INDIVIDUAL PSYCHOTHERAPY MODELS

III. SYSTEMIC APPROACHES TO TREATMENT

PART I

COMPLEX TRAUMA IN CHILDHOOD AND ADOLESCENCE

CHAPTER 1

Relational Trauma, Brain Development, and Dissociation

Allan N. Schore

Over the past two decades I have integrated findings from scientific studies and clinical data in order to construct regulation theory, a neuro-psychoanalytic model of the development, psychopathogenesis, and treatment of the implicit self (Schore, 2001, 2002). In these expositions I have suggested that in contrast to single-incident trauma from the physical environment, the intense social stressor of early relational trauma is typically ambient, cumulative, and derived from the interpersonal environment. In light of the fact that the infant's first interactions with the interpersonal environment take place within the emotional transactions of the attachment relationship, I equated developmental relational trauma with attachment trauma. Using the perspective of interpersonal neurobiology, I then described the impact of two common expressions of attachment trauma, abuse and neglect, on brain development, especially during the brain growth spurt from the last trimester through the second year of human infancy. Relational trauma thus can be understood as the quintessential expression of "complex trauma," which has been defined as "repeated interpersonal trauma occurring during crucial developmental periods" (Lanius et al., 2011, p. 2).

More recently I have expanded the model of the developmental and biological disruptions that result from relational trauma (Schore, 2009a, 2009b, 2010a, 2012). In the present chapter I continue to build on those works and provide very recent interdisciplinary data from developmental neuroscience and interpersonal neurobiology that allow for a deeper understanding of the psychological *and* biological effects of early relational trauma, especially caregiver maltreatment in the form of abuse and neglect.

Over this time period the field of developmental neuroscience has experienced "phenomenal progress" (Leckman & March, 2011, p. 333). In a recent issue of the *Journal of Child Psychology and Psychiatry* devoted to the direct relevance of these advances for both research and clinical practice, Roth and Sweatt (2011, p. 400) articulate the currently accepted view of the long-term effect of early caregiver maltreatment in psychopathogenesis:

> Abusive and neglectful experiences from the caregiver are known to leave a child particularly susceptible to cognitive and mental dysfunction. Indeed, there is a significant association of reported childhood maltreatment and the later diagnosis of adolescent and adulthood schizophrenia, borderline personality disorder, posttraumatic stress disorder, and major depression.

Leckman and March (2011) conclude: "A complex, dynamic story is unfolding of evolutionarily conserved genetic programs that guide mammalian brain development and how our in utero and our early postnatal *interpersonal worlds* shape and mold the individuals (infants, children, adolescents, adults and caregivers) we are to become" (p. 333, emphasis added).

The shaping of brain development by our early interpersonal worlds is an essential focus of the fields of interpersonal neurobiology and developmental neuropsychoanalysis. Recall that Bowlby's (1969) formulation of attachment theory attempted to integrate biology and psychoanalysis. For the past two decades a growing body of research indicates that the right hemisphere of the brain is the biological substrate of the human unconscious. This conception is echoed in recent neuroscientific writings by Tucker and Moller (2007): "The right hemisphere's specialization for emotional communication through nonverbal channels seems to suggest a domain of the mind that is close to the motivationally charged psychoanalytic unconscious" (p. 91). This chapter focuses on current studies of the enduring impact of relational trauma on the early maturing right hemisphere of the brain, and thereby on the early development of the human unconscious mind that forms an internal representation of our early interpersonal worlds.

This *interpersonal neurobiological model* explicates the mechanisms by which attachment shapes, for better of worse, the survival functions regulated by the right hemisphere of the brain. It is now clear that the developing brain is not "resilient" but "malleable" (Schore, 2012). In the following sections I offer an overview of studies on the developmental interpersonal neurobiology of secure attachment, and then on how relational trauma negatively impacts the developmental trajectory of the brain's right hemisphere and the mind and body over the course of the lifespan. Also discussed is the etiology of pathological dissociation, the bottom-line defense of all early-forming severe developmental psychopathologies.

Developmental Interpersonal Biology of Secure Attachment

The essential task of the first year of human life is the creation of a secure attachment bond of emotional communication and interactive regulation between the infant and primary caregiver (Schore & Schore, 2008). Secure attachment depends upon the caregiver's psychobiological attunement with the infant's dynamic alterations of arousal and affective states. Through nonverbal visual–facial, tactile–gestural, and auditory–prosodic communications, the caregiver and infant learn the rhythmic structure of the other and modify their behavior to fit that structure, thereby co-creating a specifically fitted interaction. During the affective communications of mutual gaze, the empathically attuned mother synchronizes the spatial–temporal patterning of her exogenous sensory stimulation with the infant's spontaneous expressions of endogenous organismic rhythms. Via this contingent responsivity, the mother appraises the nonverbal expressions of her infant's internal arousal and affective states, regulates them, and communicates them back to the infant. To accomplish this sequence, the sensitive mother must successfully modulate nonoptimal high *or* excessively low levels of stimulation that would induce extremely heightened or lowered levels of arousal in the infant.

Primary caregivers are not always able to attune to, and optimally mirror, their infants, leading to frequent moments of misattunement in the dyad and ruptures of the attachment bond. The disruption of attachment transactions leads to a transient regulatory failure and an impaired autonomic homeostasis. In the pattern of "interactive repair" or "disruption and repair" following dyadic misattunement, the "good-enough" caregiver who induces a stress response through misattunement reinvokes, in a timely fashion, a reattunement—that is, a regulation of the infant's negatively charged arousal. This repair process allows the infant to cope with stressful negatively charged affects and ultimately allows the individual to gain self-regulatory skills in the form of maintaining persistent efforts to overcome interactive stress.

In a secure attachment relationship the regulatory processes of affect synchrony that co-create positive arousal and interactive repair of negative arousal allow for the emergence of efficient self-regulation (Bradshaw & Schore, 2007). These affectively synchronized experiences trigger homeostatic alterations of neuropeptides (oxytocin, endorphins, corticotropin-releasing factor, growth factors, etc.), neuromodulators (catecholamines), and neurosteroids (cortisol) that are critical to the establishment of social bonds and to brain development (Schore, 1994, 2005; Wismer Fries, Ziegler, Kurian, Jacoris, & Pollak, 2005). Protective and growth-facilitating attachment experiences have long-term effects on the developing hypothalamic–pituitary–adrenocortical (HPA) axis, which plays a central role in the regulation of stress reactivity (Gunnar, 2000).

In this manner, the optimal interactively regulated affective communications embedded in secure attachment experiences directly imprint the postnatally maturing central nervous system (CNS) limbic system that processes and regulates social–emotional stimuli and the autonomic nervous system (ANS) that generates the somatic aspects of emotion. The limbic system derives subjective information in terms of emotional feelings that guide behavior and allow the brain to adapt to a rapidly changing environment and organize new learning. The higher regulatory systems of the right hemisphere form extensive reciprocal connections with the ANS and the limbic system. Both the ANS and the CNS continue to develop postnatally, and the assembly of these limbic–autonomic circuits (Rinaman, Levitt, & Card, 2000) in the right hemisphere, which is dominant for the human stress response (Wittling, 1997), is directly influenced by the attachment relationship.

A large body of studies now supports the proposal that the long-enduring regulatory effects of attachment are due to their impact on brain development (Schore, 1994, 2003b, 2009a, 2012). The right hemisphere is in a critical growth period from the last trimester of pregnancy through the second year (Chiron et al., 1997; Mento, Suppiej, Altoe, & Bisiacchi, 2010). Attachment transactions in the first year are occurring when total brain volume is increasing by 101% and the volume of the subcortical areas by 130% (Knickmeyer et al., 2008). Because the human limbic system myelinates in the first year and a half, and the early-maturing right hemisphere (Gupta et al., 2005; Schore, 1994; Sun et al., 2005)—which is deeply connected into the limbic system (Gainotti, 2000)—is undergoing a growth spurt at this time, attachment communications specifically impact limbic and cortical areas of the developing right brain (Ammaniti & Trentini, 2009; Cozolino, 2002; Henry, 1993; Schore, 1994, 2000, 2005; Siegel, 1999). Howard and Reggia (2007) state, "Earlier maturation of the right hemisphere is supported by both anatomical and imaging evidence" (p. 112).

In my ongoing work, I continue to present data indicating that the attachment mechanism is embedded in infant–caregiver right-brain to right-brain affective transactions (Schore, 1994, 2000, 2003b, 2009c). Consistent with this interpersonal neurobiological model, researchers in a near-infrared spectroscopy study of infant–mother attachment conclude, "our results are in agreement with that of Schore (2000) who addressed the importance of the right hemisphere in the attachment system" (Minagawa-Kawai et al., 2009, p. 289).

An essential tenet of the interpersonal neurobiological perspective of regulation theory is that affective attachment transactions shape the cortical–subcortical emotion- and stress-regulating circuits of the developing right brain during early critical periods. Indeed, basic research now establishes that optimal stress regulation is dependent on "right hemispheric specialization in regulating stress- and emotion-related processes" (Sullivan & Dufresne, 2006, p. 55). Over the first 2 years of life, a hierarchy of regulatory centers emerges in the developing right brain (Schore, 2003a, 2010b, 2012). Specifically, the subcortical amygdala, with its connections into the insula and hypothalamus, and thereby into the ANS and the HPA axis, is functional at birth. At 3–9 months of age, the anterior cingulate (medial-frontal cortex), a cortical–limbic structure that is associated with responsivity to social cues, comes online, giving the infant even greater self-regulatory capacities. From 10–12 months of age, the regulatory center in the orbital–frontal cortex begins its developmental growth period. This ventral-medial prefrontal cortex, especially in the right hemisphere, is the locus of Bowlby's attachment control system and contains the brain's most complex affect- and stress-regulating mechanisms (Schore, 1994, 2003a, 2003b). Supporting this model, developmental neurobiological research now confirms that the dendritic and synaptic maturation of the anterior cingulate and orbital-frontal cortices is specifically influenced by the social environment (Bock, Murmu, Ferdman, Leshem, & Braun, 2008). Indeed, a recent review of the functional neuroanatomy of the parent–infant relationship by Parsons, Young, Murray, Stein, and Kringelbach (2010, p. 235) concludes, "The same adult brain networks involved in emotional and social interactions are already present in immature and incomplete forms in the infant," specifically mentioning the amygdala, hypothalamus, insula, cingulate cortex, and orbitofrontal cortex.

With optimal attachment experiences, the vertical axis that connects the orbital-frontal and medial prefrontal cortices with multiple cortical and subcortical areas is well developed. This allows the right orbital-frontal cortex to efficiently regulate the subcortical amygdala, which has been shown to be centrally involved in the generation of attachment security (Lemche et al., 2006). Moreover, developmental neurobiological research reveals that coping with early life stress increases the myelination of the ventral-medial cortex, a prefrontal region that controls arousal regulation and resilience (Katz et al., 2009). For the rest of the lifespan the *right* lateralized prefrontal regions are responsible for the regulation of affects, especially stressful affects (Cerqueira, Almeida, & Sousa, 2008; Czeh, Perez-Cruz, Fuchs, & Flugge, 2008; Schore, 1994; Sullivan & Gratton, 2002; Wang et al., 2005). Attachment histories appear to be imprinted into right cortical–subcortical circuits in implicit procedural memory, thus generating an internal working model of attachment that encodes strategies of affect regulation that nonconsciously guide the individual through interpersonal contexts. These adaptive capacities are central to the dual processes of self-regulation:

interactive regulation, the ability to flexibly regulate psychobiological states of emotions with other humans in interconnected contexts, and autoregulation, which occurs apart from other humans in autonomous contexts.

Developmental Interpersonal Biology of Relational Trauma and Dissociation

In contrast to caregivers who foster secure attachment, attachment trauma occurs when the caregiver is either hyperintrusive or emotionally inaccessible and disengaged, given to inappropriate and/or rejecting responses to the infant's expressions of emotions and stress. Such responses provide minimal or unpredictable regulation of the infant's states of over- or underarousal. Instead, the caregiver induces extreme levels of stimulation and arousal (i.e., the very high stimulation of abuse and/or the very low stimulation of neglect). Due to the fact that no interactive repair of frequent significant affective ruptures of the attachment relationship is provided, the caregiver leaves the infant to endure extremely stressful and intense negative states for long periods of time. In an immature organism with undeveloped and restricted coping capacities, stress regulation, and therefore a sense of safety, must be provided by the primary caregiver. When not safety but danger emanates from the attachment relationship, the homeostatic assaults have significant short- and long-term consequences on the maturing psyche and soma.

In terms of the short-term effects, interdisciplinary evidence indicates that the infant's psychobiological reaction to severe interpersonal stressors is comprised of two separate response patterns: hyperarousal and dissociation (Perry, Pollard, Blakley, Baker, & Vigilante, 1995; Schore, 2003a). In the earliest stage of threat, the child's sudden alarm or startle reaction indicates activation of the infant's right hemisphere. This, in turn, evokes a sudden increase of the energy-expending sympathetic branch of the ANS, resulting in significantly elevated heart rate (cardiac acceleration), blood pressure, and respiration. Distress is expressed via crying and then screaming. The infant's state of frantic distress, or fear terror, is mediated by sympathetic hyperarousal that is expressed in increased secretion of corticotropin-releasing factor (CRF)—the brain's major stress hormone. CRF regulates sympathetic catecholamine activity, and thus noradrenaline, dopamine, and adrenaline levels are significantly elevated, creating a hypermetabolic state within the developing brain. Increased concentrations of cortisol and glutamate (the major excitatory neurotransmitter in the brain) also accompany the state of hyperarousal.

A second later-forming reaction to relational trauma is dissociation, in which the child disengages from stimuli in the external world—traumatized infants often are observed to be "staring off into space with a glazed look." The child's dissociation in the midst of terror involves numbing, avoidance, compliance, and restricted affect. This energy-conserving parasympathetic-dominant state of conservation–withdrawal occurs in helpless and hopeless stressful situations in which the individual becomes inhibited and strives to avoid attention in order to become "unseen" (Schore, 1994, 2003a, 2003b). This state of metabolic shutdown and cardiac deceleration is a primary regulatory process that is used throughout the lifespan. In conservation–withdrawal, the stressed individual passively disengages in order "to conserve energies . . . to foster survival by the risky posture of feigning death, to allow healing of wounds and restitution of depleted resources by immobility" (Powles, 1992, p. 213). This parasympathetic mechanism has been hypothesized to mediate the "profound detachment" (Barach, 1991) of dissociation. If early trauma is experienced as "psychic catastrophe" (Bion, 1962), then dissociation is a "detachment from an unbearable situation" (Mollon, 1996), "the escape when there is no escape" (Putnam, 1997), "a last resort defensive strategy" (Dixon, 1998).

The neurobiology of dissociative hypoarousal is different from that of hyperarousal. In this passive state of pain numbing and blunting, endogenous opiates are elevated. Serotonin dysregulation may play an important role (Pieper, Out, Bakermans-Kranenburg, & van IJzendoorn, 2011), consistent with the view that elevated parasympathetic arousal may be viewed as a survival strategy that allows the infant to maintain homeostasis in the face of the internal state of sympathetic hyperarousal. It is important to note that sympathetic energy-expending hyperarousal *and* parasympathetic energy-conserving hypoarousal are both states of "extreme emotional arousal" (Dixon, 1998).

It is now known that there are two parasympathetic vagal systems (Porges, 1997). The late-developing "mammalian" or "smart" ventral vagal system, in the nucleus ambiguus, enables contingent social interactions and secure attachment transactions via the ability to communicate with facial expressions, vocalizations, and gestures. On the other hand, the early-developing "reptilian" or "vegetative" system in the dorsal motor nucleus of the vagus shuts down metabolic activity during intense social stress, generating immobilization, death feigning, and hiding behaviors (Porges, 1997). As opposed to the mammalian ventral vagal complex that can rapidly regulate cardiac output to foster engagement and disengagement with the social environment, the dorsal vagal complex "contributes to severe emotional states and may be related to emotional states of 'immobilization' such as extreme terror" (Porges, 1997, p. 75).

The traumatized infant's sudden switch from high-energy sympathetic hyperarousal to low-energy parasympathetic dissociation is reflected in Porges's characterization of "the sudden and rapid transition from an unsuccessful strategy of struggling requiring massive sympathetic activation to the metabolically conservative immobilized state mimicking death associated with the dorsal vagal complex" (1997, p. 75). Whereas the nucleus ambiguus exhibits rapid and transitory patterns (associated with perceptive pain and unpleasantness), the dorsal vagal nucleus exhibits an involuntary and prolonged pattern of vagal outflow. This prolonged dorsal vagal parasympathetic activation could explain the lengthy "void" states that are associated with pathological dissociative detachment (Allen, Console, & Lewis, 1999).

Disorganized Attachment: The Role of Trauma and Maternal and Child Dissociation

How are the trauma-induced alterations of the developing right brain expressed in the social–emotional behavior of a traumatized toddler? Main and Solomon's (1986) classic study of attachment in traumatized infants revealed a new attachment category, type D, an insecure–disorganized/disoriented pattern that occurs in 80% of maltreated infants (Carlson, Cicchetti, Barnett, & Braunwald, 1989) and that is behaviorally similar to dissociative states (Hesse & Main, 1999). For example:

> One infant hunched her upper body and shoulders at hearing her mother's call, then broke into extravagant laugh-like screeches with an excited forward movement. Her braying laughter became a cry and distress-face without a new intake of breath as the infant hunched forward. Then suddenly she became silent, blank and dazed. (Main & Solomon, 1986, p. 119)

Main and Solomon (1986) document that type D infants often encounter disturbing and dissociative maternal behavior of two kinds: intrusive and apparently angry behavior, or maternal withdrawal and expressions of fear terror. Hesse and Main (2006) hypothesize that when the mother enters a dissociative state, a fear alarm state is triggered in the infant. In their description, the caregiver suddenly completely " 'freezes' with eyes unmoving, half-lidded, despite nearby movement and addresses the infant in an 'altered' tone with simultaneous voicing and devoicing" (2006, p. 320):

> Here the parent appears to have become completely unresponsive to, or even aware of, the external surround, including the physical and verbal behavior of their infant. . . . We observed one mother who remained seated in an immobilized and uncomfortable position with her hand in the air, blankly staring into space for 50 sec. (p. 321)

Ongoing developmental research now underscores a strong link between dissociative-like maternal behavior and disorganized infant attachment (Schuengel, Bakersmans-Kranenburg, & van IJzendoorn, 1999; MacDonald et al., 2008).

In recent writings Beebe and colleagues (2010) report studies of mothers of 4-month-old infants who later show disorganized attachment. They observe that the mothers of these infants are overwhelmed by their own unresolved abuse or trauma and therefore cannot bear to intersubjectively engage with their infant's distress. Because these mothers are unable to regulate their own distress, they cannot regulate their infant's distress. Because these mothers are unable to allow themselves to be emotionally affected by their infant's dysregulated state, they shut down emotionally, closing their faces, looking away from the infant's face, and failing to coordinate with the infant's emotional state. Beebe interprets this fearful maternal behavior as a defensive dissociation, a strategy that protects the mother from the facial and visual intimacy that would come from joining the infant's distressed moments. This type of mother thus shows disrupted and contradictory forms of affective communication (abuse intrusiveness hyperarousal *and* neglect disengagement hypoarousal), especially around the infant's need for comfort when distressed.

Over an ongoing period of relational trauma, the mother's disengagement and "detachment from an unbearable situation" is matched by the infant's disengagement, detachment, and withdrawal. Milne, Greenway, Guedeney, and Larroque (2009) describe the long-term negative developmental impact of social withdrawal and depression in 6-month-old infants. They conclude:

> A withdrawal response in infancy is problematic behavior .. . not because it leads to later withdrawal per se, but because of the compounding effects on development of not being present in the interpersonal space—the space upon which much of infant development depends. (p. 165)

Guedeney, Foucault, Bougen, Larroque, and Mentre (2008) report a study of relational withdrawal in infants ages 14–18 months. This withdrawal reaction reflects inadequate parent–infant interactions and is a feature of disorganized attachment. Guedeney et al. (2008) note: "Sustained withdrawal behavior may be viewed as a chronic diminution of the attachment system, which is gradually generalized into a diminished engagement and lowered reactivity to the environment as a whole" (p. 151). They conclude:

> Withdrawn social behavior from as early as 2 months of age, indicated by a lack of either positive (e.g., smiling, eye contact) or negative (e.g., vocal protestations) behavior, is more akin to a state of learned helplessness and should alert the clinician to the possibility that the infant is not displaying age-appropriate emotional/social behavior. (p. 151)

The developing infant/toddler who has an early history of traumatic attachment is too frequently exposed to a massively misattuning primary caregiver who triggers and does not repair long-lasting, intensely dysregulated states. The growth-inhibiting environment of relational trauma may generate dense and prolonged levels of negative affect associated with extremely stressful states of hyper- and hypoarousal. For self-protective purposes the child severely restricts her or his overt expressions of an attachment need for dyadic regulation. As discussed above, this restricted expression would be consistent with a reduction in the output of the right-lateralized emotion-processing, limbic–autonomic attachment system. When stressed, defensive functions may be rapidly initiated that quickly shift the brain from interactive regulatory modes into long-enduring, less complex autoregulatory modes that may result in dissociation.

During these episodes, the child appears to be matching the rhythmic structures of the mother's dysregulated states; this synchronization can be registered in the firing patterns of the stress-sensitive cortical and limbic regions of the infant's brain, especially in the right brain, which is in a critical period of growth (Bazhenova, Stroganova, Doussard-Roosevelt, & Posikera, 2007; Buss et al., 2003; de Haan, Belsky, Reid, Volein, & Johnson, 2004). Thus the chaotic and dysregulated alterations of state induced by relational trauma may become imprinted into the developing right brain self-system of the child.

From a developmental psychopathological viewpoint, a profound negative psychological effect of relational trauma (early abuse and neglect) is the generation of a disorganized attachment that endures over the later stages of childhood, adolescence, and adulthood and acts as a risk factor for later psychiatric and personality disorders (Schore, 2001, 2002, 2003a). From a developmental neuroscience perspective, the immediate detrimental psychobiological impact is an alteration in metabolic processes that can now only poorly sustain the critical growth period of the developing right brain, and the lasting impairment is an immature and functionally limited right-brain capacity to regulate later life stressors that, unregulated, generate intense affect states (Schore, 2003b). Montirosso, Borgatti, and Tronick (2010) conclude: "Infants cope with the emotional distress caused by unresponsive mothers through self-regulation behaviors associated with a greater activation of the right hemisphere. This finding supports the view that during a stressful condition there is a state-dependent activation of the right hemisphere" (p. 108).

Relational traumatic experiences are believed to be stored in the form of visual and procedural memories associated with the visual–spatial right hemisphere (Schiffer, Teicher, & Papanicolaou, 1995), which is dominant for the processing of unconscious emotions (Gainotti, 2012) and is the locus of implicit (Hugdahl, 1995) and autobiographical (Daselaar et al., 2007; Markowitsch, Reinkemeier, Kessler, Koyuncu, & Heiss, 2000) memory. Recent models of early-life trauma thus shift the focus from deficits in later-maturing conscious, verbal, explicit, and voluntary behavior to impairments in early-maturing nonconscious, nonverbal, implicit, and automatic adaptive social–emotional functions (Schore, 2010c). These psychological and biological perspectives converge on a basic developmental principle of regulation theory: that early traumatic sundering of attachment bonds is critical to the genesis of an enduring predisposition to a variety of early-forming severe psychopathologies that involve the autoregulating, affect-deadening defense of pathological dissociation.

A Model of the Enduring Effects of Relational Trauma: Impaired Right-Brain Emotion Processing and Stress Regulation and Pathological Dissociation

Describing the capacities of the right-lateralized "social brain," Brancucci, Lucci, Mazzatenta, and Tommasi (2009) conclude: "The neural substrates of the perception of voices, faces, gestures, smells and pheromones, as evidenced by modern neuroimaging techniques, are characterized by a general pattern of right-hemispheric functional asymmetry" (p. 895). Over all stages of the lifespan, this hemisphere is dominant not only for the processing of social interactions (Decety & Lamm, 2007; Semrud-Clikeman, Fine, & Zhu, 2011), but also for coping with negative affects (Davidson, Ekman, Saron, Senulis, & Friesen, 1990), the organization of the human stress response (Wittling, 1997), and stress regulation (Cerqueira et al., 2008; Schore, 1994; Stevenson, Halliday, Marsden, & Mason, 2008; Thayer & Lane, 2009; Wang et al., 2005). Emphasizing the essential survival functions of this (and not the left) system, Schutz (2005) noted:

> The right hemisphere operates a distributed network for rapid responding to danger and other urgent problems. It preferentially processes environmental challenge, stress and pain and manages self-protective responses such as avoidance and escape. Emotionality is thus the right brain's "red phone," compelling the mind to handle urgent matters without delay. (p. 15)

These adaptive right-brain functions often are impaired in individuals with histories of early relational trauma.

Recent neurobiological data support the proposed model of the psychopathogenetic mechanism by which attachment trauma negatively impacts right-brain development. Adamec, Blundell, and Burton (2003) reported experimental data that "implicate neuroplasticity in right-hemispheric limbic circuitry in mediating long-lasting changes in negative affect following brief but severe stress" (p. 1264). According to Gadea, Gomez, Gonzalez-Bono, and Salvador (2005), mild to moderate negative affective experiences activate the right hemisphere, but an intense experience "might interfere with right-hemisphere processing, with eventual damage if some critical point is reached" (p. 136). I suggest that this right-brain "damage" is most operative during dysregulating experiences of attachment-related hyper- and hypoarousal.

Consistent with these findings, dissociative defensive functions are initiated in attachment contexts that generate too frequent, intense, unrepaired, and enduring relational trauma. These dissociative functions may reflect a very rapid shift in the brain from interactive regulatory modes into long-enduring, less complex autoregulatory modes. These patterns are primitive strategies for survival that remain online for long intervals of time, periods in which the developing brain is in a hypometabolic state that significantly diminishes the substantial amounts of energy required for critical-period biosynthetic processes. The dysregulating events of abuse and neglect thus could create severe, chaotic biochemical alterations in the infant brain. This disruption of energy resources for the biosynthesis of right-lateralized limbic connections would be expressed in a critical period of developmental overpruning of the cortical–limbic system (see Schore, 1994, 2002, 2003a, 2009a).

It is now accepted that "psychological factors" "prune" or "sculpt" neural networks in, specifically, the postnatal frontal, limbic, and temporal cortices. Excessive pruning of cortical–subcortical limbic–autonomic circuits occurs in early histories of trauma and neglect. This severe growth impairment represents a possible mechanism of the genesis of a developmental structural defect in the "emotional" right brain. Because this defect involves limbic and autonomic circuits, the resulting functional deficit is likely to specifically affect the individual's ability to cope with intense affects. In this manner the traumatic context in which disorganized attachment arises thus could act as a growth-inhibiting environment for the experience-dependent maturation of right-lateralized CNS–ANS circuits.

The psychobiological context of disorganized attachment during the brain growth spurt of the first 2 years of life thus may alter the developmental trajectory of the right brain. The massive psychobiological stress associated with attachment trauma may not only impair the development of this system but may also set the stage for the characterological use of right-brain defensive pathological dissociation when encountering later social–emotional stressors. As noted above, converging evidence indicates that early abuse negatively impacts limbic and autonomic nervous system maturation, producing enduring neurobiological alterations that underlie affective instability, inefficient stress tolerance, memory impairment, *and* dissociative disturbances. In this manner, traumatic stress in childhood may lead to self-modulation of painful affect by directing attention away from internal emotional states (Lane, Ahern, Schwartz, & Kaszniak, 1997). The right hemisphere is dominant not only for the regulation of affects, but also for maintaining a coherent sense of one's body (Tsakiris, Costantini, & Haggard, 2008), for sustaining attention (Raz, 2004), and for pain processing (Symonds, Gordon, Bixby, & Mande, 2006). Thus, the right brain–related strategy of dissociation may represent the ultimate defense for blocking emotional body-based pain from consciousness.

Dutra, Bureau, Holmes, Lyubchik, and Lyons-Ruth (2009) observe that disrupted maternal affective communications and lack of involvement in the regulation of stressful arousal are associated with the child's use of dissociation, "one of the few available means for achieving a modicum of relief from fearful arousal." This in turn can lead to a child who does "not . . . acknowledge pain and distress within a set of caregiving relationships that are vital for survival" (p. 388). In clinical writings, Bromberg (2006) links right-brain trauma to autonomic hyperarousal, a chaotic and terrifying flooding of affect that can threaten to overwhelm sanity and imperil psychological survival. He observes that dissociation is then automatically and immediately triggered as the fundamental defense to the arousal dysregulation of overwhelming affective states.

Echoing this perspective in the neuroscience literature, Lanius and her colleagues (2005), in a functional magnetic resonance imaging (fMRI) study of traumatized patients with posstraumatic stress disorder (PTSD), show right-hemispheric activation during dissociation. These authors conclude that patients dissociate in order to escape from the overwhelming emotions associated with the traumatic memory. Using transcranial magnetic stimulation, Spitzer, Wilert, Grabe, Rizos, and Freyberger (2004) similarly report that dissociation is associated with right-hemispheric dysfunction in the form of lack of integration in the presence of emotionally distressing or threatening stimuli. Enriquez and Bernabeu (2008) also offer research showing that "dissociation is associated with dysfunctional changes in the right hemisphere which impair its characteristic dominance over emotional processing" (pp. 272–273). They document that "high dissociators" retain an ability for processing left-hemispheric verbal stimuli but show deficits in right-hemispheric perception of the emotional tone of voice (prosody).

More recently, Helton, Dorahy, and Russell (2011) report that "high dissociators" have difficulty in specifically coordinating activity within the right hemisphere and that such deficits become evident when this hemisphere is "loaded with the combined effects of a sustained attention task and negative emotional stimuli. . . . Thus, the integration of experiences, which rely heavily on right-hemispheric activation (e.g., negative emotion, sense of self with reference to the experience), may be compromised in high dissociators" (p. 700). These findings are echoed in current neurological research. Brand et al. (2009) and Stanilou, Markowitsch, and Brand (2010) document right-temporal-frontal hypometabolism in cases of dissociative amnesia, which is clinically expressed as an inability to recall important personal information of a traumatic nature: a failure to integrate consciousness, emotion, and cognition, resulting in a "constricted self" (p. 793).

Thus, both researchers and clinicians are now exploring the evolution of a developmentally impaired regulatory system and providing evidence that prefrontal cortical and limbic areas of the right hemisphere are centrally involved in the deficits in mind and body associated with a pathological dissociative response (Schore, 2002, 2009a, 2009b, 2009c). This hemisphere, more than the left, is densely and reciprocally interconnected with emotion-processing limbic regions, as well as with subcortical areas that generate both the arousal and autonomic body-based aspect of emotions.

Sympathetic ANS activity is manifest in tight engagement with the external environment and a high level of energy mobilization, whereas the parasympathetic component drives disengagement from the external environment and utilizes low levels of internal energy (Recordati, 2003). These ANS components are too frequently uncoupled for long periods of time in stressful interpersonal experiences in infants, children, adolescents, and adults who have histories of attachment trauma, and thus they are likely to be expressed in body-based visceral–somatic disturbances.

Kalsched (2005) describes operations of defensive dissociative processes used by the child during traumatic experience by which "affect in the body is severed from its corresponding images in the mind and thereby an unbearably painful meaning is obliterated" (p. 174). Nijenhuis (2000) asserts that "somatoform dissociation" is an outcome of early-onset traumatization expressed as a lack of integration of sensorimotor experiences, reactions, and functions of the individual's self-representation. Dissociatively detached individuals are not only detached from the environment, but also from the self—from their body, their actions, and their sense of identity (Allen et al., 1999). This detachment is expressed as a deficit in the right-hemispheric "corporeal self" (Devinsky, 2000). Crucian et al. (2000) describe "a dissociation between the emotional evaluation of an event and the physiological reaction to that event, with the process being dependent on intact right-hemisphere function" (p. 643).

Conclusion

In an optimal attachment scenario, a right-lateralized hierarchical prefrontal system performs an essential adaptive motivational function: the relatively fluid switching of internal body-based states in response to changes in the external environment that are nonconsciously appraised to be personally meaningful. In contrast, relational trauma elicits more than a disruption of conscious cognition and a disorganization of overt behavior, but rather, it negatively impacts the early organization of evolutionary-based right-brain mechanisms that operate beneath levels of conscious awareness. Pathological dissociation creates a maladaptive, highly defensive, rigid, closed self system, such that even low levels of intersubjective stress may lead to parasympathetic dorsal vagal hypoarousal, heart rate deceleration, and passive disengagement. This fragile unconscious system is susceptible to relational stress-induced mind–body collapse and thereby to a sudden implosion of the implicit self and a rupture of self-continuity. This collapse of the implicit self often involves the amplification of the parasympathetic-related affects of shame and disgust, and cognitions of hopelessness and helplessness. In addition, the collapse of the implicit self tends to be accompanied by an instant dissipation of a sense of safety and trust, consistent with the hypothesis that it originates in a failure of right-brain–related regulation of attachment security.

Dissociation thus may reflect an inability of the right-brain cortical–subcortical implicit self system to adaptively recognize and process external stimuli (exteroceptive information coming from the relational environment) and to integrate them, on a moment-to-moment basis, with internal stimuli (interoceptive information from the body, somatic markers, the "felt experience"). This integration failure of the higher right hemisphere with the lower right brain could thus induce an instant collapse of both subjectivity and intersubjectivity. Stressful affects, especially those associated with emotional pain, are thus not experienced in consciousness, and the individual's sense of self and of relation to others may become dissociated. The endpoint of chronically experiencing catastrophic states of relational trauma in early life is a progressive impairment of the ability to adjust, take defensive action, or act on one's own behalf, and a blocking of the capacity to register affect and pain—all critical to survival.

Psychotherapy with dissociative patients therefore needs to attend to the severe dysregulation of affect that characterizes the developmental self pathologies associated with histories of relational trauma. Experiences of relational trauma and attachment dysregulation are expressed in the therapeutic alliance as affectively stressful enactments (Schore, 2011, 2012). Bromberg (2011) observes that in the clinical encounter, pathological dissociation acts as an "early warning system" that anticipates potential affect dysregulation before the trauma arrives. Clinical work with such patients must address the early-forming dissociative defense that blocks overwhelming affects from reaching consciousness, thereby denying the possibility of interactive regulation and the organization of more complex right-brain stress regulation. With respect to the psychotherapeutic context, the clinical research of Spitzer et al. (2007) demonstrates that insecurely attached patients with dissociative defenses dissociate as a response to negative emotions arising in psychodynamic psychotherapy, leading to a less favorable treatment outcome.

The current paradigm shift from a focus on cognition to one of affect (Schore, 2012) also includes a shift in clinical work from solely a repression-based theoretical foundation to recognition of the survival strategy of dissociation. Distinguishing between early-forming dissociative defenses and later-forming repressive defenses, Diseth (2005) writes:

> As a defense mechanism, dissociation has been described as a phenomenon quite different from repression. Repression has been considered an unconscious mechanism, placing unwanted feelings away from the conscious mind because of shame, guilt or fear. . . . However, in order to repress, you must to some degree have processed the feelings, recognized their nature and the taboos connected to such feelings. Dissociation is about not having processed the inputs at all. (pp. 81, 82)

This bottom-line psychobiological defense of dissociation thus represents a major obstacle to the intersubjective change process in all affectively focused psychotherapies, but especially in patients with a history of early relational trauma. Dissociated affects are unconscious affects, and so this treatment needs to directly engage the right hemisphere, which is dominant for the processing of unconscious emotions (Gainotti, 2012), especially unconscious negative emotion (Sato & Aoki, 2006).

References

Adamec, R. E., Blundell, J., & Burton, P. (2003). Phosphorylated cyclic AMP response element bonding protein expression induced in the periaqueductal gray by predator stress: Its relationship to the stress experience, behavior, and limbic neural plasticity. *Progress in Neuro-Psychopharmacology and Biological Psychiatry, 27,* 1243–1267.

Allen, J. G., Console, D. A., & Lewis, L. (1999). Dissociative detachment and memory impairment: Reversible amnesia or encoding failure? *Comprehensive Psychiatry, 40,* 160–171.

Ammaniti, M., & Trentini, C. (2009). How new knowledge about parenting reveals the neurobiological implications of intersubjectivity: A conceptual synthesis of recent research. *Psychoanalytic Dialogues, 19,* 537–555.

Barach, P. M. M. (1991). Multiple personality disorder as an attachment disorder. *Dissociation, 4,* 117–123.

Bazhenova, O. V., Stroganova, T. A., Doussard-Roosevelt, J. A., Posikera, I. A., & Porges, S. W. (2007). Physiological responses of 5-month-old infants to smiling and blank faces. *International Journal of Psychophysiology, 63,* 64–76.

Beebe, B., Jaffe, J., Markese, S., Buck, K., Chen, H., Cohen, P., et al. (2010). The origins of 12–month attachment: A microanalysis of 4-month mother–infant interaction. *Attachment and Human Development, 12,* 3–142.

Bion, W. R. (1962). *Learning from experience.* London: Heinemann.

Bock, J., Murmu, R. P., Ferdman, N., Leshem, M., & Braun, K. (2008). Refinement of dendritic and synaptic networks in the rodent anterior cingulate and orbitofrontal cortex: Critical impact of early and late social experience. *Developmental Neurobiology, 68,* 695–698.

Bowlby, J. (1969). *Attachment and loss: Vol. 1. Attachment.* New York: Basic Books.

Bradshaw, G. A., & Schore, A. N. (2007). How elephants are opening doors: Developmental neuroethology, attachment and social context. *Ethology, 113,* 426–436.

Brancucci, A., Lucci, G., Mazzatenta, A., & Tommasi, L. (2009). Asymmetries of the human social brain in the visual, auditory and chemical modalities. *Philosophical Transactions of the Royal Society B, 364,* 895–914.

Brand, M., Eggers, C., Reinhold, N., Fujiwara, E., Kessler, J., Heiss, W.-D., et al. (2009). Functional brain imaging in 14 patients with dissociative amnesia reveals right inferolateral prefrontal hypometabolism. *Psychiatry Research: Neuroimaging, 174,* 32–39.

Bromberg, P. M. (2006). *Awakening the dreamer: Clinical journeys.* Mahwah, NJ: Analytic Press.

Bromberg, P. M. (2011). *The shadow of the tsunami and the growth of the relational mind.* New York: Routledge.

Buss, K. A., Schumacher, J. R. M., Dolski, I., Kalin, N. H., Goldsmith, H. H., & Davidson, R. J. (2003). Right frontal brain activity, cortisol, and withdrawal behavior in 6-month-old infants. *Behavioral Neuroscience, 117,* 11–20.

Carlson, V., Cicchetti, D., Barnett, D., & Braunwald, K. (1989). Disorganized/

disoriented attachment relationships in maltreated infants. *Developmental Psychology, 25,* 525–531.

Cerqueira, J., Almeida, O. F. X., & Sousa, N. (2008). The stressed prefrontal cortex: Left? Right! *Brain, Behavior, and Immunity, 22,* 630–638.

Chiron, C., Jambaque, I., Nabbout, R., Lounes, R., Syrota, A., & Dulac, O. (1997). The right brain hemisphere is dominant in human infants. *Brain, 120,* 1057–1065.

Cozolino, L. (2002). *The neuroscience of psychotherapy.* New York: Norton.

Crucian, G. P., Hughes, J. D., Barrett, A. M., Williamson, D. J. G., Bauer, R. M., Bowres, D., et al. (2000). Emotional and physiological responses to false feedback. *Cortex, 36,* 623–647.

Czeh, B., Perez-Cruz, C., Fuchs, E., & Flugge, G. (2008). Chronic stress-induced cellular changes in the medial prefrontal cortex and their clinical implications: Does hemisphere location matter? *Behavioural Brain Research, 190,* 1–13.

Daselaar, S. M., Rice, H. J., Greenberg, D. L., Cabeza, R., LaBar, K. S., & Rubin, D. C. (2007). The spatiotemporal dynamics of autobiographical memory: Neural correlates of recall, emotional intensity, and reliving. *Cerebral Cortex, 18,* 217–229.

Davidson, R. J., Ekman, P., Saron, C., Senulis, J., & Friesen, W. V. (1990). Approach/withdrawal and cerebral asymmetry: Emotional expression and brain physiology. *Journal of Personality and Social Psychology, 58,* 330–341.

Decety, J., & Lamm, C. (2007). The role of the right temporoparietal junction in social interaction: How low-level computational processes contribute to metacognition. *Neuroscientist, 13,* 580–593.

de Haan, M., Belsky, J., Reid, V., Volein, A., & Johnson, M. H. (2004). Maternal personality and infants' neural and visual responsivity to facial expressions of emotion. *Journal of Child Psychology and Psychiatry, 45,* 1209–1218.

Devinsky, O. (2000). Right cerebral hemisphere dominance for a sense of corporeal and emotional self. *Epilepsy and Behavior, 1,* 60–73.

Diseth, T. H. (2005). Dissociation in children and adolescents as reaction to trauma: An overview of conceptual issues and neurobiological factors. *Nordic Journal of Psychiatry, 59,* 79–91.

Dixon, A. K. (1998). Ethological strategies for defense in animals and humans: Their role in some psychiatric disorders. *British Journal of Medical Psychology, 71,* 417–445.

Dutra, L., Bureau, J.-F., Holmes, B., Lyubchik, A., & Lyons-Ruth, K. (2009). Quality of early care and childhood trauma: A prospective study of developmental pathways to dissociation. *Journal of Nervous and Mental Disease, 197,* 383–390.

Enriquez, P., & Bernabeu, E. (2008). Hemispheric laterality and dissociative tendencies: Differences in emotional processing in a dichotic listening task. *Consciousness and Cognition, 17,* 267–275.

Gadea, M., Gomez, C., Gonzalez-Bono, R. E., & Salvador, A. (2005). Increased cortisol and decreased right ear advantage (REA) in dichotic listening following a negative mood induction. *Psychoneuroendocrinology, 30,* 129–138.

Gainotti, G. (2000). Neuropsychological theories of emotion. In J. Borod (Ed.), *The neuropsychology of emotion.* New York: Oxford University Press.

Gainotti, G. (2012). Unconscious processing of emotions and the right hemisphere. *Neuropsychologia, 50,* 205–218.

Guedeney, A., Foucault, C., Bougen, E., Larroque, B., & Mentre, F. (2008). Screening for risk factors of relational withdrawal behavior in infants aged 14–18 months. *European Psychiatry, 23,* 150–155.

Gunnar, M. R. (2000). Early adversity and the development of stress reactivity and regulation. In C. A. Nelson (Ed.), *The Minnesota Symposium on Child Psychology: Vol. 31. The effects of early adversity on neurobehavioral development* (pp. 163–200). Mahwah, NJ: Erlbaum.

Gupta, R. K., Hasan, K. M., Trivedi, R., Pradhan, M., Das, V., Parikh, N. A., et al. (2005). Diffusion tensor imaging of the developing human cerebrum. *Journal of Neuroscience Research, 81,* 172–178.

Helton, W. S., Dorahy, M. J., & Russell, P. N. (2011). Dissociative tendencies and right-hemisphere processing load: Effects on vigilance performance. *Consciousness and Cognition, 20,* 696–702.

Henry, J. P. (1993). Psychological and physiological responses to stress: The right hemisphere and the hypothalamo–pituitary–adrenal axis—an inquiry into problems of human bonding. *Integrative Physiological and Behavioral Science, 28,* 369–387.

Hesse, E., & Main, M. M. (1999). Second-generation effects of unresolved trauma in nonmaltreating parents: Dissociated, frightened, and threatening parental behavior. *Psychoanalytic Inquiry, 19,* 481–540.

Hesse, E., & Main, M. M. (2006). Frightened, threatening, and dissociative parental behavior in low-risk samples: Description, discussion, and interpretations. *Development and Psychopathology, 18,* 309–343.

Howard, M. F., & Reggia, J. A. (2007). A theory of the visual system biology underlying development of spatial frequency lateralization. *Brain and Cognition, 64,* 111–123.

Hugdahl, K. (1995). Classical conditioning and implicit learning: The right hemisphere hypothesis. In R. J. Davidson & K. Hugdahl (Eds.), *Brain asymmetry* (pp. 235–267). Cambridge, MA: MIT Press.

Kalsched, D. (2005). Hope versus hopelessness in the psychoanalytic situation and Dante's *Divine Comedy. Spring, 72,* 167–187.

Katz, M., Liu, C., Schaer, M., Parker, K. J., Ottlet, M. C., Epps, A., et al. (2009). Prefrontal plasticity and stress inoculation-induced resilience. *Developmental Neuroscience, 31,* 293–299.

Knickmeyer, R. C., Gouttard, S., Kang, C., Evans, D., Wilber, K., Smith, J. K., et al. (2008). A structural MRI study of human brain development from birth to 2 years. *Journal of Neuroscience, 28,* 12176–12182.

Lane, R. D., Ahern, G. L., Schwartz, G. E., & Kaszniak, A. W. (1997). Is alexithymia the emotional equivalent of blindsight? *Biological Psychiatry, 42,* 834–844.

Lanius, R. A., Bluhm, R. L., & Frewen, P. A. (2011). How understanding the neurobiology of complex post-traumatic stress disorder can inform clinical practice: A social cognitive and affective neuroscience approach. *Acta Psychiatrica Scandinavica, 124*(5), 331–348.

Lanius, R. A., Williamson, P. C., Bluhm, R. L., Densmore, M., Boksman, K., Neufeld, R. W. J., et al. (2005). Functional connectivity of dissociative responses in posttraumatic stress disorder: A functional magnetic resonance imaging investigation. *Biological Psychiatry, 57,* 873–884.

Leckman, J. F., & March, J. S. (2011). Editorial: Developmental neuroscience comes of age. *Journal of Child Psychology and Psychiatry, 52,* 333–338.

Lemche, E., Giampietro, V. P., Surguladze, S. A., Amaro, E. J., Andrew, C. M., Williams, S. C. R., et al. (2006). Human attachment security is mediated by the amygdala: Evidence from combined fMRI and psychophysiological measures. *Human Brain Mapping, 27,* 623–635.

MacDonald, H. Z., Beeghly, M., Grant-Knight, W., Augustyn, M., Woods, R. W., et al. (2008). Longitudinal association between infant disorganized attachment and childhood posttraumatic stress symptoms. *Development and Psychopathology, 20,* 493–508.

Main, M., & Solomon, J. (1986). Discovery of an insecure–disorganized/disoriented attachment pattern: Procedures, findings and implications for the classification of behavior. In T. B. Brazelton & M. W. Yogman (Eds.), *Affective development in infancy* (pp. 95–124). Norwood, NJ: Ablex.

Markowitsch, H. J., Reinkemeier, A., Kessler, J., Koyuncu, A., & Heiss, W.-D. (2000).

Right amygdalar and temperofrontal activation during autobiographical, but not fictitious memory retrieval. *Behavioral Neurology, 12*, 181–190.

Mento, G., Suppiej, A., Altoe, G., & Bisiacchi, P. S. (2010). Functional hemispheric asymmetries in humans: Electrophysiological evidence from preterm infants. *European Journal of Neuroscience, 31*, 565–574.

Milne, L., Greenway, P., Guedeney, A., & Larroque, B. (2009). Long-term developmental impact of social withdrawal in infants. *Infant Behavior and Development, 32*, 159–166.

Minagawa-Kawai, Y., Matsuoka, S., Dan, I., Naoi, N., Nakamura, K., & Kojima, S. (2009). Prefrontal activation associated with social attachment: Facial-emotion recognition in mothers and infants. *Cerebral Cortex, 19*, 284–292.

Mollon, P. (1996). *Multiple selves, multiple voices: Working with trauma, violation and dissociation.* Chichester, UK: Wiley.

Montirosso, R., Borgatti, R., & Tronick, E. (2010). Lateral asymmetries in infants' regulatory and communicative gestures. In R. A. Lanius, E. Vermetten, & C. Pain (Eds.), *The impact of early life trauma on health and disease: The hidden epidemic* (pp. 103–111). Cambridge, UK: Cambridge University Press.

Nijenhuis, E. R. S. (2000). Somatoform dissociation: Major symptoms of dissociative disorders. *Journal of Trauma and Dissociation, 1*, 7–32.

Parsons, C. E., Young, K. S., Murray, L., Stein, A., & Kringelbach, M. L. (2010). The functional neuroanatomy of the evolving parent–infant relationship. *Progess in Neurobiology, 91*, 220–241.

Perry, B. D., Pollard, R. A., Blakley, T. L., Baker, W. L., & Vigilante, D. (1995). Childhood trauma, the neurobiology of adaptation, and "use-dependent" development of the brain: How states become traits. *Infant Mental Health Journal, 16*, 271–291.

Pieper, S., Out, D., Bakermans-Kranenburg, M. J., & van IJzendoorn, M. H. (2011). Behavioral and molecular genetics of dissociation: The role of the serotonin transporter gene promoter polymorphism *(5-HTTLPR). Journal of Traumatic Stress, 24*, 373–380.

Porges, S. W. (1997). Emotion: An evolutionary by-product of the neural regulation of the autonomic nervous system. *Annals of the New York Academy of Sciences, 807*, 62–77.

Powles, W. E. (1992). *Human development and homeostasis.* Madison, CT: International Universities Press.

Putnam, F. W. (1997). *Dissociation in children and adolescents: A developmental perspective.* New York: Guilford Press.

Raz, A. (2004). Anatomy of attentional networks. *Anatomical Record, 281B*, 21–36.

Recordati, G. (2003). A thermodynamic model of the sympathetic and parasympathetic nervous systems. *Autonomic Neuroscience: Basic and Clinical, 103*, 1–12.

Rinaman, L., Levitt, P., & Card, J. P. (2000). Progressive postnatal assembly of limbic-autonomic circuits revealed by central transneuronal transport of pseudorabies virus. *Journal of Neuroscience, 20*, 2731–2741.

Roth, T. L., & Sweatt, J. D. (2011). Annual research review: Epigenetic mechanism and environmental shaping of the brain during sensitive periods of development. *Journal of Child Psychology and Psychiatry, 52*, 398–408.

Sato, W., & Aoki, S. (2006). Right hemisphere dominance in processing unconscious emotion. *Brain and Cognition, 62*, 261–266.

Schiffer, F., Teicher, M., & Papanicolaou, A. (1995). Evoked potentials evidence for right brain activity during recall of traumatic memories. *Journal of Neuropsychiatry and Clinical Neuroscience, 7*, 169–175.

Schore, A. N. (1994). *Affect regulation and the origin of the self.* Mahwah, NJ: Erlbaum.

Schore, A. N. (2000). Attachment and the regulation of the right brain. *Attachment and Human Development, 2*, 23–47.

Schore, A. N. (2001). The effects of relational trauma on right brain development, affect regulation, and infant mental health. *Infant Mental Health Journal, 22,* 201–269.

Schore, A. N. (2002). Dysregulation of the right brain: A fundamental mechanism of traumatic attachment and the psychopathogenesis of posttraumatic stress disorder. *Australian and New Zealand Journal of Psychiatry, 36,* 9–30.

Schore, A. N. (2003a). *Affect regulation and the repair of the self.* New York: Norton.

Schore, A. N. (2003b). *Affect dysregulation and disorders of the self.* New York: Norton.

Schore, A. N. (2005). Attachment, affect regulation, and the developing right brain: Linking developmental neuroscience to pediatrics. *Pediatrics in Review, 26,* 204–211.

Schore, A. N. (2009a). Attachment trauma and the developing right brain: Origins of pathological dissociation. In P. F. Dell & J. A. O'Neil (Eds.), *Dissociation and the dissociative disorders: DSM-V and beyond* (pp. 107–141). New York: Routledge.

Schore, A. N. (2009b). Relational trauma and the developing right brain: An interface of psychoanalytic self psychology and neuroscience. *Annals of the New York Academy of Sciences, 1159,* 189–203.

Schore, A. N. (2009c). Right-brain affect regulation: An essential mechanism of development, trauma, dissociation, and psychotherapy. In D. Fosha, D. Siegel, & M. Solomon (Eds.), *The healing power of emotion: Affective neuroscience, development, and clinical practice* (pp. 112–144). New York: Norton.

Schore, A. N. (2010a). Relational trauma and the developing right brain: The neurobiology of broken attachment bonds. In T. Baradon (Ed.), *Relational trauma in infancy* (pp. 19–47). London: Routledge.

Schore, A. N. (2010b). A neurobiological perspective of the work of Berry Brazelton. In B. M. Lester & J. D. Sparrow (Eds.), *Nurturing families of young children building on the legacy of T. Berry Brazelton* (pp. 141–153). New York: Wiley Blackwell.

Schore, A. N. (2010c). Synopsis. In R. A. Lanius, E. Vermetten, & C. Pain (Eds.), *The impact of early life trauma on health and disease: The hidden epidemic* (pp. 1142–1147). Cambridge, UK: Cambridge University Press.

Schore, A. N. (2011). Foreword. In D. Bromberg, *The shadow of the tsunami and the growth of the relational mind* (pp. ix–xxxvii). New York: Routledge.

Schore, A. N. (2012). *The science of the art of psychotherapy.* New York: Norton.

Schore, J. R., & Schore, A. N. (2008). Modern attachment theory: The central role of affect regulation in development and treatment. *Clinical Social Work Journal, 36,* 9–20.

Schuengel, C., Bakersmans-Kranenburg, M. J., & van IJzendoorn, M. H. (1999). Frightening maternal behavior linking unresolved loss and disorganized infant attachment. *Journal of Consulting and Clinical Psychology, 67,* 54–63.

Schutz, L. E. (2005). Broad-perspective perceptual disorder of the right hemisphere. *Neuropsychology Review, 15,* 11–27.

Semrud-Clikeman, M., Fine, J. D., & Zhu, D. C. (2011). The role of the right hemisphere for processing of social interactions in normal adults using functional magnetic resonance imaging. *Neuropsychobiology, 64,* 47–51.

Siegel, D. J. (1999). *The developing mind: Toward a neurobiology of interpersonal experience.* New York: Guilford Press.

Spitzer, C., Barnow, S., Freyberger, H. J., & Grabe, H. J. (2007). Dissociation predicts symptom-related treatment outcome in short-term inpatient psychotherapy. *Australian and New Zealand Journal of Psychiatry, 41,* 682–687.

Spitzer, C., Wilert, C., Grabe, H.-J., Rizos, T., & Freyberger, H. J. (2004). Dissociation, hemispheric asymmetry, and dysfunction of hemispheric interaction: A transcranial magnetic approach. *Journal of Neuropsychiatry and Clinical Neuroscience, 16,* 163–169.

Stanilou, A., Markowitsch, H. J., & Brand, M. (2010). Psychogenic amnesia: A malady of the constricted self. *Consciousness and Cognition, 19,* 778–801.

Stevenson, C. W., Halliday, D. M., Marsden, C. A., & Mason, R. (2008). Early life programming of hemispheric lateralization and synchronization in the adult medial prefrontal cortex. *Neuroscience, 155,* 852–863.

Sullivan, R. M., & Dufresne, M. M. (2006). Mesocortical dopamine and HPA axis regulation: Role of laterality and early environment. *Brain Research, 1076,* 49–59.

Sullivan, R. M., & Gratton, A. (2002). Prefrontal cortical regulation of hypothalamic–pituitary–adrenal function in the rat and implications for psychopathology: Side matters. *Psychoneuroendocrinology, 27,* 99–114.

Sun, T., Patoine, C., Abu-Khalil, A., Visvader, J., Sum, E., Cherry, T. J., et al. (2005). Early asymmetry of gene transcription in embryonic human left and right cerebral cortex. *Science, 308,* 1794–1798.

Symonds, L. L., Gordon, N. S., Bixby, J. C., & Mande, M. M. (2006). Right-lateralized pain processing in the human cortex: An fMRI study. *Journal of Neurophysiology, 95,* 3823–3830.

Thayer, J. F., & Lane, R. D. (2009). Claude Bernard and the heart–brain connection: Further elaboration of a model of neurovisceral integration. *Neuroscience and Biobehavioral Reviews, 33,* 81–88.

Tsakiris, M., Costantini, M., & Haggard, P. (2008). The role of the right temporo-parietal junction in maintaining a coherent sense of one's body. *Neuropsychologia, 46,* 3014–3018.

Tucker, D. M., & Moller, L. (2007). The metamorphosis: Individuation of the adolescent brain. In D. Romer & E. F. Walker (Eds.), *Adolescent psychopathology and the developing brain: Integrating brain and prevention science* (pp. 85–102). Oxford, UK: Oxford University Press.

Wang, J., Rao, H., Wetmore, G. S., Furlan, P. M., Korczykowski, M., Dinges, D. F., et al. (2005). Perfusion functional MRI reveals cerebral blood flow pattern under psychological stress. *Proceedings of the National Academy of Sciences of the United States of America, 102,* 17804–17809.

Wismer Fries, A. B., Ziegler, T. E., Kurian, J. R., Jacoris, S., & Pollak, S. D. (2005). Early experience in humans is associated with changes in neuropeptides critical for regulating social behavior. *Proceedings of the National Academy of Sciences of the United States of America, 102,* 17237–17240.

Wittling, W. (1997). The right hemisphere and the human stress response. *Acta Physiologica Scandinavica, 161*(Suppl. 640), 55–59.

CHAPTER 2

Childhood Trauma, Brain Connectivity, and the Self

Ruth A. Lanius
Robyn Bluhm
Paul A. Frewen

Adult survivors of childhood abuse are at significantly higher risk of developing a variety of psychiatric disorders, including posttraumatic stress disorder (PTSD) and other anxiety disorders, depression, substance abuse, personality disorders, sexual disorders, and antisocial or violent behaviours (Caspi et al., 2002; Dube et al., 2001; Duncan, Saunders, Kilpatrick, Hanson, & Resnick, 1996; Felitti et al., 1998; Kessler, Sonnega, Bromet, Hughes, & Nelson, 1995; Krupnick et al., 2004; MacMillan et al., 2001; McCauley et al., 1997; Stein et al., 1996; Widom, 1999; Widom, Marmorstein, & White, 2006). Childhood trauma is also associated with chronic, stress-related gastrointestinal, metabolic, cardiovascular, and immunological illnesses (Cromer & Sachs-Ericsson, 2006; Felitti et al., 1998; Heim & Nemeroff, 2001; Lanius, Vermetten, & Pain, 2010).

Judith Herman described a form of complex PTSD or "disorders of extreme stress not otherwise specified" (Herman, 1997; see also van der Kolk, Roth, Pelcovitz, Sunday, & Spinazzola, 2005) in an attempt to capture the complex sequelae of chronic childhood trauma that was often not contained in the PTSD diagnosis. Symptoms of complex PTSD include persistent dysfunction in seven aspects of self-regulation and psychosocial functioning: 1) generalized affect dysregulation (in relation to anger, suicidal preoccupation, inhibited or disinhibited sexuality, and impulsivity/risk taking); alterations in (2) self-perception (e.g., believing one is ineffective, permanently damaged, or rightfully shamed), (3) relational perception (including the inability to trust others and/or revictimizing oneself and/or others), (4) meaning making (e.g., learned helplessness, hopelessness, and lack of faith), and (5) attention and consciousness (including symptoms of dissociation); and (6) somatization (i.e., physical symptoms in the absence of obvious medical etiology).

Psychiatric Disorders as Neurodevelopmental Disorders

Even though the etiology of most psychiatric diagnoses, except for PTSD, is not acknowledged in the present psychiatric diagnostic system, there has been a movement to view psychiatric disorders as having a neurodevelopmental origin—that is, as the result of alterations in brain development. As this field progresses, such a view may be particularly relevant as a framework for researching complex adaptations to psychological trauma. In general, the peak age of onset for mental disorders is 14 years (Kessler et al., 2005), though there is some variation among disorders, and there also may be differences in the age at which a disorder is likely to be diagnosed. For example, attention-deficit/hyperactivity disorder (ADHD) is often diagnosed in childhood, whereas other disorders, such as mood and anxiety disorders, eating disorders, and substance abuse, are more likely to emerge or be diagnosed during adolescence. Recent theoretical work suggests that our understanding of psychiatric disorders can be further developed using a framework that, while continuing to recognize the complex, multifactorial nature of these disorders, views them as alterations that began in the developing brain.

Research has revealed that the brain continues to develop throughout adolescence and even young adulthood. Even though total brain size appears to be constant as of approximately 5 years of age (Durston et al., 2006), many subcortical structures, including the anterior cingulate cortex, orbital–frontal cortex, basal ganglia, amygdala, and hippocampus, change in size well beyond this time (Schore, 2002). Moreover, changes occur throughout the brain in the relative proportions of gray matter (which shows an increase in volume) and white matter (which decreases). These anatomical changes occur together with altered patterns of connectivity among various regions of the brain, a point to which we return later in the chapter.

Developmental processes both influence and are influenced by psychiatric disorders. In some cases, the issue may be one of timing, so that a developmental process occurs according to its normal stages, but happens significantly earlier or later than the average age. For example, ADHD has been hypothesized to involve a maturational delay in the increase of the thickness of the cerebral cortex, particularly in prefrontal areas (Shaw et al., 2007). In other cases, the developmental process may occur to a greater or a lesser extent than is normal. An example is provided by Gogtay and colleagues (Gogtay et al., 2004, 2008), who found that schizophrenia is associated with a greater-than-normal loss of gray matter volume, which appears to be "an exaggeration" of the normal gray matter development, but that pediatric bipolar disorder appears to involve both gray matter loss (in the bilateral cingulate cortex) and increased gray matter volume (in the left temporal cortex) (Gogtay et al., 2004, 2008). Despite this diversity in the relationship between psychiatric disorders and brain development, Pavaluri and Sweeney (2008) conclude that the emergence of all psychiatric disorders during childhood and adolescence appears to involve "alterations in the developmental trajectory of functional brain systems" (p. 1274).

Challenges in Studying Brain Development and Its Relationship to Psychiatric Disorders

Investigation of the developmental alterations in neuroanatomy and physiology associated with various psychiatric disorders may therefore be a promising way to improve our understanding of these disorders, as well as leading to improvements in diagnosis and prognosis through the clearer delineation of the pathophysiology of these disorders and their subtypes. Yet this framework also faces some formidable challenges. Bluhm (in press) has argued that functional neuroimaging research in childhood psychiatric disorders faces unique challenges associated with developmental changes in both the brain and in learning and behavior, with greater variability occurring during childhood than later in life. Therefore, it often is difficult to determine if differences in brain function are related to development or to psychopathology, or both—making the drawing of conclusions about the role of brain function in children's psychiatric disorders particularly complicated.

Recall that in the proposed underlying framework these disorders are due to alterations in the developmental trajectory of brain systems. *Development* is understood in terms of alterations in neuroanatomy and neurophysiology, though these are not yet well understood, even in normal development. Development is also understood in cognitive terms, as children become more able to perform particular tasks. There is, as of yet, no clear understanding of the cognitive abnormalities associated with various psychiatric disorders, in either adults or in children and adolescents (with whom less research has been conducted). Nor is there a clear theory of the pathophysiology of any psychiatric disorder in adults, which would at least give researchers an understanding of the "end state" of the patholological developmental trajectory. In summary, as Bluhm (in press) points out:

Neuroimaging in child and adolescent psychiatry is particularly challenging because there is no overarching framework that links the anatomical, physiological, cognitive and clinical changes associated with a particular disorder. . . . It is this lack of a big picture that makes the interpretation of imaging studies in child and adolescent psychiatry difficult.

Resting-State Functional Magnetic Resonance Imaging, the Default Mode Network, and Self-Referential Processing

Because of these challenges, we suggest an alternative approach to understanding the development of PTSD in children who experience chronic trauma. This approach is based in an emerging field of neuroimaging research sometimes called "functional connectivity functional magnetic resonance imaging" (fcfMRI), or simply "resting-state functional magnetic resonance imaging (fMRI)." This research originated when scientists realized that a number of the areas of the brain that were associated with a particular cognitive or perceptual task also showed connectivity when the individual was in a resting state—that is, not attempting to think about or do anything in particular. Although the earliest studies examining resting-state connectivity investigated visual, motor, and language areas (Beckmann, DeLuca, Devlin, & Smith, 2005; Cordes et al., 2000; Lowe, Mock, & Sorenson, 1998), the majority of this work to date has focused on activity in what has been described as the default mode network (DMN) (Buckner, Andrews-Hanna, & Schacter, 2008; Fransson, 2005; Raichle, 2010; Raichle et al., 2001). In the remainder of this chapter, we show that resting-state connectivity, as studied using fMRI, may shed light on the development of childhood PTSD as well as adult PTSD that is related to prolonged childhood trauma.

The DMN is composed of a number of brain regions, including the posterior cingulate cortex (PCC), anterior cingulate cortex (ACC), medial prefrontal cortex (mPFC), and bilateral angular gyrus/inferior parietal cortex. The middle temporal gyrus has also been implicated in this network (Spreng, Mar, & Kim, 2009). Although there is no clear function assigned to this network, it has been suggested that, in the absence of task demands, the brain maintains a "default mode" that allows it to be ready to respond to environmental changes (Raichle & Gusnard, 2005).

Importantly, the default mode has also been linked to self-referential processing and the stream of consciousness (Kim, 2010; Northoff et al., 2006; Sajonz et al., 2010). *Self-referential processing* refers to how individuals think about themselves (e.g., believing that they are "bad" or "permanently damaged") and their capacity to reflect upon the personal meaning of their experience. It has been noted that the areas that make up the DMN are also involved in other self- or identity-related forms of mental activity, including theory of mind (i.e., beliefs about how the mind works), autobiographical memory, and thinking about the future (Spreng & Grady, 2010). These forms of thinking play a key role in most, if not all, of the domains of complex PTSD or disorders of extreme stress that were described above as common sequelae of exposure to trauma in early childhood.

Recent neuroimaging work has begun to characterize the development of the DMN in the maturing brain (Power, Fair, Schlaggar, & Petersen, 2010; Uddin, Supekar, Ryali, & Menon, 2011). Fransson and colleagues did not observe a fully connected DMN in lightly sedated preterm infants or in sleeping full-term neonates. They found instead that connectivity tended to occur in local areas and in parallel areas in each of the brain's two hemispheres, but that there was no connectivity between the frontal and the posterior areas of the full DMN (Fransson et al., 2007, 2009). Subsequent research showed that infants as young as 2 weeks of age may have three separate components that involve regions that will become part of the adult DMN (Gao et al., 2009). These results may be due to the anatomical immaturity of infants, who do not have well-developed white matter tracts (i.e., groups of brain cells that connect different areas of the brain) (Hermoye et al., 2006).

Integration of the areas that become the DMN appears to begin early in life, however. Gao and colleagues (2009) also found that anterior–posterior integration begins to occur in infants as young as 1 year of age. Yet the process of maturation of the DMN is prolonged. Fair and colleagues observed that in children ages 7–9, there remain significant differences from adult brain architecture (Fair et al., 2008). Furthermore, De Bie et al. (2012) reported less developed functional connectivity of the DMN in 5- to 8-year-old children and concluded that the DMN is detectable, even though it is still immature. Another study found that by 9 years of age, children show comparable DMN integration between the anterior and the posterior areas of the brain (Thomason et al., 2008).

More recently, Supekar et al. (2010) examined the maturation of the DMN from childhood to young adulthood using a multimodal imaging approach that combined resting-state fMRI, voxel-based morphometry to examine the gray matter volume of brain regions involved in the DMN, and diffusion tensor imaging-based tractography to measure white matter tracts that connect these regions of the DMN. Significant developmental changes of the DMN in functional and structural connectivity were observed in children ages 7–9, even though these changes were not uniform across all DMN nodes. Specifically, PCC–mPFC connectivity was shown to be the most immature link in the DMN of children, and both the PCC and mPFC were less fully developed in terms of gray matter volume than other brain areas. The authors suggested that this apparent later maturation of PCC–mPFC structural connectivity may play an important role in the development of self-related and social–cognitive functions that emerge later, typically not until adolescence. For example, episodic memory has been associated with increasing self-awareness (Howe & Courage, 1997; Levine, 2004; Povinelli, Landau, & Perilloux, 1996), which may be necessary for a child to be able to integrate new experiences into his or her sense of self. Similarly, children develop the capacity to move beyond purely egocentric representations in order to understand others as having a mental life similar to their own (Flavell, 1999), and also to hold multiple perspectives in mind and compare them (Perner & Wimmer, 1985). Finally, children use these capacities, which do not manifest in relatively mature form until adolescence or early adulthood, for reflection on their own and others' mental states in order to develop sophisticated representations of cognitive and emotional mental states. The potential absence or diminution of these psychological and relational capacities play an important role in PTSD, and, indeed, may be greatly altered in individuals with this disorder.

Emotional Awareness and PTSD

The sense of self-awareness and the ability to understand complex emotional states have also been shown to be impaired in adult patients with PTSD and are hypothesized to be related to alterations in neurodevelopment as a result of chronic childhood abuse (Lanius, Bluhm, & Frewen, 2011). Adults with chronic PTSD subsequent to early-life trauma often have severe difficulties with emotion recognition and emotional awareness (Frewen, Lane, et al., 2008). *Emotional awareness* is a type of self-referential processing that entails the capacity to be aware of and describe one's own emotions as well as those of others (Fridja, 2007; Lambie & Marcel, 2002). The development of this capacity, however, has been suggested to require a history of a secure attachment with one's primary caregivers (Lane & Schwartz, 1987; Winnicott, 1960). From an evolutionary perspective, our emotions have evolved, in part, to signal danger in the environment and to motivate escape. However, being unable to escape, as is the case when children grow up with a chronically abusive caregiver, can leave them unable to use their emotional responses appropriately to guide effective escape behaviors. This inability may result in a sense of learned helplessness and the conscious or unconscious belief that emotional responses are pointless. This futility, in turn, may result in individuals disconnecting themselves from their bodily experiences and emotions, so as to avoid distress that cannot be relieved through action.

Indeed, individuals with PTSD are often unaware of their own emotional responses and have difficulty identifying and expressing their emotional states in words (Frewen, Dozois, Neufeld, & Lanius, 2008). These difficulties are well described by a patient with complex PTSD, who stated, "When I get emotions and stuff like that I don't really feel them. I can say to someone I feel sadness because tears are welling in my eyes, but I do not know what that is really. They are just physical symptoms" (Lanius et al., 2011, p. 335). Clinical research studies have shown that patients with PTSD have lower levels of emotional awareness (Frewen, Lane, et al., 2008), higher levels of emotional numbing/inability to experience emotions (Frewen et al., 2012), and higher levels of alexithymia (i.e., difficulty in identifying and expressing feelings in words) (Frewen, Dozois, Neufeld, & Lanius, 2010a; Frewen, Dozois, et al., 2008) than other individuals.

Advances have also been made in terms of identifying the neural underpinnings of deficits in emotional awareness in PTSD. For example, our group has examined the relationship between trait emotional numbing symptoms and brain activation patterns during emotional imagery in individuals who suffered from PTSD related to prolonged childhood abuse (Frewen et al., 2012). A patient suffering from PTSD related to childhood abuse summed up feelings of emotional numbing by stating "It's like a blank, I think about my kids and I feel nothing for them. I'll be sitting there feeling confused and numb, and I wonder what I'm supposed to be feeling. It's like dead space . . . and when that happens, I have trouble using words, finding my words, I can't talk" (Lanius et al., 2011, p. 334). In the fMRI study, patients' emotional numbing ratings were correlated with extent of brain activation during imagery of positive (receiving others' affection/praise) and negative (rejection/criticism) scripts. Women who reported increased emotional numbing symptoms exhibited *decreased* brain activation within the dorsal-medial prefrontal cortex during imagery of both positive and negative social–emotional scripts, consistent with a role for the dorsal-medial prefrontal cortex in higher-order self-reflective functioning.

Interestingly, with healthy women completing the same task, the more an individual exhibited the capacity to "mindfully observe," referring to the intentional direction of attention to one's inner and outer stimuli and experiences (e.g., "When I'm walking, I deliberately notice the sensations of my body moving"; "I notice changes in my body, such as whether my breathing slows down or speeds up"; (Baer, Smith, & Allen, 2004; Baer, Smith, Hopkins, Krietemeyer, & Toney, 2006), the *more* activation was observed in the dorsal–medial prefrontal cortex (Frewen et al., 2010b). These findings suggest that dysfunction of the dorsal–medial prefrontal cortex may underlie the difficulties individuals with PTSD often have reflecting on and interpreting their emotional experience. It also points to the importance of teaching patients with PTSD how to mindfully observe inner and outer experiences in order to achieve an increased capacity for self-reflection and awareness of emotional states (Siegel, 2007). Future studies will need to examine patients with PTSD after treatment focusing on increasing the capacity for self-reflection, including mindful observing, in order to assess whether the deficits in the activation of the dorsal–medial prefrontal cortex can be reversed through successful psychotherapeutic intervention.

Self-Referential Processing in PTSD

Neuroimaging studies suggest that self-referential processing is partly mediated via cortical midline structures, including the mPFC, perigenual anterior cingulate cortex, posterior cingulate cortex, as well as the temporal–
parietal junction and temporal poles (Gillihan & Farah, 2005; Legrand &
Ruby, 2009; Northoff et al., 2006; Saxe, Moran, Scholz, & Gabrieli, 2006;
Schmitz & Johnson, 2007; van der Meer, Costafreda, Aleman, & David,
2010; Van Overwalle, 2009). Several of these brain regions are part of the
DMN (e.g., mPFC, PCC/precuneus, ACC), and the DMN has been implicated in self-referential processing, as described above.

In order to better study the neural underpinnings of self-reflective
functioning in PTSD related to childhood abuse, a novel cognitive paradigm, akin to mirror viewing, has been developed by our group (Frewen
et al., 2011). The neuroimaging paradigm involved the collection of self-
descriptiveness ratings for negatively (e.g., *abandoned, unlovable, despica-
ble, broken*) and positively (e.g., *lovable, special, adorable*) and later exposing participants to pictures of themselves while such words were spoken.
Results showed that patients WITH PTSD endorsed more negative and
fewer positive trait adjectives as self-descriptive, which support repeated
clinical observations that individuals with PTSD, especially related to
childhood trauma, often experience intense negative thoughts and even
self-hatred. For example, responses from individuals with PTSD to viewing their own face paired with negative adjectives included "I relate to the
negative side"; or "I noticed I was agreeing with all the negative words";
or "It made me feel bad about myself." Responses from individuals with
PTSD to seeing their own face paired with a positive word included "I did
not believe it"; or "It did not mean anything"; or "I questioned it—I did not
feel the confidence."

Brain activation patterns demonstrated that healthy women showed
an increased response within the perigenual anterior cingulate cortex when
viewing their face and listening to positive trait adjectives, whereas women
with PTSD did not show this effect. Interestingly, the perigenual anterior
cingulate cortex is one of the brain regions most responsive to emotional
manipulations, as assessed by neuroimaging (e.g., Kober et al., 2008). This
region has also been linked to self-referential processing (e.g., Kircher et
al., 2000; van der Meer et al., 2010) and is more active during negative
emotional events in healthy individuals than in individuals with PTSD (see
Etkin & Wager, 2007).

In contrast to healthy controls, in association with the degree to which
they felt positive and/or attributed positive attributes to themselves, patients
with PTSD exhibited an increased response within the right amygdala when
viewing their face and responding with positive trait adjectives adjectives
(Frewen et al., 2011). Although response within the amygdala has more
often been associated with negative emotional processing, particularly of

threat-related visual stimuli (e.g., Etkin & Wager, 2007), research also implicates the amygdala in positive emotional processing (e.g., see Murray, 2008, for review). In this study, right amygdala activation may be a sign of relatively more positive and healthier self-appraisals by women who, as a group, can be characterized by severe negative self-referential processing. It is also interesting to note that the right amygdala has been suggested to be involved in social–emotional processing, and more positive and healthier self-appraisals may be related to better social functioning (Lanius et al., 2011).

Neuroimaging Evidence for a Link between Altered DMN and PTSD Related to Early Life Trauma

To date, relatively little work has been conducted on resting-state alterations in the DMN in PTSD related to early life trauma. Given that PTSD has been associated with deficits in self-referential processing, as described above, and with altered activation in areas associated with the DMN (e.g., medial prefrontal cortex, anterior cingulate, posterior cingulate cortex; Bremner et al., 1999; Williams et al., 2006; Bryant et al., 2008; Geuze et al., 2007; Lanius et al., 2001; Liberzon et al., 1999; Shin et al., 1999; Bluhm et al., 2012), our group examined the integrity of this network in PTSD related to prolonged childhood abuse.

In these patients, significantly reduced resting-state connectivity within the DMN and, in particular, a lack of anterior–posterior integration were demonstrated (Bluhm et al., 2009). The PTSD group showed diminished connectivity between the posterior cingulate seed region and the medial prefrontal cortex, right superior frontal gyrus, and left thalamus. Furthermore, the connectivity of the medial prefrontal seed region was strictly limited to adjacent areas in the medial prefrontal cortex. It is interesting to note that the DMN connectivity described above resembles that observed in children ages 7–9, perhaps indicating interference with the development of white matter tracts due to possible toxic effects of stress hormones on the myelination process (Daniels, Frewen, McKinnon, & Lanius, 2011). We hypothesized that the negatively valenced self-loathing and often fragmented sense of self that are often experienced by individuals with highly dissociative PTSD are related to the degree of anterior–posterior integration of the DMN. Future studies will need to carefully correlate clinical symptoms of self-dysfunction with their relationship to DMN connectivity.

Conclusion

We have shown that examining resting-state brain networks, in particular the DMN, may be relevant for understanding self-referential processing (including emotional awareness) and the sense of self in individuals who have suffered from childhood abuse. In these individuals, significantly reduced resting-state connectivity within the DMN and, specifically, a lack of anterior–posterior integration were observed. Moreover, the DMN connectivity was similar to that shown in children ages 7–9 years old, perhaps indicating interference with the development of white matter tracts due to possible toxic effects of stress hormones on the myelination process.

In terms of future directions, the clinical importance of DMN connectivity assessed during rest in trauma-related disorders requires further study. Additional systematic studies that examine the relationship between clinically noted abnormalities in self-referential processing and autobiographical memory in the often complex variants of PTSD that occur following prolonged childhood abuse with brain activity patterns in the DMN across the lifespan are warranted. Moreover, it will be crucial to prospectively examine the functional connectivity of the DMN in children with and without a history of maltreatment, in order to determine if maltreatment disrupts or alters brain development in brain regions associated with the DMN. Based on the evidence that brain areas that are part of the DMN play an important role in the kinds of self-referential processing that are impaired in complex traumatic stress disorders, these studies may help scientists and clinicians to better understand if, and how, early life trauma changes not only the development of the self but also the development of areas in the brain that may make the experience of a sense of self possible.

References

Baer, R. A., Smith, G. T., & Allen, K. B. (2004). Assessment of mindfulness by self-report: The Kentucky Inventory of Mindfulness Skills. *Assessment, 11*(3), 191–206.

Baer, R. A., Smith, G. T., Hopkins, J., Krietemeyer, J., & Toney, L. (2006). Using self-report assessment methods to explore facets of mindfulness. *Assessment, 13*(1), 27–45.

Beckmann, C. F., DeLuca, M., Devlin, J. T., & Smith, S. M. (2005). Investigations into resting-state connectivity using independent component analysis. *Philosophical Transactions of the Royal Society of London. Series B: Biological Sciences, 360*(1457), 1001–1013.

Bluhm, R. L. (in press). Moving parts get broken: Neuroimaging research and child and adolescent psychiatry. In C. Perring & L. Wells (Eds.), *Classification and diagnosis in child and adolescent psychiatry.* Oxford, UK: Oxford University Press.

Bluhm, R. L., Frewen, P. A., Coupland, N. C., Densmore, M., Schore, A. N., & Lanius, R. A. (2012). Neural correlates of self-reflection in post-traumatic stress disorder. *Acta Psychiatrica Scandinavica, 125*(3), 238–246.

Bluhm, R. L., Williamson, P. C., Osuch, E. A., Frewen, P. A., Stevens, T. K., Boksman, K., et al. (2009). Alterations in default network connectivity in posttraumatic stress disorder related to early-life trauma. *Journal of Psychiatry and Neuroscience, 34*(3), 187–194.

Bremner, J. D., Staib, L. H., Kaloupek, D., Southwick, S. M., Soufer, R., & Charney, D. S. (1999). Neural correlates of exposure to traumatic pictures and sound in Vietnam combat veterans with and without posttraumatic stress disorder: A positron emission tomography study. *Biological Psychiatry, 45,* 806–816.

Bryant, R. A., Felmingham, K., Kemp, A., Das, P., Hughes, G., Peduto, A., et al. (2008). Amygdala and ventral anterior cingulate activation predicts treatment response to cognitive behaviour therapy for post-traumatic stress disorder. *Psychological Medicine, 38*(4), 555–561.

Buckner, R. L., Andrews-Hanna, J. R., & Schacter, D. L. (2008). The brain's default network: Anatomy, function, and relevance to disease. *Annals of the New York Academy of Sciences, 1124,* 1–38.

Caspi, A., McClay, J., Moffitt, T. E., Mill, J., Martin, J., Craig, I. W., et al. (2002). Role of genotype in the cycle of violence in maltreated children. *Science, 297*(5582), 851–854.

Cordes, D., Haughton, V. M., Arfanakis, K., Wendt, G. J., Turski, P. A., Moritz, C. H., et al. (2000). Mapping functionally related regions of brain with functional connectivity MR imaging. *American Journal of Neuroradiology, 21*(9), 1636–1644.

Cromer, K. R., & Sachs-Ericsson, N. (2006). The association between childhood abuse, PTSD, and the occurrence of adult health problems: Moderation via current life stress. *Journal of Traumatic Stress, 19*(6), 967–971.

Daniels, J. K., Frewen, P., McKinnon, M. C., & Lanius, R. A. (2011). Default mode alterations in posttraumatic stress disorder related to early-life trauma: A developmental perspective. *Journal of Psychiatry and Neuroscience, 36*(1), 56–59.

De Bie, H. M., Boersma, M., Adriaanse, S., Veltman, D. J., Wink, A. M., Roosendaal, S. D., et al. (2012). Resting-state networks in awake five- to eight-year old children. *Human Brain Mapping, 33*(5), 1189–1201.

Dube, S. R., Anda, R. F., Felitti, V. J., Chapman, D. P., Williamson, D. F., & Giles, W. H. (2001). Childhood abuse, household dysfunction, and the risk of attempted suicide throughout the life span: Findings from the Adverse Childhood Experiences Study. *Journal of the American Medical Association, 286*(24), 3089–3096.

Duncan, R. D., Saunders, B. E., Kilpatrick, D. G., Hanson, R. F., & Resnick, H. S. (1996). Childhood physical assault as a risk factor for PTSD, depression, and substance abuse: Findings from a national survey. *American Journal of Orthopsychiatry, 66*(3), 437–448.

Durston, S., Davidson, M. C., Tottenham, N., Galvan, A., Spicer, J., Fossella, J. A., et al. (2006). A shift from diffuse to focal cortical activity with development. *Developmental Science, 9*(1), 1–8.

Etkin, A., & Wager, T. D. (2007). Functional neuroimaging of anxiety: A meta-analysis of emotional processing in PTSD, social anxiety disorder, and specific phobia. *American Journal of Psychiatry, 164*(10), 1476–1488.

Fair, D. A., Cohen, A. L., Dosenbach, N. U., Church, J. A., Miezin, F. M., Barch, D. M., et al. (2008). The maturing architecture of the brain's default network. *Proceedings of the National Academy of Sciences of the United States of America, 105*(10), 4028–4032.

Felitti, V. J., Anda, R. F., Nordenberg, D., Williamson, D. F., Spitz, A. M., Edwards, V., et al. (1998). Relationship of childhood abuse and household dysfunction to many of the leading causes of death in adults: The Adverse Childhood Experiences (ACE) Study. *American Journal of Preventive Medicine, 14*(4), 245–258.

Flavell, J. H. (1999). Cognitive development: Children's knowledge about the mind. *Annual Review of Psychology, 50,* 21–45.

Fransson, P. (2005). Spontaneous low-frequency BOLD signal fluctuations: An fMRI investigation of the resting-state default mode of brain function hypothesis. *Human Brain Mapping, 26*(1), 15–29.

Fransson, P., Skiold, B., Engstrom, M., Hallberg, B., Mosskin, M., Aden, U., et al.

(2009). Spontaneous brain activity in the newborn brain during natural sleep: An fMRI study in infants born at full term. *Pediatric Research, 66*(3), 301–305.

Fransson, P., Skiold, B., Horsch, S., Nordell, A., Blennow, M., Lagercrantz, H., et al. (2007). Resting-state networks in the infant brain. *Proceedings of the National Academy of Sciences of the United States of America, 104*(39), 15531–15536.

Frewen, P. A., Dozois, D. J., Neufeld, R. W., Densmore, M., Lane, R. D., Stevens, T. C., et al. (2010). Individual differences in trait mindfulness predict dorsal medial prefrontal and amygdala response during emotional imagery: An fMRI study. *Personality and Individual Differences, 49*, 479–484.

Frewen, P. A., Dozois, D. J., Neufeld, R. W., Densmore, M., Stevens, T., & Lanius, R. A. (2011). Self-referential processing in women with PTSD: Affective and neural response. *Psychological Trauma: Theory, Research, Practice, and Policy, 3*(4), 318–328.

Frewen, P. A., Dozois, D. J., Neufeld, R. W., Lane, R. D., Densmore, M., Stevens, T. K., et al. (2012). Emotional numbing in posttraumatic stress disorder: A functional magnetic resonance imaging study. *Journal of Clinical Psychiatry, 73*(4), 431–436.

Frewen, P. A., Dozois, D. J., Neufeld, R. W., & Lanius, R. A. (2008). Meta-analysis of alexithymia in posttraumatic stress disorder. *Journal of Traumatic Stress, 21*(2), 243–246.

Frewen, P. A., Dozois, D. J., Neufeld, R. W., & Lanius, R. A. (2012). Disturbances of emotional awareness and expression in PTSD: Meta-mood emotion regulation mindfulness and interference of emotional expressiveness. *Psychological Trauma: Theory, Research, Practice, and Policy, 4*(2), 152–161.

Frewen, P. A., Lane, R. D., Neufeld, R. W., Densmore, M., Stevens, T., & Lanius, R. (2008). Neural correlates of levels of emotional awareness during trauma script-imagery in posttraumatic stress disorder. *Psychosomatic Medicine, 70*(1), 27–31.

Fridja, N. H. (2007). *The laws of emotion.* Mahwah, NJ: Erlbaum.

Gao, W., Zhu, H., Giovanello, K. S., Smith, J. K., Shen, D., Gilmore, J. H., et al. (2009). Evidence on the emergence of the brain's default network from 2–week-old to 2–year-old healthy pediatric subjects. *Proceedings of the National Academy of Sciences of the United States of America, 106*(16), 6790–6795.

Geuze, E., Westenberg, H. G., Jochims, A., de Kloet, C. S., Bohus, M., Vermetten, E., et al. (2007). Altered pain processing in veterans with posttraumatic stress disorder. *Archives of General Psychiatry, 64*(1), 76–85.

Gillihan, S. J., & Farah, M. J. (2005). Is self special?: A critical review of evidence from experimental psychology and cognitive neuroscience. *Psychological Bulletin, 131*, 76–97.

Gogtay, N., Ordonez, A., Herman, D. H., Hayashi, K. M., Greenstein, D., Vaituzis, C., et al. (2008). Dynamic mapping of cortical development before and after the onset of pediatric bipolar illness. *Journal of the American Academy of Child and Adolescent Psychiatry, 48*(9), 852–862.

Gogtay, N., Sporn, A., Clasen, L. S., Nugent, T. F., 3rd, Greenstein, D., Nicolson, R., et al. (2004). Comparison of progressive cortical gray matter loss in childhood-onset schizophrenia with that in childhood-onset atypical psychoses. *Archives of General Psychiatry, 61*(1), 17–22.

Heim, C., & Nemeroff, C. B. (2001). The role of childhood trauma in the neurobiology of mood and anxiety disorders: Preclinical and clinical studies. *Biological Psychiatry, 49*(12), 1023–1039.

Herman, J. (1997). *Trauma and recovery: The aftermath of violence—from domestic abuse to political terror.* New York: Basic Books.

Hermoye, L., Saint-Martin, C., Cosnard, G., Lee, S. K., Kim, J., Nassogne, M. C., et al. (2006). Pediatric diffusion tensor imaging: Normal database and observation of the white matter maturation in early childhood. *NeuroImage, 29*(2), 493–504.

Howe, M. L., & Courage, M. L. (1997). The emergence and early development of auto-biographical memory. *Psychological Review, 104*, 499–523.

Kessler, R. C., Berglund, P., Demler, O., Jin, R., Merikangas, K. R., & Walters, E. E. (2005). Lifetime prevalence and age-of-onset distributions of DSM-IV disorders in the National Comorbidity Survey Replication. *Archives of General Psychiatry, 62*(6), 593–602.

Kessler, R. C., Sonnega, A., Bromet, E., Hughes, M., & Nelson, C. B. (1995). Posttraumatic stress disorder in the National Comorbidity Survey. *Archives of General Psychiatry, 52*(12), 1048–1060.

Kim, H. (2010). Dissociating the roles of the default-mode, dorsal, and ventral networks in episodic memory retrieval. *NeuroImage, 50*(4), 1648–1657.

Kircher, T. T. J., Senior, C., Phillips, M. L., Benson, P. J., Bullmore, E. T., Brammer, M., et al. (2000). Towards a functional neuroanatomy of self processing: Effects of faces and words. *Cognitive Brain Research, 10*, 133–144.

Kober, H., Barrett, L. F., Joseph, J., Bliss-Moreau, E., Lindquist, K., & Wager, T. D. (2008). Functional grouping and cortical–subcortical interactions in emotion: A meta-analysis of neuroimaging studies. *NeuroImage, 42*(2), 998–1031.

Krupnick, J. L., Green, B. L., Stockton, P., Goodman, L., Corcoran, C., & Petty, R. (2004). Mental health effects of adolescent trauma exposure in a female college sample: Exploring differential outcomes based on experiences of unique trauma types and dimensions. *Psychiatry, 67*(3), 264–279.

Lambie, J. A., & Marcel, A. J. (2002). Consciousness and the varieties of emotion experience: A theoretical framework. *Psychological Review, 109*, 219–259.

Lane, R. D., & Schwartz, G. E. (1987). Levels of emotional awareness: A cognitive-developmental theory and its application to psychopathology. *American Journal of Psychiatry, 144*(2), 133–143.

Lanius, R. A., Bluhm, R. L., & Frewen, P. A. (2011). How understanding the neurobiology of complex post-traumatic stress disorder can inform clinical practice: A social cognitive and affective neuroscience approach. *Acta Psychiatrica Scandinavica, 124*(5), 331–348.

Lanius, R. A., Vermetten, E., & Pain, C. (Eds.). (2010). *The impact of early life trauma on health and disease: The hidden epidemic.* Cambridge, UK: Cambrige University Press.

Lanius, R. A., Williamson, P. C., Densmore, M., Boksman, K., Gupta, M. A., Neufeld, R. W., et al. (2001). Neural correlates of traumatic memories in posttraumatic stress disorder: A functional MRI investigation. *American Journal of Psychiatry, 158*, 1920–1922.

Legrand, D., & Ruby, P. (2009). What is self-specific?: Theoretical investigation and critical review of neuroimaging results. *Psychological Review, 116*, 252–282.

Levine, B. (2004). Autobiographical memory and the self in time: Brain lesion effects, functional neuroanatomy, and lifespan development. *Brain and Cognition, 55*, 54–68.

Liberzon, I., Taylor, S. F., Amdur, R., Jung, T. D., Chamberlain, K. R., Minoshima, S., et al. (1999). Brain activation in PTSD in response to trauma-related stimuli. *Biological Psychiatry, 45*, 817–826.

Lowe, M. J., Mock, B. J., & Sorenson, J. A. (1998). Functional connectivity in single and multislice echoplanar imaging using resting-state fluctuations. *NeuroImage, 7*(2), 119–132.

MacMillan, H. L., Fleming, J. E., Streiner, D. L., Lin, E., Boyle, M. H., Jamieson, E., et al. (2001). Childhood abuse and lifetime psychopathology in a community sample. *American Journal of Psychiatry, 158*(11), 1878–1883.

McCauley, J., Kern, D. E., Kolodner, K., Dill, L., Schroeder, A. F., DeChant, H. K., et al. (1997). Clinical characteristics of women with a history of childhood abuse: Unhealed wounds. *Journal of the American Medical Association, 277*(17), 1362–1368.

Murray, E. A. (2008). The amygdala, reward, and emotion. *Trends in Cognitive Sciences, 11*, 489–497.

Northoff, G., Heinzel, A., de Greck, M., Bermpohl, F., Dobrowolny, H., & Panksepp, J. (2006). Self-referential processing in our brain: A meta-analysis of imaging studies on the self. *NeuroImage, 31*(1), 440–457.

Pavaluri, M. N., & Sweeney, J. A. (2008). Integrating functional brain neuroimaging and developmental cognitive neuroscience in child psychiatry research. *Journal of the American Academy of Child and Adolescent Psychiatry, 47*(11), 1273–1288.

Perner, J., & Wimmer, H. (1985). "John thinks that Mary thinks that . . . " attribution of second-order beliefs by 5- to 10-year-old children. *Journal of Experimental Child Psychology, 39*, 437–471.

Povinelli, D. J., Landau, K. R., & Perilloux, H. K. (1996). Self-recognition in young children using delayed versus live feedback: Evidence of a developmental asynchrony. *Child Development, 67*(4), 1540–1554.

Power, J. D., Fair, D. A., Schlaggar, B. L., & Petersen, S. E. (2010). The development of human functional brain networks. *Neuron, 67*(5), 735–748.

Raichle, M. E. (2010). The brain's dark energy. *Scientific American, 302*(3), 44–49.

Raichle, M. E., & Gusnard, D. A. (2005). Intrinsic brain activity sets the stage for expression of motivated behavior. *Journal of Comparative Neurology, 493*(1), 167–176.

Raichle, M. E., MacLeod, A. M., Snyder, A. Z., Powers, W. J., Gusnard, D. A., & Shulman, G. L. (2001). A default mode of brain function. *Proceedings of the National Academy of Sciences of the United States of America, 98*, 676–682.

Sajonz, B., Kahnt, T., Margulies, D. S., Park, S. Q., Wittmann, A., Stoy, M., et al. (2010). Delineating self-referential processing from episodic memory retrieval: Common and dissociable networks. *NeuroImage, 50*(4), 1606–1617.

Saxe, R., Moran, J. M., Scholz, J., & Gabrieli, J. (2006). Overlapping and non-overlapping brain regions for theory of mind and self reflection in individual subjects. *Social Cognitive and Affective Neuroscience, 1*(3), 229–234.

Schmitz, T. W., & Johnson, S. C. (2007). Relevance to self: A brief review and framework of neural systems underlying appraisal. *Neuroscience and Biobehavioral Reviews, 31*(4), 585–596.

Schore, A. N. (2002). Dysregulation of the right brain: A fundamental mechanism of traumatic attachment and the psychopathogenesis of posttraumatic stress disorder. *Australian and New Zealand Journal of Psychiatry, 36*, 9–30.

Shaw, P., Eckstrand, K., Sharp, W., Blumenthal, J., Lerch, J. P., Greenstein, D., et al. (2007). Attention-deficit/hyperactivity disorder is characterized by a delay in cortical maturation. *Proceedings of the National Academy of Sciences of the United States of America, 104*(49), 19649–19654.

Shin, L. M., McNally, R. J., Kosslyn, S. M., Thompson, W. L., Rauch, S. L., Alpert, N. M., et al. (1999). Regional cerebral blood flow during script-driven imagery in childhood sexual abuse-related PTSD: A PET investigation. *American Journal of Psychiatry, 156*, 575–584.

Siegel, D. J. (2007). *The mindful brain: Reflection and attunement in the cultivation of well-being.* New York: Norton.

Spreng, R. N., & Grady, C. L. (2010). Patterns of brain activity supporting autobiographical memory, prospection, and theory of mind, and their relationship to the default mode network. *Journal of Cognitive Neuroscience, 22*(6), 1112–1123.

Spreng, R. N., Mar, R. A., & Kim, A. S. (2009). The common neural basis of autobiographical memory, prospection, navigation, theory of mind, and the default mode: A quantitative meta-analysis. *Journal of Cognitive Neuroscience, 21*(3), 489–510.

Stein, M. B., Walker, J. R., Anderson, G., Hazen, A. L., Ross, C. A., Eldridge, G., et al. (1996). Childhood physical and sexual abuse in patients with anxiety disorders and in a community sample. *American Journal of Psychiatry, 153*(2), 275–277.

Supekar, K., Uddin, L. Q., Prater, K., Amin, H., Greicius, M. D., & Menon, V. (2010). Development of functional and structural connectivity within the default mode network in young children. *NeuroImage, 52*(1), 290–301.

Thomason, M. E., Chang, C. E., Glover, G. H., Gabrieli, J. D., Greicius, M. D., & Gotlib, I. H. (2008). Default-mode function and task-induced deactivation have overlapping brain substrates in children. *NeuroImage, 41*(4), 1493–1503.

Uddin, L. Q., Supekar, K. S., Ryali, S., & Menon, V. (2011). Dynamic reconfiguration of structural and functional connectivity across core neurocognitive brain networks with development. *Journal of Neuroscience, 31*(50), 18578–18589.

van der Kolk, B. A., Roth, S., Pelcovitz, D., Sunday, S., & Spinazzola, J. (2005). Disorders of extreme stress: The empirical foundation of a complex adaptation to trauma. *Journal of Traumatic Stress, 18,* 389–399.

van der Meer, L., Costafreda, S., Aleman, A., & David, A. S. (2010). Self-reflection and the brain: A theoretical review and meta-analysis of neuroimaging studies with implications for schizophrenia. *Neuroscience and Biobehavioral Reviews, 34,* 935–946.

Van Overwalle, F. (2009). Social cognition and the brain: A meta-analysis. *Human Brain Mapping, 30*(3), 829–858.

Widom, C. P. (1999). Posttraumatic stress disorder in abused and neglected children grown up. *American Journal of Psychiatry, 156,* 1223–1229.

Widom, C. S., Marmorstein, N. R., & White, H. R. (2006). Childhood victimization and illicit drug use in middle adulthood. *Journal of the Society of Psychologists in Addictive Behaviors, 20*(4), 394–403.

Williams, L. M., Kemp, A. H., Felmingham, K., Barton, M., Olivieri, G., Peduto, A., et al. (2006). Trauma modulates amygdala and medial prefrontal responses to consciously attended fear. *NeuroImage, 29*(2), 347–357.

Winnicott, D. W. (Ed.). (1960). *The maturational processes and the facilitating environment.* New York: International Universities Press.

CHAPTER 3

Relational Trauma and Disorganized Attachment

Pamela C. Alexander

The concept of relational trauma is based on the notion that what is most dangerous to a child is not necessarily an *event* but instead involves threat that is directly associated with the relationship with the caregiver. Because a young child cannot survive without access to a caregiver, the caregiver need not even be abusive or frightening to the child, but instead simply emotionally unavailable, for the child to experience realistic terror (Hennighausen, Bureau, David, Holmes, & Lyons-Ruth, 2011). One striking example of this distinction was put forth by Bowlby (1973), who noted that, during the bombing of London in World War II, children who were safely removed to the countryside but without access to their parents actually exhibited more symptoms than children who stayed with their parents in the city. The long-term effects of relational trauma are pervasive and severe, encompassing physiology, brain development, cognition, affect, and behavior. The fact that the relationship with a primary caregiver is distinct from factors such as infant temperament, inborn physical characteristics, gender, or the relationship with the other parent points to its unique specificity (Lyons-Ruth, 1996; van IJzendoorn, Schuengel, & Bakermans-Kranenburg, 1999).

Attachment theory provides a framework for understanding relational trauma that emphasizes this centrality of the parent–child relationship (Bowlby, 1969/1982). This chapter focuses on attachment theory; disorganized attachment, which has been found to be associated with traumatic disruption in the caregiver–young child relationship; the neuroscience of relational trauma; and the distal antecedents and risk factors predictive of disorganized attachment. The chapter also considers factors that may influence the effects of relational trauma, including the larger family context and the child's gender and genetic vulnerabilities. Finally, implications for treatment are briefly considered.

Disclaimer about Gender of Parent

In this chapter, I use the feminine pronoun to refer to the primary caregiver with the obvious acknowledgment that men also serve as caregivers of their children. I use this convention for ease of reading. Also, because women generally are the primary caregivers in our society, research finds differences in children's reactions to mothers and fathers that more accurately reflect differences in reactions to primary and nonprimary caregivers. For example, even though mothers and fathers do not differ in their rates of behaviors that are frightening to children, infant disorganization is more likely to result from maternal than paternal disruptive behaviors (Abrams, Rifkin, & Hesse, 2006). Similarly, somatoform dissociative disorders are associated with maternal, and not paternal, abusiveness and dysfunction (Roelofs, Keijers, Hoogduin, Naring & Moene, 2002). Finally, only maternal posttraumatic stress disorder (PTSD)—and not paternal PTSD—is associated with PTSD in the offspring of Holocaust survivors, suggesting the primacy of parenting over genetics in the intergenerational transmission of this diagnosis (Yehuda, Bell, Bierer, & Schmeidler, 2008). However, the implications of research findings are undoubtedly relevant to any primary caregiver, regardless of gender.

Attachment Theory

As articulated by John Bowlby (1969/1982), attachment theory assumes that there is a biologically based bonding process that drives a child to seek access and proximity to a caregiver, especially in situations of danger or fear. Because not only abuse but also abandonment and even careless inattention by the caregiver can threaten the survival of the human infant, this relationship becomes the starting point for any discussion of trauma. In fact, the importance of the parent's availability to the child may explain why the effects of neglect appear to be more deleterious than the effects of intentional abuse (Hildyard & Wolfe, 2002; Sleed & Fonagy, 2010). In order to maintain this essential connection, the child monitors the whereabouts of the attachment figure and develops all sorts of strategies, including distortions of affect and cognition if necessary, to avoid feeling the lack of access to the attachment figure.

The child's strategies (or lack thereof) for maintaining this connection are the basis for the categorization of attachment behaviors observed in the Strange Situation, a laboratory-based series of separations and reunions between infants and primary caregivers that was validated with observations of parent–child interactions in their homes (Ainsworth, Blehar, Waters, & Wall, 1978). *Secure* attachment is marked by the child's tendency to reconnect with the parent upon reunion (or when stressed at home), to be appropriately soothed by the parent, and then to quickly return to play and exploration. From his or her experience of using the parent as a secure base from which to explore and as a safe haven during times of stress, the child learns to internalize the parent's regulation of his or her affect, to self-soothe, and to develop positive expectations of self and others. The essence of secure attachment is thus the mother's regulation of the infant's internal states, from which the child develops the capacity to self-regulate (Schore, 2010). In *avoidant* attachment, the parent is responsive to the degree that the child displays no overt need or distress (Izard & Kobak, 1991). The child thus learns that the best way to maintain contact with the rejecting parent is to suppress any expression of negative affect, with the unfortunate result that the avoidant child fails to learn to recognize and modulate his or her own negative affect. This child also learns to be highly self-sufficient and to detach as a way to ward off additional disappointment by the unresponsive caregiver. The third organized attachment strategy—*anxious–ambivalent*—refers to the child's heightened display of negative affect, which is used to get attention from an inconsistent parent. While effective in gaining the parent's attention in the moment, the parent finds the behavior annoying and tends to avoid the child, resulting in a vicious cycle of the child's fussy and demanding behavior alternating with coy, guilt-inducing, and clinging behavior (Crittenden, 1997; Moran & Pederson, 1998).

Each of these organized attachment patterns has its counterpart in the adult's state of mind or internal working model regarding attachment, assessed by means of the Adult Attachment Interview (AAI; Main & Goldwyn, 1998). By relying upon discourse analysis to assess attachment, the AAI bypasses insecure individuals' inability to accurately reflect on self-states. A meta-analysis of several longitudinal studies over a period of 20 years demonstrated a moderate correspondence between infant attachment classifications and the AAI (Fraley, 2002). Not surprisingly, the *secure/autonomous* adult has easy access to both positive and negative memories, values attachment relationships, is aware of negative affect without feeling overwhelmed by it, is less prone to anger, ruminates less, and is less avoidant (Main & Goldwyn, 1998; Mikulincer, 1998). The *dismissing* adult (comparable to the avoidant child) minimizes the importance of early attachment relationships and self-reports high levels of anger control and little overt distress, while actually exhibiting marked physiological arousal when stressed (Dozier & Kobak, 1992; Mikulincer, 1998; Spangler & Grossmann, 1993). Finally, the *preoccupied* adult (comparable to the anxious–ambivalent child) displays a passive or angry preoccupation with the attachment figure, intense and volatile emotions, high anxiety and impulsiveness, sees even ambiguous stimuli as hostile or as threatening, and tends to associate conflict and expression of anger with increased intimacy (Main & Goldwyn, 1998; Mikulincer, 1998; Pietromonaco & Barrett, 1997, 2000).

Disorganized Attachment

In addition to these organized attachment categories, a fourth category was described by researchers who found that the traditional three-category classification system did not adequately account for the Strange Situation behavior of many children with a known history of trauma (Carlson, Cicchetti, Barnett, & Braunwald, 1989). This attachment category forms the basis for most of the work on relational trauma. The *disorganized and/or disoriented* child displays odd, contradictory, approach–avoidant behaviors, trance-like dazed expressions, and apparent apprehension upon the parent's return in the Strange Situation. His or her behavior seems strikingly out of context; for example, crying and approaching the mother while looking away, or greeting the mother upon reunion and then falling prone to the floor (Main & Solomon, 1986, 1990; Solomon & George, 2011b). The disorganized classification is typically given a second classification of one of the three organized categories. The category on the AAI comparable to disorganized attachment is "unresolved" (U), given when the respondent displays lapses in reasoning or dissociated ideas or memories when asked to speak about any experiences of trauma or loss (Main & Goldwyn, 1998). As is the case for the disorganized classification in children, the U classification is given a second classification of one of the three organized categories on the AAI.

Proximal Antecedents of Disorganized Attachment

Parental behaviors empirically associated with disorganized attachment in children have understandably been the focus of much observation and theorizing. Research suggests that mothers classified as unresolved display frightening behavior toward the child or actually appear to be frightened, if not by the child him- or herself, then by some inexplicable force in the environment. In either case, the mother's fear signals a lack of protection to the child (Hesse & Main, 1999). Frequently, the child's very presence triggers a fearful reaction in the mother in which she may look to the child to help her control her anxiety (Liotti, 1992). The child thus paradoxically needs to turn for comfort to the very attachment figure who is causing the child's fear—a situation of "fright without solution" (Hesse & Main, 1999). Hesse and Main identified a number of scenarios characterized by frightening/frightened (FR) behavior by the parent. For example, the unresolved mother may display threatening behavior to the child for no particular reason, including subtle predatory or stalking behavior such as suddenly "looming" into the infant's face or placing her hands around the infant's throat from behind (Main & Hesse, 1990). She may appear to retreat in fear from the child or may appear frightened by some unseen threat. She may dissociate and thus be mentally absent, may turn to the child as a source of protection, or may display sexualized behavior toward the child. Hesse and Main emphasized that FR behaviors are not generally related to a parent's harsh discipline, which can usually be reduced by the child's compliance, or to the parent's fear of something external, but observable to the child, especially when the parent quickly reassures the child to repair the interaction.

The relationship between parental unresolved attachment, FR behaviors, and disorganized attachment is not, however, clear-cut: only 50% of disorganized children have mothers who are categorized as unresolved on the AAI (van IJzendoorn, 1995). In fact, proximal antecedents of disorganized attachment include more than FR behaviors, as made evident by Lyons-Ruth's research with at-risk samples. Lyons-Ruth and her colleagues developed a coding system of the Strange Situation (Atypical Maternal Behavior Instrument for Assessment and Classification; AMBIANCE), from which they derived five atypical maternal behaviors that are predictive of disorganized attachment in the child: (1) affective communication errors, (2) role confusion, (3) intrusiveness/negativity, (4) disorientation, and (5) withdrawal (Lyons-Ruth, Bronfman, & Parsons, 1999b). Affective communication errors are often at root of disorganized attachment and consist of the mother's contradictory communications, inappropriate responses, or the failure to respond to an infant's clear communication. For example, whereas mothers of disorganized–insecure infants exhibit hostile intrusive and role-reversing behavior, mothers of disorganized–secure children are less interactive, more fearful and inhibited in their behavior, but not frightening, dissociated, role-reversed, or actively rejecting (Lyons-Ruth, Bronfman, & Atwood, 1999a; Lyons-Ruth, Alpern, & Repacholi, 1993; Lyons-Ruth et al., 1999b; Lyons-Ruth, Repacholi, McLeod & Silva, 1991). However, similar sequelae are observed in disorganized–secure and disorganized–insecure infants, including elevated cortisol levels in reaction to stress (Lyons-Ruth, Lyubchik, Wolfe, & Bronfman, 2002). This finding suggests that a mother's *profound lack of response* may be just as damaging as FR behaviors. Even if not actively abusive, a caregiver's chronic misattunement increases the child's risk of exposure to subsequent trauma stemming from a lack of protection and from a failure to help the child resolve the emotional distress from prior exposures to trauma (Lyons-Ruth, Yellin, Melnick, & Atwood, 2005).

Consistent with this perspective, Solomon and George (1999) argued that the essence of the disorganized parent–child dynamic is parental activation of the attachment system (e.g., through prolonged separation, rejection, or threats to abandon or send the child away) combined with the parent's failure to then resolve the child's attachment behavior. *It is thus not frightening or frightened behavior per se, but more importantly the parent's abdication of caregiving that is most predictive of disorganized attachment.* Furthermore, there are several ways in which a mother might exhibit this caregiving helplessness or failure to regulate or organize the attachment–caregiving relationship (Solomon & George, 2011b). She might become enraged and punitive. She might constrict her emotions and withdraw from the child, perhaps even locking herself in a room. Or she may become dependent on her child's caregiving—the role reversal noted by Main and Hesse and by Lyons-Ruth. In each situation, the mother sees herself as helpless with regard to the child and with regard to her own strong negative emotions. She is not only abdicating her role as a parent, but also passively placing her child at risk for abuse by others. The disorganized caregiving behavior observed in the Strange Situation may thus be just a proxy for the highly dysregulated and frightening interactions within the home (Solomon & George, 1999).

The Neuroscience of Relational Trauma

The behavior of the disorganized child in relation to the mother can be understood more clearly when one considers the impact of attachment on the biological substrate of the developing brain. Through mutual gaze and the mother's interpretation of the child's facial cues, the mother monitors the child's affective states, regulates her own and her child's autonomic nervous system, and modulates the child's excessively high and excessively low levels of arousal (Schore, 2010). The concept of reflective functioning describes the same process from another perspective. Namely, the mother mirrors the child's affective state (validating and labeling the child's emotions), but then displays a different emotional state by soothing the child (exhibiting mastery of her own emotions while regulating her child's affective state). The child not only begins to understand and to regulate his or her own emotions but also comes to realize that his or her affective state is distinct from that of the mother's (Fonagy, 1999; Fonagy, Target, & Gergely, 2000). When inevitable misattunements occur, the "good-enough" parent repairs the interaction in order to re-regulate the child (Schore, 2010). This affective synchronization between mother and child leads to the release of oxytocin, catecholamines, and cortisol, all of which are necessary for the development of the brain, the development of social bonds, and the long-term development of the hypothalamic–pituitary–adrenal (HPA) axis, important for the regulation of stress (Schore, 2010). The primary site for this brain-to-brain communication between mother and child is the orbital-frontal (ventral-medial) cortex of the right hemisphere—in essence, the locus of the attachment system and "the brain's most complex affect and stress regulatory system" (Schore, 2010, p. 23), with strong connections to the limbic system (see also Schore, Chapter 1, this volume).

In contrast to the good-enough parenting described above, with relational trauma the mother actively overstimulates the child through abuse and frightening behavior and/or understimulates the child through neglect, failing to provide any repair of this misattunement, to protect the child from other sources of stress and danger, and through her inaccessibility, to regulate her child's over- and/or underarousal (Schore, 2010). There are then two phases involved in the infant's physiological reaction to this severe interpersonal stress: hyperarousal and dissociation (Schore, 2003). With hyperarousal (Bowlby's notion of "protest"), the sympathetic nervous system is activated, leading to increased secretion of the stress hormone corticotropin-releasing factor (CRF), thus accounting for the infant's behavioral symptoms of "fear-terror" (Schore, 2010, p. 29). However, when the child's intense engagement with the external environment fails to elicit a response, there is a sudden shift to a state of dissociation and hypoarousal (Schore, 2003). The infant's striking disengagement from the environment reflects the increased activation of the parasympathetic nervous system (especially the dorsal vagal complex in the brainstem medulla), characterized by metabolic shutdown and cardiac deceleration. This is, in essence, a state of conservation and withdrawal, comparable to a primitive form of defense seen in animals when they feign death and attempt to survive by remaining unnoticed (Porges, 1997; Schore, 2003). During this state of helplessness and powerlessness, endogenous opioids are released to facilitate the blunting of pain and distress, and activation of the dorsal complex in the brainstem medulla leads to decreased blood pressure, metabolic activity and heart rate. Interestingly, both chronic hyper- and hypoarousal of the HPA axis have been associated with high rates of aggression (Veenema, 2009). Given the importance of the right brain for coping with negative affect and stress (Sullivan & Dufresne, 2006), there are serious adverse effects of relational trauma on both the development of the brain (including decreased hippocampal volume; Vythilingam et al., 2002) and the child's subsequent ability to cope with stress.

Furthermore, the effects of relational trauma not only persist into adulthood but perhaps even intergenerationally due to the mechanism of epigenesis. The concept of epigenesis suggests that a child's experience, both prenatally *in utero* and postnatally in social interactions with the mother, actively alters the expression of genes through the process of DNA methylation. That is, with the addition of methyl groups (a carbon atom and two hydrogen atoms) to either adenine or cytosine—two of the four chemical bases forming DNA—the particular gene is effectively silenced, diminished, or augmented (Yehuda & Bierer, 2009). Pertinent to relational trauma, individuals with a history of maltreatment have more highly methylated glucocorticoid receptor genes leading to the release of higher amounts of stress hormones in response to stress (McGowan et al., 2009). Epigenesis thus recalibrates the system to respond differently to subsequent stress (Yehuda & Bierer, 2009) and has been associated with increased levels of attention-deficit/hyperactivity disorder (ADHD), impulsivity, aggression, and unresolved loss or trauma (Mill & Petronis, 2008; Roskam, Kinoo, & Nassogne, 2007; van IJzendoorn et al., 2010; Veenema, 2009). Moreover, although not as stable as DNA inheritance, epigenesis is not fully erased during meiosis, leading to "soft inheritance" or the intergenerational transmission of some traits (Mill & Petronis, 2008). Thus, the effects of relational trauma are not only long-lasting but may even be transmitted to subsequent generations.

Distal Antecedents of Parental Behavior

Whether described from the perspective of behavior, psychophysiology, or reflective functioning, optimal parenting is dependent upon the mother's ability to accurately read and respond to her child's inferred internal state. Therefore, it is important to ask what would lead a caregiver to view herself and/or her child as "wildly frightening, out of control and dangerous" (Solomon & George, 2011a, p. 14) and to abdicate caregiving. There appear to be multiple pathways to this cognitive representation of parenting, including a mother's history of unresolved trauma or loss, her history of hostile or helpless parenting, and her current risk environment, all of which may or may not lead her to actually maltreat her children.

Unresolved Trauma and Loss

One pathway to parenting difficulties is a mother's experience of unresolved trauma or loss, both of which predict her child's disorganized attachment (Ainsworth & Eichberg, 1991; Hughes, Turton, McGauley, & Fonagy, 2006; Main & Hesse, 1990; Moss, Bureau, St-Laurent, & Tarabulsy, 2011). Factors contributing to this lack of resolution include the mother's specific loss in childhood of her parent or attachment figure (Coffino, 2009; Lyons-Ruth et al., 1991; Main & Hesse, 1990; Schuengel, Bakermans-Kranenburg, & van IJzendoorn, 1999) as well as her experience of loss within 2 years of the birth of her child (Hesse & van IJzendoorn, 1998; Liotti, Pasquini, & the Italian Group, 2000; Solomon & George, 2011b). Trauma and loss are frequently related, especially in cases of child sexual abuse and general maltreatment (Bailey, Moran, & Pederson, 2007), and may interact with more recent traumatic experiences in predicting disorganized attachment (Hughes et al., 2006). Furthermore, whether or not a loss or trauma remains unresolved as well as its impact on the mother's relationship with her child are affected by other preexisting and current family dynamics (Solomon & George, 2011b).

The AAI and Hostile/Helpless Parenting

The failure to find a consistent pathway from unresolved attachment in the parent to disorganized attachment in the child may be due in part to several limitations of Main and Hesse's coding of the AAI. For example, the unresolved category is coded only on the portion of the AAI referring to loss or trauma and only if the individual actually reports loss or trauma, the acknowledgment of which may be absent with especially traumatized or dissociative individuals, resulting in a false negative. Second, studies conducted on at-risk samples have found upward of 80% of disorganized children with mothers who are not classified as unresolved on the AAI, suggesting that something is missed with the traditional coding of the AAI (Solomon & George, 2011b).

In an attempt to address these limitations, Lyons-Ruth developed an additional coding system of the AAI specifically for clinical populations with severe histories of chronic trauma (Lyons-Ruth, Yellin, Melnick, & Atwood, 2003, 2005). Lyons-Ruth and her colleagues derived the following codes based on discourse patterns throughout the whole interview reflecting the parent's experience of hostile or helpless (H/H) states of mind: global devaluation of a caregiver, identification with a hostile caregiver, recurrent references to fearful affect, the sense of self as bad, laughter at recollections of pain, and ruptured attachments. There is little overlap between U status and H/H states of mind in nonclinical samples (Lyons-Ruth et al., 2005), although the H/H coding system predicts disorganized–insecure attachment in infants even more than does mothers' U attachment (Lyons-Ruth et al., 2005; Melnick, Finger, Hans, Patrick, & Lyons-Ruth, 2008).

Multiple-Risk Environments

A third pathway to disorganized attachment is through the contribution of both past and current multiple-risk environments. For example, a large majority of a sample of mothers of D–insecure infants had reported histories of violence, parental substance abuse, or the loss of both parents because of out-of-home care (Lyons-Ruth et al., 1991). Thus, social risks by themselves—including marital problems, mental health problems, teen pregnancy, substance abuse, and parenting stress—may contribute directly to disorganized attachment (Bernier & Meins, 2008; Bakermans-Kranenburg, van IJzendoorn & Juffer, 2005; van IJzendoorn et al., 1999). In their meta-analysis of 69 high-risk samples, Cyr, Euser, Bakermans-Kranenburg, and van IJzendoorn (2010) found that the cumulative effects of five socioeconomic risk factors (low income, substance abuse, young maternal age at child birth, low education, and single parenthood) accounted for as much disorganization as actual child maltreatment. That is, a mother's current exposure to violence is associated with her negative evaluations of her infant and of herself as a mother; her decreased sensitivity to, or even maltreatment of, her child; and her failure to regulate her child's fear (Almqvist & Broberg, 2003; Finger, Hans, Bernstein, & Cox, 2009; Huth-Bocks, Levendosky, Theran, & Bogat, 2004; Sokolowski, Hans, Bernstein, & Cox, 2007). The effect is further exacerbated by the child's increased attachment behaviors, which trigger the mother's own posttraumatic symptoms and subsequent disengagement from her child (Almqvist & Broberg, 2003). Thus, even in the absence of abusive maternal behavior, a mother's history of loss or trauma, hostile/helpless experiences in childhood, and current experiences of multiple risks contribute to relational trauma.

Subsequent Behavior of the Disorganized Child

As opposed to the generally odd and contradictory behavior of the disorganized toddler in the Strange Situation, the behavior of the disorganized child tends to evolve by age 6 into controlling behavior toward the parent (Main & Cassidy, 1988). This apparent change in the child's strategy for interacting with the parent develops out of the child's increased physical maturity and cognitive ability to deal with the disrupted attachment. The controlling child's success in reducing the mother's stress is manifest in her decreased levels of anxiety and depression (Moss, Thibaudeau, Cyr, & Rousseau, 2001). However, although this strategy may be effective in calming and engaging her, the mother still fails to meet the child's emotional needs (Hazen, Jacobvitz, Higgins, Allen, & Jin, 2011). Furthermore, although the controlling behavior may appear organized, assessments of the children with doll play reveal highly disorganized cognitive representations of attachment relationships, with themes of danger, chaos, or inhibition present in all disorganized children, whether they are controlling or not (Hesse & Main, 1999; Solomon, George, & De Jong, 1995).

Controlling behavior typically takes one of two forms. In *controlling–punitive* behavior, the child is confrontational and combative with the parent, using verbal threats and harsh commands. The mother appears helpless, withdrawn, and intimidated by the child, is clearly stressed by this role-reversing behavior, and describes the child as moody, hyperactive, difficult, and out of control (Jacobvitz & Hazen, 1999; Moss, Bureau, et al., 2011; Moss, Cyr, & Dubois-Comtois, 2004). The child's behavior is associated with the mother's own unresolved fearful experiences and with disrupted maternal communication (Bureau, Easterbrooks, & Lyons-Ruth, 2009; Moss, Bureau, et al., 2011).

The *controlling–caregiving* child attempts to structure the interaction with the parent by being helpful or protective, trying to cheer up the parent (Hennighausen et al., 2011; Moss, Bureau, et al., 2011). However, there is a clear lack of reciprocity between the child and the mother, with the mother appearing passive and disengaged. As the child approaches school age, the mother describes increasingly more positive feelings about the child, seeing the child as precocious and taking responsibility for the mother's feelings (George & Solomon, 1996; Moss, Bureau, et al., 2011). Because the mother of the controlling–caregiving child typically did not receive comfort herself as a child, she withdraws from her child's cues of distress (Hennighausen et al., 2011; Moss, Bureau, et al., 2011). Controlling–caregiving children often have more internalizing problems, but are not typically aggressive and are therefore more likely to have positive interactions with teachers and peers (Jacobvitz & Hazen, 1999; Moss, Bureau, et al., 2011).

In research with high-risk samples, it became apparent that approximately a third of disorganized children do *not* become controlling, either because they lack the cognitive skills to do so or because the shifting alliances in their chaotic household interfere with the development of a consistent controlling strategy (Hennighausen et al., 2011; Moss, Bureau, et al., 2011). Instead, they are *behaviorally disorganized,* resembling the disorganized infant, with abrupt changes of state; fearful, disoriented, and sexualized behavior; and observable confusion and apprehension in the parent's presence (Hennighausen et al., 2011; Moss, Bureau, et al., 2011). They are the most disturbed of all the disorganized children, exhibiting odd and socially disconnected behavior when interacting with peers (Jacobvitz & Hazen, 1999; Moss, Bureau et al., 2011). Their homes are characterized by significant marital dysfunction, violence, triangulation with both parents, and hospitalization of a parent due to serious illness or accident (Hennighausen et al., 2011; Jacobvitz, Riggs, & Johnson, 1999; Moss et al., 2004).

In early and middle childhood, controlling–punitive and behaviorally disorganized children tend to exhibit externalizing problems and aggressive behavior toward peers, even controlling for gender, IQ, and socioeconomic status (SES; Lyons-Ruth et al., 1993; Moss, Bureau, et al., 2011; Munson, McMahon, & Spieker, 2001). Disorganized children in general also exhibit academic problems, poor sense of self, performance anxiety, problems in self-control, low levels of metacognition, and mental delay due in part to the parent's lack of structure and the significant attention demanded by the parent's confusing behavior (Lyons-Ruth et al., 1991; Moss, St,-Laurent & Parent, 1999; Moss, Bureau, et al., 2011).

There are implications of these behavior patterns for trajectories of subsequent relationships. For example, these unbalanced parent–child relationships continue into adolescence and range from submissive or caregiving stances to those that are controlling–punitive or disoriented (Hennighausen et al., 2011). Furthermore, these children's aggression toward peers, and their vulnerability to aggression *by* peers, lead to increased experiences of stress and limit the availability of future friendships and relationships (Alexander, 2012). The phenotypic resemblance of children's controlling behavior to adulthood relationships characterized by violence and vulnerability to violence is striking.

Potential Moderators of Relational Trauma

Not all children respond to problematic parenting with either the same degree of severity or with the same types of symptoms. Understanding the moderators of relational trauma can provide the basis for more effective preventive or treatment interventions.

The Importance of the Family Environment

As has been described, children raised in a multiple-risk family environment are much more likely to experience disorganized–insecure attachment, maltreatment, and behavioral disorganization. However, even in the absence of a chaotic violent household, family dynamics may contribute to a child's risk for relational trauma or even maltreatment. For example, a history of unresolved trauma may influence an adult's choice of a partner, as suggested by evidence of increased concordance between partners for U classification on the AAI and for other behaviors such as substance abuse or antisocial behavior often associated with a history of unresolved trauma (Galbaud du Fort, Boothroyd, Bland, Newman, & Kakuma, 2002; Low, Cui, & Merikangas, 2007; van IJzendoorn & Bakermans-Kranenburg, 1996). The result, of course, is that each parent may present with his or her own problematic history. Even the withdrawal observed in the mothers of disorganized–secure infants (Lyons-Ruth et al., 1999a) could realistically be experienced by the child as a lack of protection if some other individual inside or outside the home uses the opportunity to prey upon the child. Moreover, a role-reversing relationship with the mother frequently leads to a different form of role reversal with the father (Jacobvitz & Hazen, 1999). Similarly, marital dissatisfaction increases the risk for role-reversed parenting among trauma victims (Alexander, Teti, & Anderson, 2000). Conversely, a supportive marital relationship ameliorates the negative effect of a mother's trauma history on her parenting (Cowan & Cowan, 2007). Therefore, any discussion of relational trauma must consider the broader family context.

The Child's Gender

Gender appears to play an important moderating role in the prediction of relational trauma and in its outcomes, but only under certain conditions.

For example, gender differences in disorganized attachment have not been observed in low-risk middle-class samples, under low-FR conditions, or when the mother's behavior is characterized by withdrawal (David & Lyons-Ruth, 2005). Similarly, there are no gender differences in the overall rates of controlling punitive or caregiving behavior (Hennighausen et al., 2011; Moss et al., 2004) or in the amount of FR behaviors elicited from mothers by boys and girls (David & Lyons-Ruth, 2005).

On the other hand, gender differences do emerge in high-risk samples (Carlson et al., 1989; Solomon & George, 2011b). Namely, boys exhibit more disorganized and insecure behavior in reaction to their mothers' abusive or disrupted behavior. In contrast, girls exhibit more secure, avoidant, or disorganized–secure attachment and respond to their mothers' disorganized behavior with approach, affiliation, and compliance (Hazen et al., 2011; Lyons-Ruth et al., 1999b, 2002). David and Lyons-Ruth (2005) have interpreted these differences as evidence of Taylor's (2006) notion of fight or flight in males and tending or befriending in females. Alternatively, mothers may simply understand their daughters better, whereas boys may be more subject to their mothers' intrusiveness and negativity (Crockenberg, Leerkes, & Jo, 2008; Solomon & George, 2011b). A third possibility is that the specific mother–child dynamics may vary as a function of the mother's history. For example, Sroufe and Ward (1980) observed that mothers who had been sexually abused as children were more likely to engage in sexualized role-reversing behavior with their sons (increasing the sons' risk for disorganized attachment) while overtly rejecting their daughters (increasing the daughters' risk for avoidant but not necessarily disorganized attachment and for abuse or other exploitation by others).

Gender differences have also emerged with regard to longer-term effects of disorganized attachment: Disorganized boys are more likely than girls to exhibit externalizing behaviors, social problems, and even internalizing behaviors, although aggressive behavior may simply take different forms among boys and girls (Fearon et al., 2010; Hazen et al., 2011). Furthermore, in at-risk samples, boys are more likely to exhibit controlling–punitive behavior toward their mothers, whereas girls are more likely to exhibit controlling–caregiving behavior (Hazen et al., 2011). However, even with high-risk samples, such differences are not always consistent. For example, Munson et al. (2001) found that 9-year-old disorganized daughters exhibited more externalizing problems than did sons. The authors speculated that the higher rates of aggressive behaviors in adolescent mothers may have counteracted any gender-specific socialization of their children. In conclusion, whether due to biological predisposition, gender-specific socialization or the common absence of fathers in high-risk samples (a factor as yet unexamined in gender comparisons of disorganized attachment), gender differences appear to emerge in studies of relational trauma among mother–child dyads experiencing life stress.

Genetic Predispositions

Research on gene–environment interactions suggests that some children may be particularly vulnerable to confusing or frightening parent–child interactions because of a genetic predisposition. Lakatos et al. (2000) indeed found an association between disorganized attachment and the dopamine D4 receptor *(DRD4)* 7-repeat gene polymorphism, previously associated with impulsive behavior and substance abuse in adults and ADHD in children. Although Bakermans-Kranenburg and van IJzendoorn (2004) did not find a direct link between this genotype and disorganized attachment, they subsequently found that this polymorphism interacted with a mother's history of unresolved loss or trauma to heighten the risk, by 18.8-fold, for her child's disorganized attachment status, compared to children without this genotype (van IJzendoorn & Bakermans-Kranenburg, 2006).

In addition to research focused on the dopaminergic system, other research has focused on serotonin (5-hydroxytryptamine, or 5-HT) functioning due to its role in the regulation of mood, social behavior, impulsivity, and eating behavior. More specifically, the presence of a short-allele copy of the 5-HT transporter promoter region polymorphism *(5HTTLPR)* has been found to interact with a history of child maltreatment in predicting increased risks for stimulus seeking, insecure attachment, depression, and PTSD (Aguilera et al., 2009; Steiger et al., 2007; Xie et al., 2009). Other researchers have observed disorganized attachment in a sample of low-risk children with this serotonergic polymorphism only if their mothers displayed low responsiveness, highlighting the comparability of outcomes between this type of maternal behavior and other types of maltreatment (Spangler, Johann, Ronai, & Zimmermann, 2009). These findings were bolstered by Caspers et al.'s (2009) finding of an association between the *5HTTLPR* polymorphism and unresolved attachment in adults. While these studies suggest a genetic vulnerability to the effects of abuse, the results could also reflect children's increased risk for abuse due to their parents' genetic predisposition for impulsive or pathological behavior or due to the children's own impulsivity or risk-taking behavior that may elicit maltreatment (Steiger et al., 2008).

Implications for Treatment

A number of interventions has been developed to reduce the risk for disorganized attachment as a strategy for preventing future mental health problems. A meta-analysis of 51 randomized controlled studies (Bakermans-Kranenburg, van IJzendoorn, & Juffer, 2003) as well as a subsequent meta-analysis of 15 preventive interventions (Bakermans-Kranenburg et al., 2005) both concluded that relatively brief, behavioral dyadic parent–child interventions that focus explicitly on increasing maternal sensitivity are the most successful in reducing disorganized attachment. Consistent with this perspective, Madigan, Hawkins, Goldberg, and Benoit (2006) demonstrated the success of an attachment-based intervention, consisting of an assessment feedback session and three intervention sessions, in decreasing disrupted caregiver behavior. Using videotaped interactive free play, therapists identified adaptive and positive caregiver behaviors as well as insensitive or disruptive caregiver behaviors in response to infants' behavioral cues. A similar six-session intervention titled "Video-Feedback Intervention to Promote Positive Parenting and Sensitive Discipline" (VIPP-SD) for middle-class Dutch families also proved effective in enhancing maternal sensitivity and sensitive discipline (Van Zeijl et al., 2006). Yet another efficacious program consisted of 8 weeks of home visitation with maltreating families, combining the use of video feedback with discussions of attachment and emotion regulation (Moss, Dubois-Comtois, et al., 2011).

However, Lyons-Ruth's work with high-risk families highlighted the complexity of working with multiproblem families. Although 0–18 months of weekly home visits for children referred for treatment because of community agencies' concerns about caregiving quality did indeed subsequently lead to day care workers'/teachers' reports of reduced aggressive behavior, results were variable (Lyons-Ruth & Easterbrooks, 2006; Lyons-Ruth & Melnick, 2004). Namely, the behavior of infants who received fewer services deteriorated over time, perhaps because the full developmental effects of the dysfunctional family environment were not yet evident by 18 months when the home visits ceased. On the other hand, longer-served families developed generalized family communication or problem-solving skills that seemed to stabilize the rates of problem behaviors that came and went over time. Moreover, conflict arising within high-risk and non-co-residing partners may need to be addressed to enhance maternal sensitivity and reduce the child's exposure to frightening parental behavior (Finger et al., 2009). In summary, consistent with the research on behaviorally disorganized children and multiple-risk environments, the dyadic parent–child interaction cannot be divorced from the broader family and community context.

Interventions focused on caregiver sensitivity are also less effective for mothers with histories of unresolved trauma (Moran, Pederson, & Krupka, 2005). For example, Forough and Muller (2011) noted that dyadic parent–child therapy may inadvertently trigger early attachment-related concerns in parents with a history of childhood trauma, thereby necessitating the processing of parents' trauma experiences along with the dyadic interactions. In fact, the VIPP intervention referred to earlier proved to be even more effective when it included discussions of mothers' childhood attachment experiences with regard to their current caregiving (Velderman, Bakermans-Kranenburg, Juffer, & van IJzendoorn, 2006). Lyons-Ruth and Spielman (2004) described the utility of therapists explicitly addressing mothers' experiences of hostile–helpless parenting in order to help them learn to balance the needs of the self with the needs of the infant. Koren-Karie, Oppenheim, and Getzler-Yosef (2008) stressed the importance of mothers' resolution of trauma in predicting their sensitivity in guiding their children's conversations about emotional events. Polansky, Lauterbach, Litzke, Coulter, and Sommers (2006) described an attachment-based parenting group for drug-addicted mothers. Group participants reflected on their experiences of being parented by their own mothers with the goal of using their self-empathy to learn to empathize with, and better care for, their own children. For mothers with a history of traumatic loss, mourning the loss may be essential to allow them to be more available to their new infants (Hughes et al., 2006). Therefore, although Webster and Hackett (2011) underscored the need to intervene with mothers regarding their caregiving as distinct from their own attachment system, it is doubtful that unresolved mothers will be able to fully benefit from dyadic parent–child interventions without also attending to their own attachment histories and unresolved issues.

Finally, it is important to not ignore the role of the child in the attachment relationship. Research on disorganized attachment and relational trauma has implications for treating children suffering from traumatic loss (Crenshaw, 2006) and for intervening with adolescents (Hilburn-Cobb, 2004). Marvin and Whelan (2003) reflected upon their work with the Circle of Security Project to emphasize that children with problematic attachments miscue their caregivers about their attachment needs. This remains a significant challenge for even securely attached adoptive or foster parents, let alone biological parents who share the same genes, the same histories, and the same current circumstances.

Conclusion

Traditional definitions of trauma frequently fail to capture what is most dangerous and frightening, and hence, most traumatizing, to an infant. The most potentially terrifying experiences for a child occur within the context of his or her most important relationship—that with the primary caregiver. Therefore, the best way to ameliorate the child's experience of trauma is to intervene, when possible, in that relationship, focusing on ways to foster the caregiver's sensitivity and responsiveness, both directly and by addressing those historical and current conditions that interfere with the caregiver's responsiveness.

References

Abrams, K. Y., Rifkin, A., & Hesse, E. (2006). Examining the role of parental frightened/frightening subtypes in predicting disorganized attachment within a brief observational procedure. *Development and Psychopathology, 18,* 345–361.
Aguilera, M., Arias, B., Wichers, M., Barrantes-Vidal, N., Moya, J., Villa, H., et al.

(2009). Early adversity and 5-HTT/BDNF genes: New evidence of gene–environment interactions on depressive symptoms in a general population. *Psychological Medicine, 39*, 1425–1432.

Ainsworth, M. D. S., Blehar, M., Waters, E., & Wall, S. (1978). *Patterns of attachment.* Hillsdale, NJ: Erlbaum.

Ainsworth, M. D. S., & Eichberg, C. G. (1991). Effects on infant–mother attachment of mother's unresolved loss of an attachment figure, or other traumatic experience. In C. M. Parkes & J. Stevenson-Hinde (Eds.), *Attachment across the life cycle* (pp. 160–183). New York: Tavistock/Routledge.

Alexander, P. C. (2012). Retraumatization and revictimization: An attachment perspective. In M.P. Duckworth & V. M. Follette (Eds.), *Retraumatization: Assessment, treatment and prevention* (pp. 191–220). New York: Routledge.

Alexander, P. C., Teti, L., & Anderson, C. L. (2000). Child sexual abuse history and role reversal in parenting. *Child Abuse and Neglect, 24*, 829–838.

Almqvist, K., & Broberg, A. G. (2003). Young children traumatized by organized violence together with their mothers: The critical effects of damaged internal representations. *Attachment and Human Development, 5*, 367–380.

Bailey, H. N., Moran, G., & Pederson, D. R. (2007). Childhood maltreatment, complex trauma symptoms, and unresolved attachment in an at-risk sample of adolescent mothers. *Attachment and Human Development, 9*, 139–161.

Bakermans-Kranenburg, M. J., & van IJzendoorn, M. H. (2004). No association of the dopamine D4 receptor (DRD4) and -521 C/T promoter polymorphisms with infant attachment disorganization. *Attachment and Human Development, 6*, 211–218.

Bakermans-Kranenburg, M. J., van IJzendoorn, M. H., & Juffer, F. (2003). Less is more: Meta-analyses of sensitivity and attachment interventions in early childhood. *Psychological Bulletin, 129*, 195–215.

Bakermans-Kranenburg, M. J., van IJzendoorn, M. H., & Juffer, F. (2005). Disorganized infant attachment and preventive interventions: A review and meta-analysis. *Infant Mental Health Journal, 26*, 191–216.

Bernier, A., & Meins, E. (2008). A threshold approach to understanding the origins of attachment disorganization. *Developmental Psychology, 44*, 969–982.

Bowlby, J. (1973). *Attachment and loss: Vol. 2. Separation: Anger and anxiety.* New York: Basic Books.

Bowlby, J. (1982). *Attachment and loss: Vol. 1. Attachment.* New York: Basic Books. (Original work published 1969)

Bureau, J.-F., Easterbrooks, E. A., & Lyons-Ruth, K. (2009). Attachment disorganization and role-reversal in middle childhood: Maternal and child precursors and correlates. *Attachment and Human Development, 11*, 1–20.

Carlson, V., Cicchetti, D., Barnett, D., & Braunwald, K. (1989). Disorganized/disoriented attachment relationships in maltreated infants. *Developmental Psychology, 25*, 525–531.

Caspers, K. M., Paradiso, S., Yucuis, R., Troutman, B., Arndt, S., & Philibert, R. (2009). Association between the serotonin transporter promoter polymorphism *(5-HTTLPR)* and adult unresolved attachment. *Developmental Psychology, 45*, 64–76.

Coffino, B. (2009). The role of childhood parent figure loss in the etiology of adult depression: Findings from a prospective longitudinal study. *Attachment and Human Development, 11*, 445–470.

Cowan, P. A., & Cowan, C. P. (2007). Attachment theory: Seven unresolved issues and questions for future research. *Research in Human Development, 4*, 181–201.

Crenshaw, D. A. (2006). An interpersonal neurobiological-informed treatment model for childhood traumatic grief. *Omega: Journal of Death and Dying, 54*, 319–335.

Crittenden, P. M. (1997). Toward an integrative theory of trauma: A dynamic-maturation approach. In D. Cicchetti & S. L. Toth (Eds.), *Developmental perspectives on trauma: Theory, research, and intervention* (pp. 33–84). Rochester, NY: University of Rochester Press.

Crockenberg, S. C., Leerkes, E. M., & Jo, P. S. B. (2008). Predicting aggressive behavior in the third year from infant reactivity and regulation as moderated by maternal behavior. *Development and Psychopathology, 20,* 37–54.

Cyr, C., Euser, E. M., Bakermans-Kranenburg, M. J., & van IJzendoorn, M. H. (2010). Attachment security and disorganization in maltreating and high-risk families: A series of meta-analyses. *Development and Psychopathology, 22,* 87–108.

David, D. H., & Lyons-Ruth, K. (2005). Differential attachment responses of male and female infants to frightening maternal behavior: Tend or befriend versus fight or flight? *Infant Mental Health Journal, 26,* 1–18.

Dozier, M., & Kobak, R. (1992). Psychophysiology in attachment interviews: Converging evidence for deactivating strategies. *Child Development, 63,* 1473–1480.

Fearon, R. P., Bakermans-Kranenburg, M. J., van IJzendoorn, M. H., Lapsley, A.-M., & Roisman, G. I. (2010). The significance of insecure attachment and disorganization in the development of children's externalizing behavior: A meta-analytic study. *Child Development, 81,* 435–456.

Finger, B., Hans, S. L., Bernstein, V. J., & Cox, S. M. (2009). Parent relationship quality and infant–mother attachment. *Attachment and Human Development, 11,* 285–306.

Fonagy, P. (1999). Male perpetrators of violence against women: An attachment theory perspective. *Journal of Applied Psychoanalytic Studies, 1,* 7–27.

Fonagy, P., Target, M., & Gergely, G. (2000). Attachment and borderline personality disorder: A theory and some evidence. *Psychiatric Clinics of North America, 23,* 103–122.

Foroughe, M. F., & Muller, R. T. (2011). Dismissing (avoidant) attachment and trauma in dyadic parent–child psychotherapy. *Psychological Trauma, 3,* 1–8.

Fraley, R. C. (2002). Attachment stability from infancy to adulthood: Meta-analysis and dynamic modeling of developmental mechanisms. *Personality and Social Psychology Review, 6,* 123–151.

Galbaud du Fort, G., Boothroyd, L. J., Bland, R. C., Newman, S. C., & Kakuma, R. (2002). Spouse similarity for antisocial behavior in the general population. *Psychological Medicine, 32,* 1407–1416.

George, C., & Solomon, J. (1996). Representational models of relationships: Links between caregiving and attachment. *Infant Mental Health Journal, 17,* 198–216.

Hazen, N. L., Jacobvitz, D., Higgins, K. N., Allen, S., & Jin, M. K. (2011). Pathways from disorganized attachment to later social–emotional problems: The role of gender and parent–child interaction patterns. In J. Solomon & C. George (Eds.), *Disorganized attachment and caregiving* (pp. 167–206). New York: Guilford Press.

Hennighausen, K. H., Bureau, J.-F., David, D. H., Holmes, B. M., & Lyons-Ruth, K. (2011). Disorganized attachment behavior observed in adolescence: Validation in relation to Adult Attachment Interview classifications at age 25. In J. Solomon & C. George (Eds.), *Disorganized attachment and caregiving* (pp. 207–244). New York: Guilford Press.

Hesse, E., & Main, M. (1999). Second-generation effects of unresolved trauma in non-maltreating parents: Dissociated, frightening, and threatening parental behavior. *Psychoanalytic Inquiry, 19,* 481–540.

Hesse, E., & van IJzendoorn, M. H. (1998). Parental loss of close family members and propensities towards absorption in offspring. *Developmental Science, 1,* 299–305.

Hilburn-Cobb, C. (2004). Adolescent psychopathology in terms of multiple behavioral systems: The role of attachment and controlling strategies and frankly disorganized behavior. In L. Atkinson & S. Goldberg (Eds.), *Attachment issues in psychopathology and intervention* (pp. 95–135). Mahwah, NJ: Erlbaum.

Hildyard, K. L., & Wolfe, D. A. (2002). Child neglect: Developmental issues and outcomes. *Child Abuse and Neglect, 26,* 679–695.

Hughes, P., Turton, P., McGauley, G. A., & Fonagy, P. (2006). Factors that predict infant disorganization in mothers classified as U in pregnancy. *Attachment and Human Development, 8,* 113–122.

Huth-Bocks, A. C., Levendosky, A. A., Theran, S. A., & Bogat, G. A. (2004). The impact of domestic violence on mothers' prenatal representations of their infants. *Infant Mental Health Journal, 25,* 79–98.

Izard, C., & Kobak, R. (1991). Emotion system functioning and emotion regulation In J. Garber & K. Dodge (Eds.), *The development of affect regulation* (pp. 303–321). Cambridge, UK: Cambridge University Press.

Jacobvitz, D., & Hazen, N. (1999). Developmental pathways from infant disorganization to childhood peer relationships. In J. Solomon & C. George (Eds.), *Attachment disorganization* (pp. 127–159). New York: Guilford Press.

Jacobvitz, D., Riggs, S., & Johnson, E. M. (1999). Cross-sex and same-sex family alliances: Immediate and long-term effects on daughters and sons. In N. D. Chase (Ed.), *Parentified children: Theory, research and treatment* (pp. 34–55). Thousand Oaks, CA: Sage.

Koren-Karie, N., Oppenheim, D., & Getzler-Yosef, R. (2008). Shaping children's internal working models through mother–child dialogues: The importance of resolving past maternal trauma. *Attachment and Human Development, 10,* 465–483.

Lakatos, K., Toth, I., Nemoda, Z., Ney, K., Sasvari-Szekely, M., & Gervai, J. (2000). Dopamine D4 receptor *(DRD4)* gene polymorphism is associated with attachment disorganization in infants. *Molecular Psychiatry, 5,* 633–637.

Liotti, G. (1992). Disorganized/disoriented attachment in the etiology of the dissociative disorders. *Dissociation, 5,* 196–204.

Liotti, G., Pasquini, P., & the Italian Group for the Study of Dissociation. (2000). Predictive factors for borderline personality disorder: Patients' early traumatic experiences and losses suffered by the attachment figure. *Acta Psychiatrica Scandinavica, 102,* 282–289.

Low, N., Cui, L., & Merikangas, K. R. (2007). Spousal concordance for substance use and anxiety disorders. *Journal of Psychiatric Research, 41,* 942–951.

Lyons-Ruth, K. (1996). Attachment relationships among children with aggressive behavior problems: The role of disorganized early attachment patterns. *Journal of Consulting and Clinical Psychology, 64,* 64–73.

Lyons-Ruth, K., Alpern, L., & Repacholi, B. (1993). Disorganized infant attachment classification and maternal psychosocial problems as predictors of hostile-aggressive behavior in the preschool classroom. *Child Development, 64,* 572–585.

Lyons-Ruth, K., Bronfman, E., & Atwood, G. (1999a). A relational diathesis model of hostile–helpless states of mind: Expressions in mother–infant interaction. In J. Solomon & C. George (Eds.), *Attachment disorganization* (pp. 33–70). New York, NY: Guilford Press.

Lyons-Ruth, K., Bronfman, E., & Parsons, E. (1999b). Maternal frightened, frightening or atypical behavior and disorganized infant attachment patterns. *Monographs of the Society for Research on Child Development, 64,* 67–96.

Lyons-Ruth, K., & Easterbrooks, M. A. (2006). Assessing mediated models of family change in response to infant home visiting: A two-phase longitudinal analysis. *Infant Mental Health Journal, 27,* 55–69.

Lyons-Ruth, K., Lyubchik, A., Wolfe, R., & Bronfman, E. (2002). Parental depression and child attachment: Hostile and helpless profiles of parent and child behavior among families at risk. In S. H. Goodman & I. H. Gotlib (Eds.), *Children of depressed parents: Mechanisms of risk and implications for treatment* (pp. 89–120). Washington, DC: American Psychological Association.

Lyons-Ruth, K., & Melnick, S. (2004). Dose–response effect of mother–infant clinical home visiting on aggressive behavior problems in kindergarten. *Journal of the American Academy of Child Adolescent Psychiatry, 43,* 699–707.

Lyons-Ruth, K., Repacholi, B., McLeod, S., & Silva, E. (1991). Disorganized attachment behavior in infancy: Short-term stability, maternal and infant correlates, and risk-related subtypes. *Development and Psychopathology, 3,* 377–396.

Lyons-Ruth, K., & Spielman, E. (2004). Disorganized infant attachment strategies and helpless–fearful profiles of parenting: Integrating attachment research with clinical intervention. *Infant Mental Health Journal, 25,* 318–335.

Lyons-Ruth, K., Yellin, C., Melnick, S., & Atwood, G. (2003). Childhood experiences of trauma and loss have different relations to maternal unresolved and hostile–helpless states of mind on the AAI. *Attachment and Human Development, 5,* 330–352.

Lyons-Ruth, K., Yellin, C., Melnick, S., & Atwood, G. (2005). Expanding the concept of unresolved mental states: Hostile/helpless states of mind on the Adult Attachment Interview are associated with disrupted mother–infant communication and infant disorganization. *Development and Psychopathology, 17,* 1–23.

Madigan, S., Hawkins, E., Goldberg, S., & Benoit, D. (2006). Reduction of disrupted caregiver behavior using modified interaction guidance. *Infant Mental Health Journal, 27,* 509–527.

Main, M., & Cassidy, J. (1988). Categories of response to reunion with the parent at age 6: Predictable from infant attachment classifications and stable over a 1-month period. *Developmental Psychology, 24,* 415–426.

Main, M., & Goldwyn, R. (1998). *Adult attachment scoring and classification system, Version 6.3.* Unpublished manuscript, University of California at Berkeley.

Main, M., & Hesse, E. (1990). Parents' unresolved traumatic experiences are related to infant disorganized attachment status: Is frightened and/or frightening parental behavior the linking mechanism? In M. T. Greenberg, D. Cicchetti, & E. M. Cummings (Eds.), *Attachment in the preschool years* (pp. 161–182). Chicago: University of Chicago Press.

Main, M., & Solomon, J. (1986). Discovery of a new, insecure–disorganized/disoriented attachment pattern. In T. B. Brazelton & M. W. Yogman (Eds.), *Affective development in infancy* (pp. 95–124). Norwood, NJ: Ablex.

Main, M., & Solomon, J. (1990). Procedures for identifying infants as disorganized/disoriented during the Ainsworth Strange Situation. In M. T. Greenberg, D. Cicchetti, & E. M. Cummings (Eds.), *Attachment in the preschool years* (pp. 121–160). Chicago: University of Chicago Press.

Marvin, R. S., & Whelan, W. F. (2003). Disordered attachments: Toward evidence-based clinical practice. *Attachment and Human Development, 5,* 283–288.

McGowan, P. O., Sasaki, A., D'Alessio, A. C., Dymov, S., Labonte, B., Szyf, M., et al. (2009). Epigenetic regulation of the glucocorticoid receptor in human brain associates with childhood abuse. *Nature Neuroscience, 12,* 342–348.

Melnick, S., Finger, B., Hans, S., Patrick, M., & Lyons-Ruth, K. (2008). Hostile–helpless states of mind in the AAI: A proposed additional AAI category with implications for identifying disorganized infant attachment in high-risk samples. In H. Steele & M. Steele (Eds.), *Clinical applications of the Adult Attachment Interview* (pp. 399–423). New York: Guilford Press.

Mikulincer, M. (1998). Adult attachment style and individual differences in functional versus dysfunctional experiences of anger. *Journal of Personality and Social Psychology, 74,* 513–524.

Mill, J., & Petronis, A. (2008). Pre- and peri-natal environmental risks for attention-deficit hyperactivity disorder (ADHD): The potential role of epigenetic processes in mediating susceptibility. *Journal of Child Psychology and Psychiatry, 49,* 1020–1030.

Moran, G., & Pederson, D. R. (1998). Proneness to distress and ambivalent relationships. *Infant Behavior and Development, 21,* 493–503.

Moran, G., Pederson, D. R., & Krupka, A. (2005). Maternal unresolved attachment status impedes the effectiveness of interventions with adolescent mothers. *Infant Mental Health Journal, 26,* 231–249.

Moss, E., Bureau, J.-F., St.-Laurent, D., & Tarabulsy, G. M. (2011). Understanding disorganized attachment at preschool and school age: Examining divergent pathways of disorganized and controlling children. In J. Solomon & C. George (Eds.), *Disorganized attachment and caregiving* (pp. 52–79). New York: Guilford Press.

Moss, E., Cyr, C., & Dubois-Comtois, K. (2004). Attachment at early school age and developmental risk: Examining family contexts and behavior problems of controlling–caregiving, controlling–punitive, and behaviorally disorganized children. *Developmental Psychology, 40,* 519–532.

Moss, E., Dubois-Comtois, K., Cyr, C., Tarabulsy, G. M., St.-Laurent, D., & Bernier, A. (2011). Efficacy of a home-visiting intervention aimed at improving maternal sensitivity, child attachment, and behavioral outcomes for maltreated children: A randomized control trial. *Development and Psychopathology, 23,* 195–210.

Moss, E., St.-Laurent, D., & Parent, S. (1999). Disorganized attachment and developmental risk at school age. In J. Solomon & C. George (Eds.), *Attachment disorganization* (pp. 160–186). New York, NY: Guilford Press.

Moss, E., Thibaudeau, P., Cyr, C., & Rousseau, D. (2001, April). *Controlling attachment and child management of parental emotion.* Paper presented at the biennial meeting of the Society for Research in Child Development, Minneapolis, MN.

Munson, J. A., McMahon, R. J., & Spieker, S. J. (2001). Structure and variability in the developmental trajectory of children's externalizing problems: Impact of infant attachment, maternal depressive symptomatology, and child sex. *Development and Psychopathology, 13,* 277–296.

Pietromonaco, P. R., & Barrett, L. (1997). Working models of attachment and daily social interactions. *Journal of Personality and Social Psychology, 73,* 1409–1423.

Pietromonaco, P. R., & Barrett, L. F. (2000). The internal working models concept: What do we really know about the self in relation to others? *Review of General Psychology, 4,* 155–175.

Polansky, M., Lauterbach, W., Litzke, C., Coulter, B., & Sommers, L. (2006). A qualitative study of an attachment-based parenting group for mothers with drug addictions: On being and having a mother. *Journal of Social Work Practice, 20,* 115–131.

Porges, S. W. (1997). Emotion: An evolutionary by-product of the neural regulation of the autonomic nervous system. *Annals of the New York Academy of Sciences, 807,* 62–77.

Roelofs, K., Keijers, G. P., Hoogduin, K. A., Naring, G. W., & Moene, F. C. (2002). Childhood abuse in patients with conversion disorder. *American Journal of Psychiatry, 159,* 1908–1913.

Roskam, I., Kinoo, P., & Nassogne, M.-C. (2007). Children displaying externalizing behavior: Epigenetic and developmental framework. *Neuropsychiatrie de l'Enfance et de l'Adolescence, 55,* 204–213.

Schore, A. N. (2003). Early relational trauma, disorganized attachment, and the development of a predisposition to violence. In M. F. Solomon & D. J. Siegel (Eds.), *Healing trauma: Attachment, mind, body, and brain* (pp. 107–167). New York: Norton.

Schore, A. N. (2010). Relational trauma and the developing right brain. In T. Baradon (Ed.), *Relational trauma in infancy* (pp. 19–47). New York: Routledge.

Schuengel, C., Bakermans-Kranenburg, M. J., & van IJzendoorn, M. (1999). Frightening maternal behavior linking unresolved loss and disorganized infant attachment. *Journal of Consulting and Clinical Psychology, 67,* 54–63.

Sleed, M., & Fonagy, P. (2010). Understanding disruptions in the parent–infant relationship: Do actions speak louder than words? In T. Baradon (Ed.), *Relational trauma in infancy: Psychoanalytic, attachment, and neuropsychological contributions to parent–infant psychotherapy* (pp. 136–162). New York: Routledge/Taylor & Francis.

Sokolowski, M. S., Hans, S. L., Bernstein, V. J., & Cox, S. M. (2007). Mothers' representations of their infants and parenting behavior: Associations with personal and social–contextual variables in a high-risk sample. *Infant Mental Health Journal, 28,* 344–365.

Solomon, J., & George, C. (1999). The place of disorganization in attachment theory: Linking classic observations with contemporary findings. In J. Solomon & C. George (Eds.), *Attachment disorganization* (pp. 3–32). New York: Guilford Press.

Solomon, J., & George, C. (2011a). The disorganized attachment–caregiving system: Dysregulation of adaptive processes at multiple levels. In J. Solomon & C. George (Eds.), *Disorganized attachment and caregiving* (pp. 1–24). New York: Guilford Press.

Solomon, J., & George, C. (2011b). Disorganization of maternal caregiving across two generations: The origins of caregiving helplessness. In J. Solomon & C. George (Eds.), *Disorganized attachment and caregiving* (pp. 25–51). New York: Guilford Press.

Solomon, J., George, C., & De Jong, A. (1995). Children classified as controlling at age six: Evidence of disorganized representational strategies and aggression at home and at school. *Development and Psychopathology, 7,* 447–463.

Spangler, G., & Grossmann, K. E. (1993). Biobehavioral organization in securely and insecurely attached infants. *Child Development, 64,* 1439–1450.

Spangler, G., Johann, M., Ronai, Z., & Zimmermann, P. (2009). Genetic and environmental influence on attachment disorganization. *Journal of Child Psychology and Psychiatry, 50,* 952–961.

Sroufe, L. A., & Ward, M. J. (1980). Seductive behavior of mothers of toddlers: Occurrence, correlates, and family origins. *Child Development, 51,* 1222–1229.

Steiger, H., Richardson, J., Joober, R., Gauvin, L., Israel, M., Bruce, K. R., et al. (2007). The *5HTTLPR* polymorphism, prior maltreatment, and dramatic–erratic personality manifestations in women with bulimic syndromes. *Journal of Psychiatry and Neuroscience, 32,* 354–362.

Steiger, H., Richardson, J., Joober, Israel, M., Bruce, K. R., & Kin, N. M. K. (2008). Dissocial behavior, the *5HTTLPR* polymorphism, and maltreatment in women with bulimic syndromes. *American Journal of Medical Genetics: Part B, 147B,* 128–130.

Sullivan, R. M., & Dufresne, M. M. (2006). Mesocortical dopamine and HPA axis regulation: Role of laterality and early environment. *Brain Research, 1076,* 49–59.

Taylor, S. (2006). Tend and befriend: Biobehavioral bases of affiliation under stress. *Current Directions in Psychological Science, 15,* 273–277.

van IJzendoorn, M. (1995). Adult attachment representations, parental responsiveness, and infant attachment: A meta-analysis on the predictive validity of the Adult Attachment Interview. *Psychological Bulletin, 117,* 387–403.

van IJzendoorn, M. H., & Bakermans-Kranenburg, M. J. (1996). Attachment representations in mothers, fathers, adolescents, and clinical groups: A meta-analytic search for normative data. *Journal of Consulting and Clinical Psychology, 64,* 8–21.

van IJzendoorn, M. H., & Bakermans-Kranenburg, M. J. (2006). *DRD4* 7-repeat polymorphism moderates the association between maternal unresolved loss or trauma and infant disorganization. *Attachment and Human Development, 8,* 291–307.

van IJzendoorn, M. H., Caspers, K., Bakermans-Kranenburg, M. J., Beach, S. R. H.,

& Philibert, R. (2010). Methylation matters: Interaction between methylation density and serotonin transporter genotype predicts unresolved loss or trauma. *Biological Psychiatry, 68,* 405–407.

van IJzendoorn, M. H., Schuengel, C., & Bakermans-Kranenburg, M. J. (1999). Disorganized attachment in early childhood: Meta-analysis of precursors, concomitants, and sequelae. *Development and Psychopathology, 11,* 225–249.

Van Zeijl, J., Mesman, J., van IJzendoorn, M. H., Bakermans-Kranenburg, M. J., Juffer, F., Stolk, M. N., et al., (2006). Attachment-based intervention for enhancing sensitive discipline in mothers of 1- to 3-year-old children at risk for externalizing behavior problems: A randomized controlled trial. *Journal of Consulting and Clinical Psychology, 74,* 994–1005.

Veenema, A. H. (2009). Early life stress, the development of aggression, and neuroendocrine and neurobiological correlates: What can we learn from animal models? *Frontiers in Neuroendocrinology, 30,* 497–518.

Velderman, M. K., Bakermans-Kranenburg, M. J., Juffer, F., & van IJzendoorn, M. H. (2006). Effects of attachment-based interventions on maternal sensitivity and infant attachment: Differential susceptibility of highly reactive infants. *Journal of Family Psychology, 20,* 266–274.

Vythilingam, M., Heim, C., Newport, J., Miller, A. H., Anderson, E., Bronen, R., et al. (2002). Childhood trauma associated with smaller hippocampal volume in women with major depression. *American Journal of Psychiatry, 159,* 2072–2080.

Webster, L., & Hackett, R. K. (2011). An exploratory investigation of the relationships among representational security, disorganization, and behavior ratings in maltreated children. In J. Solomon & C. George (Eds.), *Disorganized attachment and caregiving* (pp. 292–317). New York: Guilford Press.

Xie, P., Kranzler, H. R., Poling, J., Stein, M. B., Anton, R. F., Brady, K., et al. (2009). Interactive effect of stressful life events and the serotonin transporter *5-HTTLPR* genotype on posttraumatic stress disorder diagnosis in 2 independent populations. *Archives of General Psychiatry, 66,* 1201–1209.

Yehuda, R., Bell, A., Bierer, L. M., & Schmeidler, J. (2008). Maternal, not paternal, PTSD is related to increased risk for PTSD in offspring of Holocaust survivors. *Journal of Psychiatric Research, 42,* 1104–1111.

Yehuda, R., & Bierer, L. M. (2009). The relevance of epigenetics to PTSD: Implications for the DSM-V. *Journal of Traumatic Stress, 22,* 417–434.

CHAPTER 4

Betrayal Trauma

Laura A. Kaehler
Rebecca Babcock
Anne P. DePrince
Jennifer J. Freyd

An estimated 6 million children and adolescents in the United States were referred to child protective services (CPS) in 2010 for experiences of maltreatment, including abuse (physical, sexual, and emotional) and/or neglect (U.S. Department of Health and Human Services [USDHHS], 2010). In an estimated 81% of those cases, perpetrators were caregivers. Due to variations in legal and research definitions of child maltreatment as well as false negatives in reporting (Chu, Pineda, DePrince, & Freyd, 2011), the prevalence of caregiver maltreatment is likely underestimated by federal numbers. Moreover, the terms *child maltreatment* and *child sexual abuse* are used in ways that obscure the fact that perpetrators are often relatives or those otherwise in positions of responsibility or known to the child. In the case of sexual abuse, *incest* is the more accurate terminology (Courtois, 2010). Children and adolescents mistreated by those in positions of trust (e.g., caregivers) are at high risk for a range of deleterious outcomes, including depression (Putnam, 2003), dissociation (Putnam, 1997), cognitive deficits (DePrince, Weinzierl, & Combs, 2009), and difficulties in emotional processing (Reichmann-Decker, DePrince, & McIntosh, 2010). For clinicians and researchers seeking to understand the adverse outcomes associated with caregiver maltreatment, betrayal trauma theory (BTT) offers a potentially useful theoretical framework (Freyd, Klest, & DePrince, 2009, p. 20). At its heart, "BTT is an approach to conceptualizing trauma that points to the importance of social relationships in understanding posttraumatic outcomes, including 'reduced recall' " (Freyd, DePrince, & Gleaves, 2007, p. 297; see also Freyd, 1994, 1996, 2001).

This chapter first offers a review of relevant issues from attachment theory as they relate to BTT and child maltreatment. Next, we describe BTT research conducted with adult samples and discuss the importance of studying BTT with child and adolescent samples. We then present the BTT research conducted with children and adolescents. Next, the clinical implications of BTT research with children and adults are discussed in terms of the theory's relevance for revictimization prevention and therapeutic intervention. The chapter concludes with recommendations for future BTT-related clinical and research directions.

Attachment Theory and Maltreatment

Attachment theory, developed by Bowlby (1973, 1988), posits that infants are biologically programmed to develop and maintain an attachment to a caregiver early in life in order to ensure survival. The attachment system supports two major functions: a protective and coping function when the child is faced with dangerous situations ("safe haven") and an exploratory function by ensuring the availability of the attachment figure (the "secure base"). The attachment system becomes activated under stressful conditions: perceived threats to the availability of an attachment figure, perceived danger in the environment, and perceived challenges when exploring new and challenging situations (Kobak, Cassidy, Lyons-Ruth, & Ziv, 2006). Yet, when the parent is the source of the danger (e.g., in maltreatment or incest), there is a paradox of approach–avoidance needs. The parent's frightening behavior places the child in an unsolvable situation because the attachment figure acts as both the safe haven and the source of the threat. When frightened, the child will have the urge to move toward the parent (safe haven) as well as away from the source of threat; however, if the child moves away from the source of the threat, he or she then will want to move toward the parent (safe haven). Hesse and Main (1999, 2006) term this paradox the "fright without solution."

Mary Ainsworth and colleagues (Ainsworth, Blehar, Waters, & Wall, 1978) identified three styles of attachment: securely attached infants (type B) and two insecurely attached groups: anxious–avoidant (type A) and anxious–ambivalent (type C). Main and Solomon (1986) developed a fourth category, disorganized (type D) because the behaviors displayed by many children could not be classified using the three "organized" categories. These children demonstrated contradictory approach–avoidance behaviors and appeared to present an inconsistent behavioral and attentional strategy. In a literature review based on 13 studies, on average 76% of maltreated infants were classified as being insecurely attached compared to 34% of controls (Morton & Browne, 1998). Maltreated children are more likely than nonmaltreated children to exhibit insecure attachment styles during their preschool (Cicchetti & Barnett, 1991; Crittenden, 1988) and school-age years (Lynch & Cicchetti, 1991). Of great significance is the fact that between half (van IJzendoorn, Schuengel, & Bakermans-Kranenburg, 1999) to more than three quarters (Barnett, Ganiban, & Cicchetti, 1999; Beeghly & Cicchetti, 1994; Carlson, Cicchetti, Barnett, & Braunwald, 1989; Cicchetti & Barnett, 1991) of maltreated children have been found to have disorganized attachment styles.

Betrayal Trauma Theory

Bowlby (1988, p. 121) suggested that the attachment relationship "has a key survival function of its own, namely protection." Betrayal traumas involve a violation of the trust that children innately have in their protective caregivers, thus constituting a threat to these children's survival. BTT posits that in order to maintain a necessary attachment to a caregiver, a survivor of parental maltreatment must remain blind to that betrayal—that is, "betrayal blindness" (Freyd, 1996). Ordinarily it would be advantageous to detect betrayal in order to prevent a future violation; however, if detecting that betrayal could damage the security of attachment to an essential caregiver, it may be psychologically necessary to remain unaware of that violation (Freyd, 1996). Awareness of the betrayal caused by abuse may lead to withdrawal from that caregiver; however, by doing so, the child may risk further harm if the parent no longer continues to protect or meet the child's needs. Therefore, in order to preserve a sense of security and ensure survival, the child may remain unaware of the betrayal. This unawareness allows the child to avoid the "fright without solution" paradox (Hesse & Main, 1999, 2006). One mechanism by which this betrayal blindness may occur is dissociation, which Bernstein and Putnam (1986, p. 727) define as "a lack of normal integration of thoughts, feelings, and experiences into the stream of consciousness and memory." It is for this reason that research studies derived from a BTT framework have focused on associations between betrayal and dissociation, as well as related alterations in cognition, mental health symptoms, and problems in social and relationship functioning.

Empirical Research on BTT with Adult Samples

Freyd, Martorello, Alvarado, Hayes, and Christman (1998), using a college sample, found that "high dissociators" had difficulty in consciously controlling attentional focus. In a follow-up study, DePrince and Freyd (1999) again compared high and "low dissociators" and found that high dissociators had more difficulty than low dissociators when trying to ignore information (i.e., selective attention), but less difficulty when trying to remember to pay attention. Furthermore, high dissociators were less able to recall trauma-related than neutral information, whereas low dissociators showed the opposite pattern. These results have been replicated in follow-up research (DePrince & Freyd, 2001; DePrince & Freyd, 2004), which linked high levels of dissociation to more trauma history (Freyd & DePrince, 2001) and more betrayal trauma (DePrince & Freyd, 2004). These results support the BTT premise that interpersonally traumatized individuals may use dissociation as a mechanism for betrayal blindness.

Research conducted by Freyd, DePrince, and Zurbriggen (2001) further explored this tenet by looking at memory for abuse based on the relationship to the perpetrator. They showed that although most participants reported no memory impairment, the impairment occurred more frequently if the perpetrator was a caretaker, even after controlling for the age and duration effects of the abuse. Relatedly, in a sample of adult survivors of childhood sexual abuse, Ullman (2007) found that those who were victimized by relatives were more likely to disbelieve that the documented abuse occurred compared to participants victimized by strangers or acquaintances.

When formulating BTT, Freyd (1996) drew a distinction between two independent aspects of trauma: a terror-inducing or fear dimension associated with immediate life threat, and a social-betrayal dimension associated with threats to security in protective relationships (see Figure 4.1). She later suggested that these two dimensions may account for posttraumatic stress disorder (PTSD) symptom clusters, with the hyperarousal and intrusive symptoms arising from the fear dimension, and the avoidance/numbing symptoms (including dissociation) being evoked by the social-betrayal aspect of the trauma (Freyd, 1999).

Although not focusing specifically on these two dimensions in relation to PTSD, Tang and Freyd (2012), using both a college and a community sample, demonstrated that traumas high in betrayal (i.e., perpetrated by a close other) had the strongest association with symptoms of PTSD (as well as to depression and anxiety) compared to traumas lower in betrayal. Similarly, Ullman (2007) found that those for whom family members were perpetrators (which the authors designate as a betrayal trauma) had more PTSD symptoms than those abused by nonrelatives in an adult sample of child sexual abuse survivors. Looking at general mental health symptoms, Freyd, Klest, and Allard (2005) explored betrayal trauma history and mental health symptoms in a community sample of chronically medically ill patients. Results showed that experiencing traumas high in betrayal predicted anxiety, dissociation, and depression symptoms assessed by the Trauma Symptom Checklist (TSC; Briere,

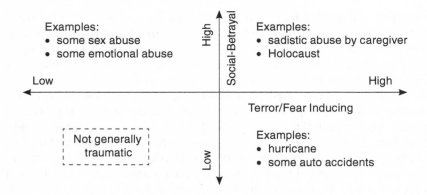

FIGURE 4.1. Two-dimensional model of trauma. Copyright 1996 by Jennifer J. Freyd. Reprinted by permission.

1996). Goldsmith, Freyd, and DePrince (2012) replicated these findings in a nonclinical sample.

In addition to being connected to what DSM-IV (and earlier editions of DSM) referred to as Axis I symptoms, betrayal traumas have also been associated with Axis II symptoms. Kaehler and Freyd (2009) demonstrated that traumas high in betrayal predicted borderline personality disorder characteristics, while traumas low in betrayal did not. In a follow-up study with community participants (Kaehler & Freyd, 2012), a significant gender effect was revealed: Traumas higher in betrayal predicted borderline personality characteristics for both men and women; however, traumas lower in betrayal also predicted these characteristics for men (but not for women). Belford, Kaehler, and Birrell (2012) showed that strong relational health weakened the association between betrayal trauma experiences and borderline personality characteristics. In sum, a history of betrayal trauma has been linked to a broad range of psychopathological symptoms in adults.

BTT (Freyd, 1996) suggests that experiencing traumas high in betrayal may damage trust mechanisms, resulting in either insufficient or excessive trust. Consequently, the survivor may not able to protect him- or herself when confronted with subsequent betrayals. In their prospective study of college women, Messman-Moore and Brown (2006) found that prior victimization and delayed responses to danger cues increased women's vulnerability to rape and sexual revictimization. Zurbriggen and Freyd (2004) proposed that traumas high in betrayal impair cognitive mechanisms that would typically help an individual make advantageous relationship decisions. This premise has been supported by the work of DePrince (2005), who showed that undergraduates who had been revictimized made significantly more cognitive errors when it came social or safety issues than students who had not been revictimized. Furthermore, there were no group differences for more abstract problems, indicating that the cognitive impairments are not attributable to general reasoning differences. Interestingly, pathological dissociation significantly predicted errors in the social and safety rules.

Recent research has explored the impact that a history of high-betrayal trauma (i.e., abuse perpetrated by someone with whom the survivor was "very close") has on survivors' interpersonal relationships. Gobin and Freyd (2009) found that high-betrayal trauma survivors reported more everyday betrayals than those who had not experienced a high-betrayal trauma. These survivors also had lower levels of trust, a decreased awareness of betrayals in their intimate relationships, and were more likely to remain in a relationship after a betrayal occurred. Thus, survivors of high-betrayal trauma are more likely to experience betrayals in their intimate relationships and maintain these violating relationships despite having lower levels of trust. The authors suggest that these factors are indicative of a continued pattern of betrayal blindness later in life that may increase survivors' risk of revictimization. In fact, Gobin and Freyd (2009) found that 69% of participants with a childhood history of high-betrayal traumas were revictimized as adolescents and 49% were revictimized as adults; however, only 9% of participants without this history were victimized as adults. For those with an adolescent history of high-betrayal traumas, 41% later experienced at least one high-betrayal trauma as an adult, whereas only 7% of participants without such histories were victimized as adults.

Owen, Quirk, and Manthos (2012) revealed a positive association between childhood high-betrayal traumas and both avoidance and anxious attachment. Furthermore, participants with this history perceived their romantic partners as less respectful, compared to partners of participants with a history of interpersonal trauma perpetrated by someone not close. Moreover, this association between high-betrayal traumas and perceived partner respect was mediated by psychological well-being and anxious attachment, such that those who had higher well-being or less anxious attachment had more (perceived) respectful partners. Gobin (2012) demonstrated that experiencing a high-betrayal trauma resulted in a devaluation of loyalty in a romantic partner. Being revictimized was associated with less desire for a sincere or trustworthy partner and stronger attraction to verbally aggressive partners. In a community sample of women survivors of intimate partner abuse (IPA), Babcock and DePrince (2012b) showed that IPA survivors with high-betrayal trauma histories were more likely to be revictimized over the course of 6 months after the domestic violence incident by the same intimate partner. Interestingly, IPA survivors who experienced trauma high in betrayal during their childhoods were also more likely to blame themselves for a domestic violence incident reported to the police, compared to women who had not experienced betrayal trauma (Babcock & DePrince, 2012a).

Importance of Studying BTT in Children and Adolescents

Studying BTT with child and adolescent samples is critical in order to better understand the nature and consequences of betrayal trauma experiences and to inform and target interventions toward these younger age groups. Though research studies utilizing adult participants have greatly advanced the field's understanding of childhood betrayal trauma, retrospective accounts of betrayal trauma experiences are subject to potential reporting biases. Thus, studying betrayal trauma and its sequelae in childhood could provide a clearer test of the relationships between it and dissociation and revictimization postulated by BTT.

Previous research (Brewin, Andrews, & Gotlib, 1993; Hardt & Rutter, 2004) demonstrated that when study participants retrospectively report that abuse or neglect has occurred, their reports are most often correct. Despite evidence about the accuracy of retrospective reporting of trauma history, research has shown that children's memories of traumatic experiences can be fragmented or nonlinear, especially if the child dissociated during the traumatic event. As BTT (Freyd, 1996) posits, the closer the child is to the abuser, the more adaptive it may for the child to dissociate or distance him- or herself psychologically from the abuse in order to maintain a necessary attachment for survival. Dissociation at the time of the traumatic experience can result in partial or full amnesia of the abuse.

Dissociative amnesia limits the data that researchers are able to collect, in that participants can report only on experiences they can recall, and dissociation interferes with memory encoding and recall. In fact, Hardt and Rutter's (2004) review of literature involving abuse revealed that false negative reports of abuse and measurement error were the two most common threats to validity coming from retrospective reports. Even in the cases where abuse and neglect were substantiated through documentation, rates of denying abuse have ranged from approximately 33% (Hardt & Rutter, 2004) to 50% (Fergusson, Horwood, & Woodward, 2000). Other factors such as long-term memory accuracy, infantile amnesia, and mood may also influence retrospective self-reports of abuse (Hardt & Rutter, 2004; Goldsmith & Freyd, 2005).

Given the limitations of retrospective self-reports, prospective research on the impact of childhood betrayal trauma is needed. Asking children and adolescents about their abuse experiences shortly after the abuse occurred may provide more accurate information about the traumatic event, and a clearer account of how the traumatic experience impacted the youth. Moreover, conducting research about betrayal trauma with children and adolescents can inform intervention strategies and hopefully prevent future incidences of abuse. Such studies could also provide invaluable information for the treatment of youth who have experienced betrayal trauma. By providing early interventions to these children and adolescents, the long-term consequences of betrayal trauma, like increased risk for revictimization and trauma-related psychopathology, may be prevented.

Empirical Research on BTT with Child Samples

Similar to the research with adults, cognitive aspects of BTT have been examined in children as well. Becker-Blease, Freyd, and Pears (2004) found that abused preschool-age children with high levels of dissociation showed poorer memory recognition for emotionally charged, threatening pictures compared to a group of nonabused children with low dissociation in a divided attention state. These results are consistent with the findings from the DePrince and Freyd (1999, 2001, 2004) studies, suggesting that those who have been exposed to betrayal traumas and dissociation may have difficulty processing distressing information.

DePrince et al. (2009) more directly replicated the DePrince and Freyd (1999, 2001, 2004) studies and found that higher levels of dissociation per children's self-report were associated with less interference when trying to remember rather than to ignore information; however, children with lower levels of dissociation showed the opposite pattern. An important limitation of this study, however, is that it did not include trauma or threat-related stimuli.

Research has also investigated detection of rule violations among children who have been maltreated. As mentioned previously, work by DePrince (2005) showed that young adults who reported histories of revictimization made significantly more errors detecting violations of social and safety rules compared to their peers who had not been revictimized, but the groups did not differ in abstract reasoning. Pathological dissociation scores predicted these errors. DePrince, Chu, and Combs (2008) explored dissociation and rule violation errors in school-age children. In this study, unlike the DePrince (2005) experiment, there were no significant differences among groups (no trauma, noninterpersonal, or interpersonal) for any of the rules (abstract, social, or safety). However, as in the DePrince (2005) study, dissociation did predict errors in social and safety rules, even after controlling for estimated IQ, socioeconomic status, and child age. Thus, children as well as adults who dissociate appear to be at risk of insufficiently perceiving social and physical dangers at the time and later.

DePrince et al. (2009) examined executive functioning (EF) in children who had not experienced trauma versus children who had experienced either familial (higher-betrayal) or nonfamilial (lower-betrayal) traumas. Regression analyses revealed an association between familial trauma exposure and an EF composite (consisting of working memory, inhibition, auditory attention, and processing speed). For trauma-exposed participants, an increasing number of familial events significantly predicted worse EF performance; however, the number of nonfamilial events was not significantly associated with EF ability.

Looking specifically at attention-deficit/hyperactivity disorder (ADHD), Becker-Blease and Freyd (2008) showed that abused children (defined as experiencing physical, sexual, or emotional abuse or neglect) had higher levels of impulsivity and inattention, but not hyperactivity, compared to nonabused children. This study had a small sample size, prohibiting further exploration of other potentially relevant variables associated with trauma exposure. However, there does seem to be emerging evidence that exposure to traumas higher in betrayal results in poorer overall cognitive functioning. As with the adult samples, BTT has also been utilized to explain symptoms of psychopathology in children.

Comparing a maltreated, preschool-age, foster care sample to a community, nonmaltreated control group, Hulette et al. (2008) demonstrated that children in a foster care sample had significantly higher levels of dissociation and PTSD symptomatology. Hulette, Freyd, and Fisher (2011), studying the same sample of children when they were school-age, showed that the children who had been in foster care continued to have significantly higher levels of dissociation. Moreover, foster children were more likely to be *pathologically* dissociative than their nonmaltreated peers. Unfortunately, PTSD symptoms were not assessed in that research. Given that the children were placed in foster care, they were more likely to have been exposed to high-betrayal traumas. However, because both of these studies relied on CPS case files for information regarding maltreatment, no definitive conclusions can be made regarding the betrayal aspects of the events. Yet, these are important first steps in understanding how betrayal traumas may be related to psychopathology.

Looking at intergenerational effects, Chu and DePrince (2006) found that a mother's own betrayal trauma history predicted her school-age children's dissociation levels, even when controlling for children's own betrayal trauma exposure. Hulette, Kaehler, and Freyd (2011) showed that there was a significant association between a mother's history of interpersonal trauma and her child's history of interpersonal trauma—that is, more children who experienced interpersonal trauma had a mother who had experienced her own interpersonal trauma. Moreover, more revictimized mothers had children with interpersonal trauma experiences, while nonrevictimized mothers were more likely to have children with no interpersonal trauma experiences. This finding is in line with research on disorganized attachment that has found that the primary caregiver is likely to have had a history of unresolved interpersonal trauma or loss (Lyons-Ruth, Dutra, Schuder, & Bianchi, 2006).

Clinical Implications

Extensive research reveals that experiencing betrayal trauma during childhood places survivors at increased risk of entering relationships in which they will be additionally victimized. By understanding the mechanisms that lead to the revictimization of betrayal trauma survivors, intervention strategies can be developed that teach specific skills to children and adolescents to prevent them from further experiences of betrayal or abuse in their interpersonal relationships as adults.

Gobin and Freyd (2009) explain that child maltreatment involving betrayal may damage certain social and cognitive mechanisms that are necessary to detect potential harm in interpersonal relationships. For example, a cognitive mechanism impacted by betrayal trauma experiences is the *cheater detector* (Cosmides & Tooby, 1992), which refers to people's ability to detect trustworthiness (or its absence) in other people. Studies have shown that experiencing childhood betrayal trauma is associated with a less well-developed ability to detect cheaters, making it difficult for survivors to determine whether or not someone is trustworthy in their interpersonal relationships (Gobin & Freyd, 2009; Zurbriggen & Freyd, 2004). By not recognizing interpersonal betrayals or identifying whether someone is trustworthy, victims of betrayal trauma become vulnerable to experiencing continued acts of betrayal and abuse by their intimate partners later in life. Not only can the inability to determine whether someone is trustworthy increase a survivor's risk of being revictimized by an untrustworthy partner, it can also prevent the survivor from identifying *trustworthy* people as well—people who could provide him or her with support and help to leave exploitive and abusive relationships (Gobin & Freyd, 2009).

In addition to lack of awareness of interpersonal betrayals and difficulty detecting trustworthiness in people, investigators have found that betrayal trauma survivors have trouble detecting risk in social situations (Soler-Baillo, Marx, & Sloan, 2005). DePrince (2005) found that survivors of child sexual abuse (CSA) had significantly greater difficulty detecting violations in social exchange rules. Furthermore, Cloitre, Scarvalone, and Difede (1997) found that CSA survivors failed to identify threat triggers, and as result, were unable to accurately perceive interpersonal violence as an actual violation when these occurred in their intimate relationships. These difficulties in risk detection are compounded by the tendency of perpetrators of IPA to slowly escalate the severity of the betrayal and abuse (e.g., verbal abuse building to physical abuse) they inflict over time (Platt, Barton, & Freyd, 2009). In order for a survivor to recognize this slow progression of violations, he or she must be able to detect less obvious forms of risk or betrayal. If this ability is not developed, it is likely that survivors will adapt behaviors to preserve the relationship with partners, and will not become aware of their partner's betrayal until the risk of harm is severe.

High-betrayal trauma survivors also report higher levels of dissociation and trauma-related distress (Gobin & Freyd, 2009). Dissociation may render a survivor unaware of betrayal and abuse from his or her intimate partner, thus potentially preserving the relationship in the same manner (with similar emotional and physical costs and dangers) that he or she did when betrayed as a child. Dissociation has been linked to a decreased capacity of victims to feel fear and anxiety that typically accompany dangerous situations (Noll, Trickett, & Putnam, 2003), which may in turn prevent a survivor from attempting to avoid or flee the situation when IPA is imminent. Higher levels of dissociation and trauma-related distress actually distinguish survivors of betrayal trauma who were revictimized from those who were not revictimized (Gobin & Freyd, 2009). Additionally, Ullman and colleagues found that PTSD numbing symptoms, which Freyd (1999) suggests may arise from the betrayal aspects of the trauma, directly predicted further interpersonal revictimization (Ullman, Najdowski, & Filipas, 2009). These findings underscore the significant role that betrayal blindness and associated PTSD symptoms play in increasing a survivor's risk of being revictimized. Research on how long-term consequences of childhood betrayal trauma increase survivors' risk of revictimization highlights how essential it is to treat young survivors of betrayal trauma to prevent them from experiencing lifelong abuse.

Sociocognitive deficits, dissociation, and trauma-related distress can also thwart survivors' abilities to function adaptively in their social relationships. As a result, survivors are often unable to differentiate between appropriate and inappropriate social behavior, establish healthy boundaries for themselves, or engage in self-protection by avoiding or withdrawing from relationships that are harmful. These difficulties may serve as risk factors for survivors' children as well. Survivors may be unable to (1) differentiate appropriate and inappropriate behavior regarding interactions with their children, (2) establish healthy boundaries around their children, or (3) engage in protective behaviors by ending relationships harmful to their children. Further, survivors' increased risk of experiencing revictimization in their intimate relationships may also, in turn, increase the likelihood that their children will be exposed to, or witness, IPA. Chu and DePrince (2006) showed that children who experienced betrayal traumas had mothers who experienced more betrayal traumas compared to children with no betrayal traumas. Hulette, Kaehler, et al. (2011) expanded this work by demonstrating associations among maternal dissociation, revictimization status, and their child's trauma history. Revictimized mothers had higher levels of dissociation (which may have contributed to their being revictimized) compared to nonrevictimized mothers. Furthermore, the children who experienced interpersonal traumas were more likely to have a revictimized mother. Thus, parental betrayal trauma history and posttraumatic sequelae may increase children's vulnerability of experiencing betrayal as well. Clearly, it is important to assess for potential intergenerational effects of betrayal trauma and to provide appropriate interventions at the parent level to prevent trauma at the child level. This can be done as part of a family therapy model (e.g., child–parent psychotherapy; Lieberman & Van Horn, 2008) or as part of the parent's individual treatment (e.g., see Ford, Steinberg, & Zhang, 2011).

Findings from these studies point to several mechanisms that can be targeted in the treatment of child and adolescent survivors. In addition to treating trauma-related distress in the form of PTSD, depression, and dissociation, interventions that focus on sociocognitive skills training in detecting interpersonal violations, betrayal, and trustworthiness, along with assertiveness, may help young survivors avoid entering unhealthy relationships. Child and adolescent survivors must become aware of and understand the nature of the betrayal they experienced as a child, and be taught methods to identify whether a person is trustworthy or not. Problem-solving and assertiveness skills could be invaluable in teaching young survivors adaptive options of "what to do" in risky or unhealthy interpersonal scenarios in order to protect themselves and avoid harm. If child and adolescent survivors can learn to identify risky situations and recognize what constitutes interpersonal betrayal, they will be better equipped to avoid unhealthy relationships and utilize self-protective strategies if violations do occur. By making prevention of revictimization a priority for survivors of betrayal trauma, we can help to ensure that young survivors will grow up to have healthy interpersonal relationships rather than relationships characterized by more betrayal and abuse.

Conclusion

BTT provides a useful framework for understanding cognitive, emotional, and social consequences of child abuse perpetrated by someone on whom the victim depends. Further, the theory sets the stage for several lines of clinical and research inquiry.

Nonoffending Family Members

As noted by DePrince and colleagues (2012), researchers have focused primarily on victims, particularly when seeking to understand the effects of trauma on memory. However, nonoffending relatives situated in the family system where abuse occurs may also experience pressure to remain unaware, leading to similar psychological consequences as occur in victims. Future research is needed to investigate this possibility. This research could go hand in hand with exploring clinical interventions that target nonoffending parents and children together, such as in trauma-focused cognitive-behavioral therapy (e.g., Cohen, Deblinger, Mannarino, & Steer, 2004) and child–parent psychotherapy (e.g., Lieberman & Van Horn, 2008).

Fear and/or Betrayal?

Following traumas, including child maltreatment, researchers and clinicians have frequently focused on the fear-inducing aspects of these events (for a review, see DePrince & Freyd, 2002). Fear is important, but it is not the only dimension of danger in trauma. BTT points to the need for researchers and clinicians to consider the social and relational context in which abuse occurs, with important implications for understanding problems such as complex PTSD. The sorts of chronic interpersonal traumas that precede complex PTSD, such as familial sexual abuse/incest or emotional abuse and neglect, also include significant betrayals. As children navigate betrayal in caregiving relationships, their attempts at coping with this untenable situation may give rise to the symptoms of complex PTSD, including problems in affect and impulse regulation, attention and consciousness, self-perception, relations with others, somatic functioning, and systems of meaning (see Dorahy et al., 2009; Ford et al., 1999; Herman, 1992; Taylor, Asmundson, & Carleton, 2006). BTT offers researchers and clinicians a road map for formulating and testing questions about the role that betrayal and attachment play in serious posttraumatic responses, such as complex PTSD.

References

Ainsworth, M. D. S., Blehar, M. C., Waters, E., & Wall, S. (1978). *Patterns of attachment: A psychological study of the strange situation.* Oxford, UK: Erlbaum.

Babcock, R., & DePrince, A. P. (2012a). Childhood betrayal trauma and self-blame appraisals among survivors of intimate partner abuse. *Journal of Trauma and Dissociation, 13,* 526–538.

Babcock, R., & DePrince, A. P. (2012b, December 24). Factors contributing to ongoing intimate partner abuse: Childhood betrayal trauma and dependence on one's perpetrator. *Journal of Interpersonal Violence.* Advance online publication doi:10.1177/0886260512468248.

Barnett, D., Ganiban, J., & Cicchetti, D. (1999). Maltreatment, negative expressivity, and the development of type D attachments from 12- to 24-months of age. *Society for Research in Child Development Monograph, 64,* 97–118.

Becker-Blease, K. A., & Freyd, J. J. (2008). A preliminary study of ADHD symptoms and correlates: Do abused children differ from non-abused children? *Journal of Aggression, Maltreatment, and Trauma, 17,* 133–140.

Becker-Blease, K. A., Freyd, J. J., & Pears, K. C. (2004). Preschoolers' memory for threatening information depends on trauma history and attentional context: Implications for the development of dissociation. *Journal of Trauma and Dissociation, 5,* 113–131.

Beeghly, M., & Cicchetti, D. (1994). Child maltreatment, attachment, and the self system: Emergence of an internal state lexicon in toddlers at high social risk. *Development and Psychopathology, 6,* 5–30.

Belford, B., Kaehler, L. A., & Birrell, P. (2012). Relational health as a mediator between betrayal trauma and borderline personality disorder. *Journal of Trauma and Dissociation, 13,* 244–257.

Bernstein, E. M., & Putnam, F. W. (1986). Development, reliability, and validity of a dissociation scale. *Journal of Nervous and Mental Disease, 174,* 727–735.

Bowlby, J. (1973). *Attachment and loss: Vol. 2. Separation: Anxiety and anger.* New York: Basic Books.

Bowlby, J. (1988). *A secure base: Parent–child attachments and healthy human development.* New York: Basic Books.

Brewin, C. R., Andrews, B., & Gotlib, I. H. (1993). Psychopathology and early experience: A reappraisal of retrospective reports. *Psychological Bulletin, 113*, 82–98.

Briere, J. (1996). Psychometric review of the Trauma Symptom Checklist–40. In B. H. Stamm (Ed.), *Measurement of stress, trauma, and adaptation*. Lutherville, MD: Sidran Press.

Carlson, V., Cicchetti, D., Barnett, D., & Braunwald, K. (1989). Disorganized/disoriented attachment relationships in maltreated infants. *Developmental Psychology, 25*, 525–531.

Chu, A. T., & DePrince, A. P. (2006). Development of dissociation: Examining the relationship between parenting, maternal trauma, and child dissociation. *Journal of Trauma and Dissociation, 7*, 75–89.

Chu, A. T., Pineda, A. S., DePrince, A. P., & Freyd, J. J. (2011). Vulnerability and protective factors for child abuse and maltreatment. In J. W. White, M. P. Koss, & A. E. Kazdin (Eds.), *Violence against women and children: Vol. 1. Mapping the terrain* (pp. 55–75). Washington, DC: American Psychological Association.

Cicchetti, D., & Barnett, D. (1991). Attachment organization in pre-school-aged maltreated children. *Development and Psychopathology, 3*, 397–411.

Cloitre, M., Scarvalone, P., & Difede, J. (1997). Posttraumatic stress disorder, self- and interpersonal dysfunction among sexually retraumatized women. *Journal of Traumatic Stress, 10*, 437–452.

Cohen, J. A., Deblinger E., Mannarino, A. P., & Steer, R. A. (2004). A multisite randomized control trial for sexually abused children with PTSD symptoms. *Journal of the American Academy of Child and Adolescent Psychiatry, 43*, 393–402.

Cosmides, L., & Tooby, J. (1992). Cognitive adaptations for social exchange. In J. H. Barkow, L. Cosmides, & J. Tooby (Eds.), *The adapted mind: Evolutionary psychology and the generation of culture* (pp. 163–228). New York: Oxford University Press.

Courtois, C. A. (2010). *Healing the incest wound: Adult survivors in therapy* (2nd ed.). New York: Norton.

Crittenden, P. M. (1988). Relationships at risk. In J. Belsky & T. Nezworski (Eds.), *Clinical implications of attachment theory* (pp. 136–174). Hillsdale, NJ: Erlbaum.

DePrince, A. P. (2005). Social cognition and revictimization risk. *Journal of Trauma and Dissociation, 6*, 125–141.

DePrince, A. P., Brown, L., Cheit, R., Freyd, J. J., Gold, S., Pezdek, K., et al. (2012). Motivated forgetting and misremembering: Perspectives from betrayal trauma theory. In R. F. Belli (Ed.), *True and false recovered memories: Toward a reconciliation of the debate: Vol. 58. Nebraska Symposium on Motivation* (pp. 193–243). New York: Springer.

DePrince, A. P., Chu, A. T., & Combs, M. D. (2008). Trauma-related predictors of deontic reasoning: A pilot study in a community sample of children. *Child Abuse and Neglect, 32*, 732–737.

DePrince, A. P., & Freyd, J. J. (1999). Dissociative tendencies, attention, and memory. *Psychological Science, 10*, 449–452.

DePrince, A. P., & Freyd, J. J. (2001). Memory and dissociative tendencies: The roles of attentional context and word meaning in a directed forgetting task. *Journal of Trauma and Dissociation, 2*, 67–82.

DePrince, A. P., & Freyd, J. J. (2002). The harm of trauma: Pathological fear, shattered assumptions or betrayal? In J. Kauffman (Ed.), *Loss of the assumptive world* (pp. 71–82). New York: Taylor & Francis.

DePrince, A. P., & Freyd, J. J. (2004). Forgetting trauma stimuli. *Psychological Science, 15*, 488–492.

DePrince, A. P., Weinzierl, K. M., & Combs, M. D. (2009). Executive function performance and trauma exposure in a community sample of children. *Child Abuse and Neglect, 33*, 353–361.

Dorahy, M. J., Corry, M., Shannon, M., MacSherry, A., Hamilton, G., McRobert, G., et al. (2009). Complex PTSD, interpersonal trauma and relational consequences: Findings from a treatment-receiving Northern Irish sample. *Journal of Affective Disorders, 112,* 71–80.

Fergusson, D. M., Horwood, L. J., & Woodward, L. J. (2000). The stability of child abuse reports: A longitudinal study of the reporting behavior of young adults. *Psychological Medicine, 30,* 529–544.

Ford, J. D., Racusin, R., Daviss, W. B., Ellis, C. G., Thomas, J., Rogers, K., et al. (1999). Trauma exposure among children with oppositional defiant disorder and attention deficit-hyperactivity disorder. *Journal of Consulting and Clinical Psychology, 67,* 786–789.

Ford, J. D., Steinberg, K. L., & Zhang, W. (2011). A randomized clinical trial comparing affect regulation and social problem-solving psychotherapies for mothers with victimization-related PTSD. *Behavior Therapy, 42,* 560–578.

Freyd, J. J. (1994). Betrayal trauma: Traumatic amnesia as an adaptive response to childhood abuse. *Ethics and Behavior, 4,* 307–329.

Freyd, J. J. (1996). *Betrayal trauma: The logic of forgetting childhood abuse.* Cambridge, MA: Harvard University Press.

Freyd, J. J. (1999). Blind to betrayal: New perspectives on memory for trauma. *Harvard Mental Health Letter, 15,* 4–6.

Freyd, J. J. (2001). Memory and dimensions of trauma: Terror may be 'all-too-well remembered' and betrayal buried. In J. R. Conte (Ed.), *Critical issues in child sexual abuse: Historical, legal, and psychological perspectives* (pp. 139–173). Thousand Oaks, CA: Sage.

Freyd, J. J., & DePrince, A. P. (2001). Perspectives on memory for trauma and cognitive processes associated with dissociative tendencies. *Journal of Aggression, Maltreatment, and Trauma, 4,* 137–163.

Freyd, J. J., DePrince, A. P., & Gleaves, D. (2007). The state of betrayal trauma theory: Reply to McNally (2007)—Conceptual issues and future directions. *Memory, 15,* 295–311.

Freyd, J. J., DePrince, A. P., & Zurbriggen, E. L. (2001). Self-reported memory for abuse depends upon victim–perpetrator relationship. *Journal of Trauma and Dissociation, 2,* 5–16.

Freyd, J. J., Klest, B., & Allard, C. B. (2005). Betrayal trauma: Relationship to physical health, psychological distress, and a written disclosure intervention. *Journal of Trauma and Dissociation, 6,* 83–104.

Freyd, J. J., Klest, B., & DePrince, A. P. (2010). Avoiding awareness of betrayal: Comment on Lindblom and Gray (2009). *Applied Cognitive Psychology, 24,* 20–26.

Freyd, J. J., Martorello, S. R., Alvarado, J. S., Hayes, A. E., & Christman, J. C. (1998). Cognitive environments and dissociative tendencies: Performance on the standard Stroop task for high versus low dissociators. *Applied Cognitive Psychology, 12,* S91–S103.

Gobin, R. L. (2012). Partner preferences among survivors of betrayal trauma. *Journal of Trauma and Dissociation, 13,* 152–174.

Gobin, R. L., & Freyd, J. J. (2009). Betrayal and revictimization: Preliminary findings. *Psychological Trauma: Theory, Research, Practice, and Policy, 1,* 242–257.

Goldsmith, R. E., & Freyd, J. J. (2005). Awareness of emotional abuse. *Journal of Emotional Abuse, 5,* 95–123.

Goldsmith, R. E., Freyd, J. J., & DePrince, A. P. (2012). Betrayal trauma: Associations with psychological and physical symptoms in young adults. *Journal of Interpersonal Violence, 27,* 547–567.

Hardt, J., & Rutter, M. (2004). Validity of adult retrospective reports of adverse childhood experiences: Review of the evidence. *Journal of Child Psychology and Psychiatry, 45,* 260–273.

Herman, J. L. (1992). *Trauma and recovery.* New York: Basic Books.

Hesse, E., & Main, M. (1999). Second-generation effects of unresolved trauma in non-maltreating parents: Dissociated, frightened, and threatening parental behavior. *Psychoanalytic Inquiry, 19,* 481–540.

Hesse, E., & Main, M. (2000). Disorganized infant, child and adult attachment: Collapse in behavioral and attentional strategies. *Journal of the American Psychoanalytic Association, 48,* 1097–1127.

Hesse, E., & Main, M. (2006). Frightened, threatening, and dissociative (FR) parental behavior as related to infant D attachment in low-risk samples: Description, discussion, and interpretations. *Development and Psychopathology, 18,* 309–343.

Hulette, A. C., Freyd, J. J., & Fisher, P. A. (2011). Dissociation in middle childhood among foster children with early maltreatment experiences. *Child Abuse and Neglect, 35,* 123–126.

Hulette, A. C., Freyd, J. J., Pears, K. C., Kim, H. K., Fisher, P. A., & Becker-Blease, K. A. (2008). Dissociation and posttraumatic symptoms in maltreated preschool children. *Journal of Child and Adolescent Trauma, 1,* 93–108.

Hulette, A. C., Kaehler, L. A., & Freyd, J. J. (2011). Intergenerational associations between trauma and dissociation. *Journal of Family Violence, 26,* 217–225.

Kaehler, L. A., & Freyd, J. J. (2009). Borderline personality characteristics: A betrayal trauma approach. *Psychological Trauma: Theory, Research, Practice, and Policy, 1,* 261–268.

Kaehler, L. A., & Freyd, J. J. (2012). Betrayal trauma and borderline personality characteristics: Gender differences. *Psychological Trauma: Theory, Research, Practice, and Policy, 4,* 379–385.

Kobak, R., Cassidy, J., Lyons-Ruth, K., & Ziv, Y. (2006). Attachment, stress, and psychopathology: A developmental pathways model. In D. Cicchecti & D. J. Cohen (Eds.), *Developmental psychopathology: Vol. 1. Theory and method* (2nd ed., pp. 333–369). Hoboken, NJ: Wiley.

Lieberman, A. F., & Van Horn, P. (2008). *Psychotherapy with infants and young children: Repairing the effects of stress and trauma on early attachment.* New York: Guilford Press.

Lynch, M., & Cicchetti, D. (1991). Patterns of relatedness in maltreated and nonmaltreated children: Connections among multiple representational models. *Development and Psychopathology, 3,* 207–226.

Lyons-Ruth, K., Dutra, L., Schuder, M. R., & Bianchi, I. (2006). From infant attachment disorganization to adult dissociation: Relational adaptations or traumatic experiences? *Psychiatric Clinics of North America, 29,* 63–86.

Main, M., & Hesse, E. D. (1990). Parents' unresolved traumatic experiences are related to infant disorganized attachment status: Is frightened and/or frightening parental behavior the linking mechanism? In M. Greenberg, D. Cichetti, & M. Cummings (Eds.), *Attachment in the preschool years* (pp. 161–184). Chicago: Chicago University Press.

Main, M., & Solomon, J. (1986). Discovery of an insecure–disorganized/disoriented attachment pattern. In T. B. Brazelton & M. W. Yogman (Eds.), *Affective development in infancy* (pp. 95–124). Norwood, NJ: Ablex.

Messman-Moore, T. L., & Brown, A. L. (2006). Risk perception, rape, and sexual revictimization: A prospective study of college women. *Psychology of Women Quarterly, 30,* 159–172.

Morton, N., & Browne, K. D. (1998). Theory and observation of attachment and its relation to child maltreatment: A review. *Child Abuse and Neglect, 22,* 1093–1104.

Noll, J. G., Trickett, P. K., & Putnam, F. W. (2003). A prospective investigation of the impact of childhood sexual abuse on the development of sexuality. *Journal of Consulting and Clinical Psychology, 71,* 575–586.

Owen, J., Quirk, K., & Manthos, M. (2012). I get no respect: The relationship between betrayal trauma and romantic relationship functioning. *Journal of Trauma and Dissociation, 13,* 175–189.

Platt, M., Barton, J., & Freyd, J. J. (2009). A betrayal trauma perspective on domestic violence. In E. Stark & E. S. Buzawa (Eds.), *Violence against women in families and relationships: Vol. 1* (pp. 185–207). Westport, CT: Greenwood Press,

Putman, F. (1997). *Dissociation in children and adolescents: A developmental perspective.* New York: Guilford Press.

Putman, F. (2003). Ten-year research update: Child sexual abuse. *Journal of American Academy of Child and Adolescent Psychiatry, 42,* 269–278.

Reichmann-Decker, A., DePrince, A. P., & McIntosh, D. N. (2009). Affective responsiveness, betrayal, and childhood abuse. *Journal of Trauma and Dissociation, 10,* 276–296.

Soler-Baillo, J. M., Marx, B. P., & Sloan, D. M. (2005). The psychophysiological correlates of risk recognition among victims and non-victims of sexual assault. *Behavior Research and Therapy, 43,* 169–181.

Tang, S. S., & Freyd, J. J. (2012). Betrayal trauma and gender differences in posttraumatic stress. *Psychological Trauma: Theory, Research, Practice, and Policy, 4,* 469–478.

Taylor, S., Asmundson, G. J., & Carleton, R. N. (2006). Simple versus complex PTSD: A cluster analytic investigation. *Journal of Anxiety Disorders, 20,* 459–472.

Ullman, S. E. (2007). Relationship to perpetrator, disclosure, social reactions, and PTSD symptoms in child sexual abuse survivors. *Journal of Child Sexual Abuse, 16,* 19–36.

Ullman, S. E., Najdowski, C. J., & Filipas, H. H. (2009). Child sexual abuse, posttraumatic stress disorder, and substance use: Predictors of revictimization in adult sexual assault survivors. *Journal of Child Sexual Abuse, 18,* 367–385.

U. S. Department of Health and Human Services. (2010). *Child maltreatment 2010: Reports from the states to the National Child Abuse and Neglect Data System.* Washington, DC: U.S. Government Printing Office.

van IJzendoorn, M. H. (1995). Adult attachment representations, parental responsiveness, and infant attachment: A meta-analysis on the predictive validity of the Adult Attachment Interview. *Psychological Bulletin, 117,* 387–403.

van IJzendoorn, M. H., Schuengel, C., & Bakermans-Kranenburg, M. J. (1999). Disorganized attachment in early childhood: Meta-analysis of precursors, concomitant, and sequelae. *Development and Psychopathology, 11,* 225–250.

Zurbriggen, E. L., & Freyd, J. J. (2004). The link between childhood sexual abuse and risky sexual behavior: The role of dissociative tendencies, information-processing effects, and consensual sex decision mechanisms. In L. J. Koenig, L. S. Doll, A. O'Leary, & W. Pequegnat (Eds.), *From child sexual abuse to adult sexual risk: Trauma, revictimization, and intervention* (pp. 135–157). Washington, DC: American Psychological Association.

CHAPTER 5

Cumulative Trauma in Childhood

Damion Grasso
Carolyn Greene
Julian D. Ford

Maria is a 14-year-old girl who has been involved with child protective services (CPS) for most of her life. From 2 to 4 years of age she was sexually abused by her mother's boyfriend. When it was discovered, CPS placed her with an aunt, who turned out to be both emotionally and physically abusive. She returned to live with her biological mother once, but was removed again due to her mother's drug use and eventual incarceration. When her mother completed her sentence, she left the state without notifying CPS or seeing Maria. Maria remained with her aunt, in a neighborhood characterized by criminal activity and violence. In the home, Maria's aunt and uncle often fought physically, and to escape, Maria began to spend more time away from the house, with a group of older adolescents who frequently abused alcohol and drugs. At age 13, one of the older teenagers raped her. She remained a part of the group, and later referred to the perpetrator as her boyfriend. Her teachers were concerned that she seemed to change from outgoing, popular, and studious to angry, defiant, and at times even apparently purposefully vengeful and cruel toward peers and adults. Maria became involved with the juvenile justice system after she and these peers were fleeing from police and crashed their car into a telephone pole. One of the girls in the group died in the accident.

Maria made three serious suicide attempts prior to the age of 14—each following an alcohol binge and prescription drug use. The last attempt resulted in residential treatment for more than a year. When asked about feelings of depression, Maria claims that she has been "this way" all of her life and often finds herself thinking that the hurt and pain are just not worth living through. Maria engages in self-mutilation and often uses this means to "get back at" others who hurt or disappoint her. In school, Maria reportedly has difficulty paying attention in class and frequently skips class and leaves school grounds without permission, often saying that being in school "makes me so sick that I get migraines or have to puke." Her teachers complain that she seems lost in thought, as though she is mentally someplace else. Maria reportedly experiences frequent nightmares of being attacked by "monsters with no faces," and she endorses symptoms that are characteristic of posttraumatic stress disorder (PTSD), including intrusive thoughts about past abuse, feeling "on edge" and unsafe, and using marijuana to escape these thoughts and feelings. Also prominent are Maria's problems with interpersonal relationships, which tend to be unstable and filled with conflict. Maria claims that she cannot trust anyone because everyone she has tried to be close to has "stabbed her in the back." According to residential treatment facility staff, Maria is quick to anger, and her behavior is difficult to manage. Staff often has to implement hands-on restraints to stop her from physically attacking peers when she feels "disrespected."

This case is based on the real stories of numerous girls (and boys) who come into the Child Trauma Clinic where we work, having developed severe behavioral, medical, school, family, peer group, and legal problems after experiencing a lifetime of repeated and cumulative adversity and traumatic stressors. Although these experiences cut across virtually every aspect of Maria's life, they are most notable for the almost nonexistent primary attachment bonds, multiple forms of violence and abuse, violation of her physical and psychological self, and the disruption of primary attachment bonds that occurred within the context of her familial and other intimate and peer relationships. Maria's experiences may sound extreme, but unfortunately Maria is not alone. According to research findings, about a fifth of youth nationwide (United States) have been exposed to more than one type of victimization (Saunders, 2003; Turner, Finkelhor, & Ormrod, 2010), and many are exposed to multiple types involving multiple perpetrators. These are interpersonal victimizations, such as physical and/or sexual abuse; emotional abuse and neglect; witnessing domestic violence; and separation from, abandonment by, or impairment of (due to drugs, illness, or incarceration) caregivers. They tend to accumulate as one victimization experience leads to another (referred to as *cumulative* trauma); to involve many types of victimization rather than only a single form (referred to as *polyvictimization*); and to involve a complex combination of frightening, alienating, and demoralizing experiences in the absence of adequate response or protection *(complex trauma)*. In this chapter we summarize research findings concerning cumulative, polyvictimization, and complex trauma that have direct implications for clinicians treating children and adolescents such as Maria.

Much of the contemporary understanding of complex trauma and its impact on development over the course of childhood, adolescence, and the entire lifespan has grown out of three separate, but closely related, lines of work on (1) adverse childhood experiences (ACEs; Felitti et al., 1998), (2) polyvictimization (Finkelhor, Ormrod, & Turner, 2007a), and (3) cumulative trauma (Briere & Spinazzola, 2005; Cloitre et al., 2009). Although these three conceptualizations of complex trauma share commonalities, each is unique in terms of the population type and demographic makeup of the samples used in the studies as well as in the operational definitions used to measure adverse or traumatic events and high exposure. Despite these differences, these researchers and others have consistently found that multiple adversities in childhood are associated with an increased risk for psychiatric and behavioral symptoms and impairment in childhood (Cloitre et al., 2009), adolescence (Finkelhor, Ormrod, & Turner, 2007b), and adulthood (Felitti et al., 1998) when compared to their nontraumatized counterparts. Further, in clinical (Cloitre et al., 2009; Ford, Wasser, & Connor, 2011) and community (Anda et al., 2006; Briere, Kaltman, & Green, 2008; Finkelhor et al., 2007b; Ford, Elhai, Connor, & Frueh, 2010) populations, a dose–response relationship between adversity and impairment has been found, such that the more categories of adversity endorsed, the more severe the impairment and the broader the spectrum of symptoms. Factors such as a younger age of onset, a close relationship to the perpetrator(s), nonresponse by bystander(s), and insufficient protection and support from caregivers within and outside the family can coalesce to create circumstances ripe for retraumatization at the time and throughout the life course (Follette & Duckworth, 2011).

As the recognition of the substantial impact that multiple adversities have on psychological development has grown, it has become clear that, at the present time, no single current diagnosis accounts for the cluster of symptoms frequently associated with such a history (D'Andrea, Ford, Stolbach, Spinazzola, & van der Kolk, 2012). The reactions of victims of repeated and extensive childhood trauma often do not fit well into the traditional PTSD symptom triad of reexperiencing, avoidance, and hyperarousal (Courtois, 2004). Rather, as is evident with Maria, the sequelae of multiple adversities in childhood are more likely to involve problems associated with self-regulation and interpersonal relatedness that manifest as difficulties with emotion regulation, somatization, attention, impulse control, dissociation, interpersonal relationships, and self-attributions (Cook et al., 2005; D'Andrea et al., 2012). This symptom cluster has been described elsewhere as *complex posttraumatic stress disorder* (Herman, 1992) in adults or *developmental trauma disorder* (D'Andrea et al., 2012; van der Kolk, 2005) in children.

In this chapter we provide a foundation for understanding the impact of exposures to multiple potentially traumatic adversities on development in childhood and throughout the lifespan by exploring the key findings of each of the major bodies of research in this area. In the final section we review the clinical implications of this research. We refer to the case illustration of Maria throughout to emphasize some of the key points of the chapter.

Defining and Measuring Exposure to Multiple Adversities: Three Approaches

ACEs Study

The Adverse Childhood Experiences (ACEs) Study is a large-scale, longitudinal, epidemiological study that has yielded a wealth of data connecting physical and mental health problems in adulthood with traumatic experiences that occur in childhood and adulthood. The study originally was based on information obtained from more than 17,000 young and midlife adults who completed a routine health screening while receiving health care services in the California Kaiser Permanente Health Maintenance Organization. Subsequently, the 11 questions that were used to assess ACEs were included by the Centers for Disease Control and Prevention (2010) in a random sampling of the adult populations of five states in the United States, replicating the key findings from the initial health care sample. Whereas the majority of prior studies examined a single type of childhood abuse, the ACEs Study was one of the first to simultaneously assess multiple categories of childhood maltreatment and adversity and to explore the cumulative impact of these experiences (Anda & Brown, 2010). It also examined a wider range of ACEs than most of the studies predating it, most of which had focused on one or two categories of maltreatment (i.e., physical abuse, sexual abuse, or domestic violence). As the name implies, the ACEs Study greatly expanded the study to include other forms of adverse experiences in childhood, including exposure to maltreatment (emotional abuse or neglect, physical abuse or neglect, sexual abuse) as well as to household dysfunction and parental impairment (domestic violence, parental separation or divorce, incarceration of a household member, family mental illness, or family substance use disorder).

This broader conceptualization of potentially traumatic adversity reflects the growing body of research documenting the impact on development and functioning of childhood experiences not included in traditional definitions of trauma, such as emotional abuse and parental separation or impairment due to drugs, mental illness, or incarceration (Turner & Lloyd,

1995). The authors also note that each of the experiences included in the study is interpersonal in nature and represents an event for which public- and private-sector efforts have been made to reduce their occurrence (Anda & Brown, 2010). Accidents and natural disasters do not fall into the class of interpersonal trauma and so were not included.

More than 17,000 middle-class adults seeking preventive medical care at a California health maintenance organization (80% white; 54% female; average age = 57 years old) participated in the study by simply indicating on a brief questionnaire which of the ACEs they recalled having experienced before the age of 18. Each participant was assigned a score based on the number of ACEs categories endorsed. Even among this middle-class sample, ACEs were common: nearly two-thirds of the participants reported at least one ACE, and one in six people experienced four or more (Anda & Brown, 2010). Women were 50% more likely than men to have experienced five or more ACEs categories (Felitti & Anda, 2009). Rates for individual categories experienced occurred at frequencies consistent with national population studies: 18% of men and 25% of women had experienced childhood sexual abuse; 22% of men and 20% of women had experienced childhood physical abuse; 12% of men and 15% of women had witnessed maternal battering (Edwards, Holden, Felitti, & Anda, 2003).

The research study showed that ACEs, in addition to being common, are highly interrelated. Of those people who endorsed one category of ACE, 81–98% (median = 87%) reported at least one additional category (Dong et al., 2004), suggesting that ACEs tend to co-occur with high frequency. For example, 65% of individuals who had witnessed domestic violence also reported growing up in a home where substance abuse was present (compared to 23% of respondents who had not witnessed domestic violence). Likewise, 81% of individuals reporting emotional abuse also reported physical abuse (compared with 20% of individuals who did not report emotional abuse). Therefore, assessing and examining the effects of just one or two categories of ACEs risk overestimating the impact of any one category and missing the cumulative effect of co-occurring childhood traumatic stressors.

The ACEs Study also explored the relationship of these childhood adverse experiences to a wide variety of outcomes associated with the leading causes of morbidity and mortality in adulthood (Felitti et al., 1998). These measures included self-rated health as well as risk factors (smoking, obesity, physical inactivity, depressed mood, suicide attempts, alcoholism, drug abuse, sexual promiscuity, sexually transmitted disease) and disease conditions (heart disease, cancer, stroke, chronic bronchitis, chronic obstructive pulmonary disease (COPD), diabetes, hepatitis and skeletal fractures). Confirming the cumulative effect of adverse experiences, the researchers found a dose–response relationship such that the more categories of ACEs an individual experienced, the greater his or her risk for the health risk behaviors and diseases examined in the study (Felitti et al., 1998).

Adjusting for the adverse effect of having a household member with a psychiatric disorder during childhood, women who experienced 5 or more ACEs were five times as likely to have a lifetime history of depressive disorders, and men were 2.4 times more likely, compared to participants with no history of adverse experiences (Chapman et al., 2004). An even stronger relationship was found for self-reported suicide attempts, in which individuals reporting five or more ACEs were 10 times as likely to report having attempted suicide in childhood, adolescence, or adulthood, and those reporting seven or more ACEs were 30 times more likely to attempt suicide. When other known risk factors for suicide were accounted for (alcoholism, depressed mood, and illicit drug use), individuals with an ACEs score of seven or higher continued to be 17 times more likely to attempt suicide than their counterparts who reported no ACEs (Dube, 2001).

Although these initial reports stemming from the ACE Study were based on retrospective recall of ACEs by adults, newer studies report findings from prospective follow-up data collected between 1998 and 2005. These longitudinal outcomes confirm and greatly strengthen the initial findings of the ACE Study. The studies have found, for example, that the complexity and severity of psychiatric problems (as measured indirectly by the number of psychotropic medications prescribed for an individual), as well as the risk for developing lung cancer or autoimmune diseases, are associated with the number of ACEs experienced in childhood (Anda et al., 2007; Brown et al., 2010; Dube et al., 2009). In study after study, growing up with ACEs has been found to be associated with behavioral, health, and social problems as well as with high-risk behaviors including chronic medical diseases; premature mortality; cigarette, alcohol, and drug use; high-risk sexual behaviors; and depression and suicidality (Anda & Brown, 2010). These relationships point to a common pathway from childhood adversity to adult health and psychosocial problems that may reflect the neurological impact of cumulative exposure to traumatic stress on the developing brain and the body's stress response and immune systems (Anda et al., 2006).

The ACEs studies offer substantial evidence that suggests that chronic and repeated stress overtaxes biological systems and alters a host of stress-related bodily responses that promote adaptation and survival, as well as preserve the integrity of crucial regulatory processes in the body—*biological business as usual*—or homeostasis (McEwen, 2000). When the body's capacity to adapt is overwhelmed, psychophysiological changes and psychological as well as physical illness may occur due to a breakdown of the body's stress response and immune systems, which McEwen (2000) described as creating a state of constant overload, or "allostasis." Allostasis may alter the brain systems implicated in cognitive and emotional functions such as memory, learning, motivation, information processing, problem solving, and distress tolerance—all crucial for healthy development (Belsky & de Haan, 2011). The developing brain is particularly susceptible during so-called sensitive periods (or developmental epochs), when an overabundance of neural connections undergoes a process called *pruning;* neural connections reinforced by experiences become stronger, whereas inactive neurons die off (Belsky & de Haan, 2011). ACEs may compromise the body and brain's basic foundation, potentially undermining the progressive building of the complex neural networks necessary to accomplish the developmental tasks of adolescence and adulthood (Cicchetti, 2006). Support for this view comes from recent studies that suggest that ACEs may alter not only the biology of the body's basic systems, but also the very genes that regulate those bodily systems—a process referred to as *epigenetics* (Skelton, Ressler, Norrholm, Jovanovic, & Bradley-Davino, 2011). Thus, when a child must cope with multiple adversities, he or she may develop not only problems with emotions, self-control, relationships, and learning, but with the basic biological systems that are necessary throughout the rest of life for self-regulation and healthy development (Ford, 2009).

Let's return to our case example, Maria, who had experienced at least 7 of the 10 ACE categories by the age of only 14 years old, and who is already experiencing many of the problems and engaging in many of the high-risk behaviors that would be predicted on the basis of these study findings. Maria abuses alcohol and other substances, suffers from depression, and has made several suicide attempts. She describes physical symptoms that may lead to, or place her at risk for, numerous potentially chronic physical health problems and illnesses. Beyond these outcomes that would be predicted by the ACEs studies, Maria's disregard for personal safety and her tendency to be defiant and to react in an aggressive manner when she feels challenged/attacked or disrespected, portend serious social and legal problems and place her in danger of being exposed to recurrent victimization. Maria's difficulty developing interpersonal relationships and trusting others; her struggles to regulate her emotions (as exemplified by her deliberate self-harm and her quick temper); and her dissociative symptoms and related difficulty concentrating, following through, and staying engaged in school are common sequelae of complex trauma not assessed in the ACEs Study (D'Andrea et al., 2012). Therefore, we turn next to a line of research that conceptualizes multiple childhood adversities in a slightly different manner: in terms of polyvictimization.

Polyvictimization

The term *polyvictimization* grew out of a large, nationally representative random digit-dial survey conducted with caregivers of children ages 2 to 9 years old and adolescents ages 10 to 17 years old (Finkelhor, Ormrod, Turner, & Hamby, 2005). Victimization experienced in the past year was measured using the Juvenile Victimization Questionnaire (JVQ), which surveyed 34 different types of victimization. Although noninterpersonal events (e.g., accident, natural disaster) could be viewed as "victimizing" survivors or witnesses, in these studies victimization was defined as including only interpersonal events (e.g., physical or sexual assault, abuse, or witnessed violence).

Consider for example, that Maria's traumatic experiences included being the victim of a tragic accident in which her life was in jeopardy and she witnessed the death of a friend. As terrifying and grief-rending as that experience may have been, it differed in clinically important ways from the many intentional assaults that Maria had sustained and witnessed. When traumatic victimization is inflicted by other human beings, especially those who ordinarily are expected to protect rather than harm (whether purposefully or by omission) vulnerable persons such as children, the adverse impact tends to be profound and persistent. Betrayal of trust by others who should be trustworthy is a key feature that differentiates interpersonal forms of victimization from noninterpersonal events such as accidents or natural disasters that do not involve the intentional acts of other people (Freyd, DePrince, & Gleaves, 2007; see also Kaehler et al., Chapter 4, this volume). While non-interpersonal traumatic events have been associated with the development of PTSD, specific phobia, and other internalizing disorders in children (Briggs-Gowan et al., 2010; Kim et al., 2009; Luthra et al., 2009) as well as adults (Baranyi et al., 2010; Birmes, Daubisse, & Brunet, 2008; Bui et al., 2010; Kassam-Adams, Fleisher, & Winston, 2009), exposure to intentional interpersonal trauma has been empirically linked to a broader spectrum of internalizing and externalizing disorders than noninterpersonal trauma (D'Andrea et al., 2012).

The JVQ study demonstrated the clinical utility of considering the total number of victimization *types* when estimating risk by determining its ability to predict PTSD symptomatology significantly better than any single type alone (Finkelhor et al., 2005). Specifically, youth were defined as having been polyvictimized if they endorsed exposure to four or more victimization types on the JVQ. This is similar to the ACEs score, in that it is based on the number of different *types* of victimization rather than the number of times or chronicity or severity of any single type of victimization (although both are important and contribute to layered or cumulative trauma). However, a much larger number of more specifically defined types of victimization were assessed than the 10 fairly general types of adversities assessed as ACEs. Victimization also was assessed based only on the past year of each respondent, rather than as recalled several decades later. Despite these definitional and methodological differences, the findings regarding polyvictimization were remarkably similar to the findings for ACEs.

In their sample of 2,030 children and adolescents, polyvictims comprised nearly a quarter, with the largest portion of the polyvictims being older and male (Finkelhor et al., 2005). Polyvictims were on average 4 times more likely to be revictimized in the year following the study, and nearly half of polyvictims at baseline were categorized as polyvictims again in the second year (Finkelhor, Ormrod, & Turner, 2007b). This was referred to as *persistent polyvictimization,* for which youth were at greater risk if they had resided in a family inflicted with violence, experienced child maltreatment, been exposed to familial alcohol and drug abuse, or had a parent who was unemployed (Finkelhor et al., 2007b)—findings that are consistent with those of the ACEs studies. The most robust predictor of repeat polyvictimization was having higher scores on a measure of anger and aggression (Finkelhor et al., 2007b), consistent with the findings of another study that found that children and adolescents in intensive psychiatric treatment who had had multiple forms of victimization were particularly prone to problems with anger, aggression, and impulsivity (Ford, Connor, & Hawke, 2009). Polyvictimized children encounter adversity across multiple contexts where violence is pervasive, inflicted by a variety of perpetrators: physical and emotional maltreatment by caregivers; bullying by peers; sexual abuse by caregivers, mentors, or acquaintances; and witnessing a host of violent and traumatic incidents in the home, school, and community (Cuevas, Finkelhor, Clifford, Ormrod, & Turner, 2010; Holt, Finkelhor, & Kantor, 2007; Saunders, 2003). Although aggressive behavior may be adaptive for a polyvictim as an attempt to gain control in the face of actual or perceived threat, these findings suggest that it also puts youth at higher risk of being victimized in the future.

On the other hand, youth who reported having more friends had a lower risk of being categorized as a polyvictim in the second year (Finkelhor et al., 2007b). This finding is consistent with literature showing that social support is a potent protective factor against victimization and PTSD chronicity (Brewin, Andrews, & Valentine, 2000; Charuvastra & Cloitre, 2008; Pynoos, Steinberg, & Piacentini, 1999). Unfortunately, however, polyvictims tend to seek social support from peers who are involved in deviant or delinquent behavior (Chen, 2009; Cuevas, Finkelhor, Turner, & Ormrod, 2007; Ford et al., 2010), thus remaining at risk for further victimization, while, at the same time, seeking protection and support from peers.

Consistent with these findings, four primary precipitants of polyvictimization have been identified: (1) residing in a dangerous community, (2) living in a dangerous family, (3) living in a nondangerous but chaotic and multiproblem family environment, and (4) having emotional problems that increase risk behavior, foster antagonism, and increase the likelihood of being victimized (Finkelhor, Ormrod, Turner, & Holt, 2009). The latter pathway was particularly salient for youth in the sample who were less than 10 years of age. Interestingly, polyvictimization onset was disproportionately likely to occur either in the year prior to turning 7 years old or prior to turning 15 years old (Finkelhor, Ormrod, Turner, et al., 2009). The authors note that these years approximate a youth's entry into elementary and high school, respectively, and are known to be challenging social adjustment periods when emotional and behavioral problems are likely to manifest (Finkelhor, Ormrod, Turner, et al., 2009).

Finally, Finkelhor et al. examined lifetime victimization data to derive a lifetime polyvictimization classification. Polyvictims represented the top 10% of youth with the highest victimization scores. When polyvictimization was defined this way, polyvictims showed significantly more distress and noninterpersonal adversity and were less likely to reside in an intact family (Finkelhor, Ormrod, & Turner, 2009). Additionally, the best linear predictor of psychological distress on the basis of polyvictimization emerged when child maltreatment and sexual assault were weighted by 4 and 3, respectively, suggesting a greater psychological impact of these types of victimization (Finkelhor, Ormrod, & Turner, 2009).

Maria would more than satisfy the criteria for being classified as a polyvictim, given that 13 out of 34 items on the JVQ were positive in Maria's history. Consistent with the polyvictimization perspective, Maria suffered from not only PTSD and emotional distress, but she also had severe difficulty with anger and aggression, substance abuse and suicidality, and she sought protection and support from delinquent peers. However, neither the ACEs nor polyvictimization frameworks fully account for Maria's impairments with self-regulation, such as her tendency to self-harm and her dissociative symptoms. We now turn to a third line of research on multiple adversities, which focuses on cumulative exposure to traumatic stressors.

Cumulative Trauma

Over the past two decades, a diverse set of studies has provided a growing body of evidence that the number of traumatic stressors experienced over the lifespan predicts the severity of a broad range of symptoms and disorders, including PTSD, depression, dissociation, somatization, sleep and sexual problems, substance abuse, eating and body image problems, anger and emotion dysregulation, and interpersonal problems (Follette & Vijay, 2008; Follette & Duckworth, 2011), especially (but not only) when the onset of traumatic stressors occurs in early childhood (Ford, 2010). Follette, Polusny, Bechtle, and Naugle (1996) found that in addition to anxiety, depression, and sleep problems, sexual problems and dissociation also were directly related to the number of trauma categories reported (including childhood sexual abuse, adult sexual assault, and adult physical abuse by a partner). Other studies show that adults with multiple traumatic exposures report elevated levels of guilt, dissociation, shame, anger, and interpersonal sensitivity (Hagenaars, Fisch, & van Minnen, 2011), and problems with emotion regulation when the cumulative exposure occurred in childhood (Ehring & Quack, 2010; Ford & Smith, 2008; Ford, Stockton, Kaltman, & Green, 2006).

Expanding on this evidence, recent studies have demonstrated a dose–response relationship between the number of types of interpersonal traumatic exposures and the number of different symptoms endorsed in a number of affective, cognitive, psychosomatic, and interpersonal domains

(Briere et al., 2008; Cloitre et al., 2009). Briere et al. (2008) surveyed 2,453 female university students and found a direct relationship between the number of different types of childhood traumatic events reported and the number of domains of current symptoms reported (i.e., anxious arousal, depression, anger irritability, intrusive experiences, defensive avoidance, dissociation, sexual concerns, dysfunctional sexual behavior, impaired self-reference, and tension reduction behaviors). Although exposure to five of the trauma types each independently predicted symptom complexity, cumulative trauma was associated with symptom complexity over and above the contribution of these trauma types. Thus, exposure to multiple types of childhood traumatic stressors may lead to multiple types of symptoms independent of the specific type(s) of traumatic stressors that have occurred.

Cloitre et al. (2009) replicated these findings among clinical samples of women and children, and extended them by examining the impact of adult as well as childhood traumatic experiences. Similar to the Briere et al. (2008) findings, Cloitre et al. (2009) showed that cumulative childhood traumatic exposure was associated with symptom complexity in both adults and children, but adult cumulative trauma was not. Although these findings suggest that multiple types of childhood traumatic exposure may be more strongly associated with multifaceted symptom problems than multiple types of adult traumatic exposure, a close examination of the numerous studies on cumulative trauma exposure (or "retraumatization"; Follette & Vijay, 2008) indicates that adults who experience multiple types of traumatic stressors are likely to have particularly severe and persistent symptoms, even if they do not necessarily develop as wide a variety of symptoms as multiply traumatized children. One possibility that warrants further scientific and clinical study is that the cumulative impact of multiple traumas on children may disrupt the development of core self-regulation capacities and lead to a variety of symptomatic problems (Ford et al., 2006), whereas multiply traumatized adults may experience a range of symptoms that reflect their adaptation to the stressors despite intact self-regulation capacities.

Finally, a recent study examining lifetime victimization data from the Finnish Child Victim Survey, with a sample of 13,459 sixth- and ninth-grade students, found that being older; female; using alcohol, drugs, or tobacco; being exposed to parental alcohol abuse or domestic violence; receiving child welfare services; spending less time with family; and having more unsupervised time predicted a greater number of endorsed victimization types (Ellonen & Salmi, 2011). The findings suggest that there may be an accumulation of risk factors for youth exposed to multiple adversities such that these youth not only are prone to additional severe or traumatic stressors but also to large numbers of other life stressors and negative experiences.

Returning again to Maria, we see that she clearly demonstrates the symptom complexity described in the cumulative trauma studies. She displays a wide range of symptoms consistent with severe anxiety and dysphoria (e.g., PTSD, depression, substance abuse, suicidality). In addition, she also has several symptoms consistent with more fundamental problems in several domains of self-regulation (Ford et al., 2006): self-mutilation; reactive aggression; dissociation; proneness to, and difficulty in recovering from, extreme emotional states (notably anger, but potentially also grief, despair, guilt, and shame); somatic complaints; and interpersonal relationships characterized by poor choice, mistrust, and conflict. Thus, Maria's difficulties tragically illustrate the cumulative adverse impact that exposure to multiple types of interpersonal traumatic stressors can have not only on a child or adolescent's psychosocial functioning and well-being, but also on the development of core capacities for self-regulation that are the foundation for adjustment across the lifespan.

Converging Evidence

In our case illustration, Maria qualifies for at least 7 of the 10 ACEs categories, 13 of the 34 JVQ items, and 6 of the 7 predictors used in the child and adolescent cumulative trauma studies. In each instance, she would fall into the group of children who had faced the highest number of adversities: high ACEs, polyvictim, and cumulative trauma. Despite this consistent finding, it is important to consider how each framework's approach to defining and measuring complex trauma can add to the clinical or scientific understanding of trauma history. For example, the three ACEs of having an incarcerated parent, having a parent dependent on alcohol and drugs, and being abandoned would constitute only two items on the JVQ (neglect and emotional maltreatment) and two cumulative trauma categories (impaired caregiver and out-of-home placement). Moreover, these adversities would not necessarily be considered traumatic stressors according to the *Diagnostic and Statistical Manual of Mental Disorders, Fifth Edition* (American Psychiatric Association, 2013), and therefore might not count toward a cumulative trauma index if that standard were rigorously applied. On the other hand, the ACEs do not provide the same degree of specificity as the JVQ in defining exact types of victimization, and neither the ACEs nor the JVQ assess whether adverse events were life-threatening or violations of bodily integrity, as is done in assessing traumatic stressors.

Clearly none of these surveys provides a comprehensive list, nor are the items on any list assumed to confer equal risk. Rather, each provides a proxy measure for the extent of adversity—and therefore, the allostatic load—experienced by multiply victimized children and adolescents. None of the surveys specifically assesses the loss or disruption of primary relational bonds with caregivers early in life, which has been found to be associated with biological as well as psychosocial vulnerability to stressors and trauma throughout the rest of the lifespan (D'Andrea et al., 2012; Ford et al., 2006; see also Schore, Chapter 1, this volume). Measuring trauma histories in this way provides useful epidemiological information about the relative frequency with which different types of victimization and violence experiences occur, the interrelationship between different categories of childhood victimization, and the impact of these experiences on development and functioning throughout the lifespan. The definitions and measures provide clinicians with examples that can be adapted for use in formulating and conducting trauma-informed clinical assessments with youth such as Maria.

Next Steps: Developing Victimization Profiles

There are, however, limitations to the measurement approach used in these studies. Because each category of adversity is given equal weight in the summary scores, recording the number of categories of adversity experienced does not take into account other abuse characteristics, such as the relative impact of the type, frequency, severity, or duration of victimization experiences (Scott-Storey, 2011). Finkelhor et al. (2005) attempted to utilize a weighting system to acknowledge the differing impact of varied types of abuse, but did not find that this weighting provided any improvement over the simple counting method.

To address some of these measurement issues, a few studies have begun to empirically identify subgroups of children and adolescents with distinct profiles of victimization experiences. In a large national sample of adolescents, for example, Ford and colleagues (2010) used latent class analyses (LCA) to identify six distinct subgroups based on their trauma history profiles: (1) sexual abuse/assault polyvictimization; (2) physical abuse/assault polyvictimization; (3) assault witness; (4) accident/disaster victim; (5) community violence polyvictimization; and (6) sexual and physical assault polyvictimization. Members of each of the polyvictimization subgroups were more likely than nontraumatized adolescents to have PTSD, major depression, or a substance use disorder. Their risk for these comorbid or co-occurring conditions also far exceeded that of adolescents with trauma histories who were not polyvictimized. Similar results have been found among child and adolescent psychiatric outpatients, identifying a distinct polyvictimized subgroup of clients whose members experienced nearly 4 times as many types of maltreatment as other child clients and had more severe parent-rated externalizing behavior and clinician-rated impairment (Ford et al., 2011). The vast majority of children and adolescents in the polyvictimized subgroup had trauma histories consistent with high ACEs and cumulative trauma, including substance abusing or psychiatrically impaired parents, and had experienced violence or other traumatic stressors, as well as physical and sexual abuse.

Employing cluster analysis, a study with 689 urban fifth graders identified three profiles: (1) minimally victimized children, (2) children victimized by peers, and (3) polyvictims. Polyvictims reported significantly more psychosocial distress and demonstrated poorer academic performance in comparison to those in the other classifications (Holt et al., 2007). Another study used LCA on data containing lifetime endorsement of 41 discrete incidents belonging to five broader categories of violence exposure, as well as lifetime status of PTSD and major depressive disorder (MDD) in children referred to the U.S. Navy's Family Advocacy Program due to parent-inflicted child sexual abuse, physical abuse, or intimate partner violence (Grasso et al., 2011). Three classes of children best fit the data: children with exposure to multiple forms of violence and greater than 70% prevalence of PTSD and MDD, children with moderate exposure and less than a 35% prevalence of these disorders, and children with considerably less exposure and less than a 10% prevalence of these disorders (Grasso et al., 2011). Children in the class with the highest exposure to violence had less perceived parental and teacher support, were less likely to view themselves as competent and others as trustworthy, and were more likely to exhibit symptomatic alcohol and substance use and delinquent behavior at a 3-year follow-up, compared to the less cumulatively exposed (and likely lower ACEs) children. Thus, findings from studies using statistical approaches to identifying children with complex trauma histories replicate those of the studies that defined ACEs, polyvictimization, and cumulative trauma on a logical or a priori basis.

Clinical Implications

Since research on ACEs, polyvictimization, and cumulative trauma is still in early stages, there are no set guidelines for how clinicians should assess and utilize information about their clients' histories of exposure to multiple adversities. However, there are a number of implications that clinicians may consider. It is clear that exposure to multiple types of adversities tells us more about a client than simply knowing that the client has been exposed to any single type of adversity. First, a client with a history of multiple adversities is at elevated risk for high-risk behaviors, such as suicide, self-injury, and alcohol/drug abuse and dependence, which must be carefully assessed at intake and monitored throughout treatment.

Second, a traumatized client with multiple adversities may present with symptoms that are not fully captured by the current DSM diagnosis of PTSD, and that result in multiple psychiatric diagnoses that are difficult to treat without an encompassing conceptualization such as developmental trauma disorder and multiple psychotherapeutic and pharmacological interventions. Maria, for example, had received prescriptions for more than 15 different medications, ranging from antidepressants to stimulants to mood regulators to antipsychotics, and had been seen (unsuccessfully) by more than 10 different psychotherapists who used psychodynamic, cognitive-behavioral (for depression, substance abuse, and PTSD), parent behavior management, family systems, motivational enhancement, and in-home multidimensional and multisystemic therapies. However, neither she nor her caregivers had received trauma-informed education or psychotherapy focused on emotion regulation skills to manage biological and psychological stress reactivity. This would be the approach taken if the proposed developmental trauma disorder were used as a treatment framework (see Ford, Blaustein, Habib, & Kagan, Chapter 14, this volume), in order to focus treatment on addressing profound dysregulation in emotional, cognitive, behavioral, and relational domains (D'Andrea et al., 2012).

Third, knowing a child or adolescent has been exposed to multiple adversities should raise serious concern regarding possible subsequent exposure to adversity and trauma. Thus, clinicians might join with the family, child welfare workers, and other professionals in the community toward reducing the youth's risk of future exposure. Because adversity, polyvictimization, and cumulative exposure to traumatic stressors are pervasive in these youth's lives in the home, school, neighborhood, and community, there is a need to intervene at multiple levels—which further points to the need to establish collaborative relationships among adults responsible for these youth in each of these contexts (see Navalta, Brown, Nisewaner, Ellis, & Saxe, Chapter 18, this volume). While a large portion of this mandate falls under child protection, we should also be cognizant of other, less salient forms of adversity that contribute to the increased risk for psychopathology and repeat exposure yet are often undetected or unaddressed. Often overlooked or discounted is emotional abuse and neglect that occur in the home. This includes a parent repeatedly telling a child that he or she is no good, unworthy, and unloved, as well as being emotionally unavailable to the child, ignoring the child's bids for attention, and being insensitive to the child's emotional needs. In addition to having a direct, negative effect on mental health, an emotionally abusive family environment has been found to exacerbate the impact of other types of child maltreatment (Edwards et al., 2003). Nonphysical bullying and online bullying are also often missed, yet have serious implications for emotional well-being, as recent tragic cases of youth and young-adult suicide illustrate. Finally, witnessing violence in the home and in the community is also often overlooked as a sressor, yet living in a virtual "warzone," as Maria's story shows, can be a major contributor to the emotional, behavioral, and relational problems caused by ACEs, polyvictimization, or cumulative trauma exposure.

In addition to taking steps toward preventing future exposure, efforts should be made to help these children and adolescents establish protective resources within these contexts to help them cope with future exposure to adversity and potential trauma. Protective resources can be interpersonal (e.g., perceived social support; Charuvastra & Cloitre, 2008) or intrapersonal in nature (e.g., protective cognitions; Cohen & Mannarino, 2000; Walter, Horsey, Palmieri, & Hobfoll, 2010). Relevant to this topic is the conservation of resources theory (COR theory; Hobfoll, 1989), which posits that an individual exposed to a potentially traumatic event experiences a loss of resources and is faced with the option of replacing or substituting resources, or to succumb to what Hobfoll (2001) refers to as a *loss spiral,* in which loss begets more loss. Indeed, regaining resources following a significant stressor is costly, as it demands utilization of existing resources to do so. Although this investment is feasible for those with sufficient resources to facilitate maintenance, acquisition, and enhancement of resources following trauma, individuals whose resources are depleted and insufficient are often unsuccessful. The majority of children and adolescents who have been exposed to multiple adversities do not have sufficient resources to facilitate these proactive steps toward reinforcing protective resources; thus, it is up to clinicians, child welfare professionals, and other adults to foster protective resource enhancement.

The value of having information about a client's history of adversity and trauma clearly indicates the importance of adequately assessing it early in treatment. As reviewed elsewhere (Ford, 2011; Stover & Berkowitz, 2005; Strand, Sarmiento, & Pasquale, 2005), there are several instruments available to survey exposure to adversity and potential trauma in children and adolescents. The Traumatic Events Screening Inventory (TESI; Ford et al., 2000) and Violence Exposure Scales—Revised (VEX-R; Fox & Levitt, 1995) assess a wide variety of childhood traumas, and both have caregiver and child-report versions. The Child Trauma Questionnaire (CTQ; Bernstein, Ahluvalia, Pogge, & Handelsman, 1997) provides an excellent assessment of a range of maltreatment experiences. In addition to the JVQ, other detailed measures of intimate partner or family violence can be obtained with the Revised Conflict Tactics Scale (CTS-R; Straus, Hamby, Boney-McCoy, & Sugarman, 1996) or the Partner Violence Inventory (PVI; Bernstein, 1998). Lastly, reliable methods have also been developed to extract and rate severity of maltreatment experiences from case records (Barnett, Manly, & Cicchetti, 1993) and to integrate trauma data from multiple informants (Hawkins & Radcliffe, 2006; Kaufman, Jones, Stieglitz, Vitulano, & Mannarino, 1994).

Conclusion

As understanding of the way in which exposure to multiple types of traumatic experiences in childhood and adolescence can interfere with adjustment and the development of self-regulatory capacities grows, clinicians and researchers will be able to take a transdiagnostic approach to assessment, case formulation, and treatment planning and monitoring, rather than attempting to diagnose and treat an overwhelming array of symptoms and comorbid disorders. Although the biopsychosocial problems facing clients with a history of ACEs, polyvictimization, or cumulative exposure to

traumatic stressors—and the corresponding challenges facing clinicians—
are undeniably complex and daunting, taking a complex trauma framework derived from those three lines of research can paradoxically provide a
degree of simplicity to assessment and treatment that is the result of an integrative understanding of the importance of focusing on addressing stress
reactivity and self-regulation.

References

American Psychiatric Association. (2013). *Diagnostic and statistical manual of mental disorders* (5th ed.). Arlington, VA: Author.

Anda, R. F., & Brown, D. W. (2010). *Adverse childhood experiences and population health in Washington: The face of a chronic public health disaster.* Olympia, WA: Family Policy Council.

Anda, R. F., Brown, D. W., Felitti, V. J., Bremner, J. D., Dube, S. R., & Giles, W. H. (2007). Adverse childhood experiences and prescribed psychotropic medications in adults. *American Journal of Preventive Medicine, 32*(5), 389–394.

Anda, R. F., Felitti, V. J., Bremner, J. D., Walker, J. D., Whitfield, C., Perry, B. D., et al. (2006). The enduring effects of abuse and related adverse experiences in child-hood. *European Archives of Psychiatry and Clinical Neuroscience, 256,* 174–186.

Baranyi, A., Leithgob, O., Kreiner, B., Tanzer, K., Ehrlich, G., Hofer, H. P., et al. (2010). Relationship between posttraumatic stress disorder, quality of life, social support, and affective and dissociative status in severely injured accident victims 12 months after trauma. *Psychosomatics, 51*(3), 237–247.

Barnett, D., Manly, J., & Cicchetti, D. (1993). Defining child maltreatment: The inter-face between policy and research. In D. Cicchetti & S. Toth (Eds.), *Advances in applied developmental psychology: Vol. 8. Child abuse, child development, and social policy* (pp. 7–74).

Belsky, J., & de Haan, M. (2011). Annual research review: Parenting and children's brain development: The end of the beginning. *Journal of Child Psychology and Psychiatry, and Allied Disciplines, 52*(4), 409–428.

Bernstein, D. (1998). A new screening measure for detecting "hidden" domestic vio-lence. *Psychiatric Times, 15*(11), 448–453.

Bernstein, D., Ahluvalia, T., Pogge, D., & Handelsman, L. (1997). Validity of the Child-hood Trauma Questionnaire in an adolescent psychiatric population. *Journal of the American Academy of Child and Adolescent Psychiatry, 36*(3), 340–348.

Birmes, P. J., Daubisse, L., & Brunet, A. (2008). Predictors of enduring PTSD after an industrial disaster. *Psychiatric Services, 59*(1), 116.

Brewin, C. R., Andrews, B., & Valentine, J. D. (2000). Meta-analysis of risk factors for posttraumatic stress disorder in trauma-exposed adults. *Journal of Consulting and Clinical Psychology, 68*(5), 748–766.

Briere, J., Kaltman, S., & Green, B. L. (2008). Accumulated childhood trauma and symptom complexity. *Journal of Traumatic Stress, 21*(2), 223–226.

Briere, J., & Spinazzola, J. (2005). Phenomenology and psychological assessment of complex posttraumatic stress. *Journal of Traumatic Stress, 18*(5), 401–412.

Briggs-Gowan, M. J., Carter, A. S., Clark, R., Augustyn, M., McCarthy, K. J., & Ford, J. D. (2010). Exposure to potentially traumatic events in early childhood: Differ-ential links to emergent psychopathology. *Journal of Child Psychology and Psy-chiatry, 51*(10), 1132–1140.

Brown, D. W., Anda, R. F., Felitti, V. J., Edwards, V. J., Malarcher, A. M., Croft, J. B., et al. (2010). Adverse childhood experiences are associated with the risk of lung cancer: A prospective cohort study. *BioMed Central Public Health, 10*(20), 12.

Bui, E., Joubert, S., Manetti, A., Camassel, C., Charpentier, S., Ribereau-Gayon, R., et al. (2010). Peritraumatic distress predicts posttraumatic stress symptoms in older people. *Internatioinal Journal of Geriatric Psychiatry, 25*(12), 1306–1307.

Centers for Disease Control and Prevention. (2010). Adverse childhood experiences reported by adults—five states, 2009. *Morbidity and Mortality Weekly Report, 59*(49), 1609–1613.

Chapman, D. P., Whitfield, C. L., Felitti, V. J., Dube, S. R., Edwards, V. J., & Anda, R. F. (2004). Adverse childhood experiences and the risk of depressive disorders in adulthood. *Journal of Affective Disorders, 82*(2), 217–225.

Charuvastra, A., & Cloitre, M. (2008). Social bonds and posttraumatic stress disorder. *Annual Review of Psychology, 59*, 301–328.

Chen, X. (2009). The linkage between deviant lifestyles and victimization: An examination from a life course perspective. *Journal of Interpersonal Violence, 24*(7), 1083–1110.

Cicchetti, D. (2006). Development and psychopathology. In D. Ciccheti & D. J. Cohen (Eds.), *Developmental psychopathology: Theory and method* (2nd ed., pp. 1–23). New York: Wiley.

Cloitre, M., Stolbach, B. C., Herman, J. L., van der Kolk, B., Pynoos, R., Wang, J., et al. (2009a). A developmental approach to complex PTSD: Childhood and adult cumulative trauma as predictors of symptom complexity. *Journal of Traumatic Stress, 22*(5), 399–408.

Cohen, J. A., & Mannarino, A. B. (2000). Predictors of treatment outcome in sexually abused children. *Child Abuse and Neglect, 24*(7), 983–994.

Cook, A., Spinazzola, J., Ford, J., Lanktree, C., Blaustein, M., Cloitre, M., et al. (2005). Complex trauma in children and adolescents. *Psychiatric Annals, 35*(5), 390–398.

Courtois, C. A. (2004). Complex trauma, complex reactions: Assessment and treatment. *Psychotherapy, 41*(4), 412–425.

Cuevas, C. A., Finkelhor, D., Clifford, C., Ormrod, R. K., & Turner, H. A. (2010). Psychological distress as a risk factor for re-victimization in children. *Child Abuse and Neglect, 34*(4), 235–243.

Cuevas, C. A., Finkelhor, D., Turner, H. A., & Ormrod, R. K. (2007). Juvenile delinquency and victimization: A theoretical typology. *Journal of Interpersonal Violence, 22*(12), 1581–1602.

D'Andrea, W., Ford, J. D., Stolbach, B., Spinazzola, J., & van der Kolk, B. A. (2012). Understanding interpersonal trauma in children: Why we need a developmentally appropriate trauma diagnosis. *American Journal of Orthopsychiatry, 82*, 187–200.

Dong, M., Anda, R. F., Felitti, V. J., Dube, S. R., Williamson, D. F., Thompson, T. J., et al. (2004). The interrelatedness of multiple forms of childhood abuse, neglect, and household dysfunction. *Child Abuse and Neglect, 28*(7), 771–784.

Dube, S. R. (2001). Childhood abuse, household dysfunction, and the risk of attempted suicide throughout the life span: Findings from the Adverse Childhood Experiences Study. *Journal of the American Medical Association, 286*(24), 3089–3096.

Dube, S. R., Fairweather, D., Pearson, W. S., Felitti, V. J., Anda, R. F., & Croft, J. B. (2009). Cumulative childhood stress and autoimmune diseases in adults. *Psychosomatic Medicine, 17*, 243–250.

Edwards, V., Holden, G. W., Felitti, V. J., & Anda, R. F. (2003). Relationship between multiple forms of childhood maltreatment and adult mental health in community respondents: Results from the Adverse Childhood Experiences Study. *American Journal of Psychiatry, 160*(8), 1453–1460.

Ehring, T., & Quack, D. (2010). Emotion regulation difficulties in trauma survivors:

The role of trauma type and PTSD symptom severity. *Behavior Therapy, 41*(4), 587–598.

Ellonen, N., & Salmi, V. (2011). Poly-victimization as a life condition: Correlates of poly-victimization among Finnish children. *Journal of Scandinavian Studies in Criminology and Crime Prevention, 12*(1), 20–44.

Felitti, V. J., & Anda, R. F. (2009). The relationship of adverse childhood experiences to adult medical disease, psychiatric disorders, and sexual behavior: Implications for healthcare. In R. Lanius & E. Vermetten (Eds.), *The hidden epidemic: The impact of early life trauma on health and disease.* New York: Cambridge University Press.

Felitti, V. J., Anda, R. F., Nordenberg, D., Williamson, D. F., Spitz, A. M., Edwards, V., et al. (1998). Relationship of childhood abuse and household dysfunction to many of the leading causes of death in adults. *American Journal of Preventive Medicine, 14*(4), 245–258.

Finkelhor, D., Ormrod, R., Turner, H., & Holt, M. (2009). Pathways to poly-victimization. *Child Maltreatment, 14*(4), 316–329.

Finkelhor, D., Ormrod, R. K., & Turner, H. A. (2007a). Poly-victimization: A neglected component in child victimization. *Child Abuse and Neglect, 31*(1), 7–26.

Finkelhor, D., Ormrod, R. K., & Turner, H. A. (2007b). Re-victimization patterns in a national longitudinal sample of children and youth. *Child Abuse and Neglect, 31*(5), 479–502.

Finkelhor, D., Ormrod, R. K., & Turner, H. A. (2009). Lifetime assessment of poly-victimization in a national sample of children and youth. *Child Abuse and Neglect, 33*(7), 403–411.

Finkelhor, D., Ormrod, R. K., Turner, H. A., & Hamby, S. L. (2005). Measuring poly-victimization using the Juvenile Victimization Questionnaire. *Child Abuse and Neglect, 29*(11), 1297–1312.

Follette, V., & Duckworth, M. (2011). *Retraumatization.* New York: Taylor & Francis.

Follette, V. M., Polusny, M. A., Bechtle, A. E., & Naugle, A. E. (1996). Cumulative trauma: The impact of child sexual abuse, adult sexual assault, and spouse abuse. *Journal of Traumatic Stress, 9*(1), 25–35.

Follette, V., & Vijay, A. (2008). Retraumatization. In G. Reyes, J. Elhai, & J. D. Ford (Eds.), *Encyclopedia of psychological trauma* (pp. 586–589). Hoboken, NJ: Wiley.

Ford, J. D. (2009). Neurobiological and developmental research: Clinical implications. In C. A. Courtois & J. D. Ford (Eds.), *Treating complex traumatic stress disorders: An evidence-based guide* (pp. 31–58). New York: Guilford Press.

Ford, J. D. (2010). Complex adult sequelae of early life exposure to psychological trauma. In R. A. Lanius, E. Vermetten, & C. Pain (Eds.), *The hidden epidemic: The impact of early life trauma on health and disease* (pp. 69–76). New York: Cambridge University Press.

Ford, J. D. (2011). Assessing child and adolescent complex traumatic stress reactions. *Journal of Child and Adolescent Trauma, 4*(3), 217–232.

Ford, J. D., Connor, D. F., & Hawke, J. (2009). Complex trauma among psychiatrically impaired children: A cross-sectional, chart-review study. *Journal of Clinical Psychiatry, 70*(8), 1155–1163.

Ford, J. D., Elhai, J. D., Connor, D. F., & Frueh, B. C. (2010). Poly-victimization and risk of posttraumatic, depressive, and substance use disorders and involvement in delinquency in a national sample of adolescents. *Journal of Adolescent Health, 46*(6), 545–552.

Ford, J. D., Racusin, R., Ellis, C. G., Daviss, W. B., Reiser, J., Fleischer, A., et al. (2000). Child maltreatment, other trauma exposure, and posttraumatic symptomatology among children with oppositional defiant and attention deficit hyperactivity disorders. *Child Maltreatment, 5*(3), 205–217.

Ford, J. D., & Smith, S. (2008). Complex posttraumatic stress disorder in trauma-exposed adults receiving public sector outpatient substance abuse disorder treatment. *Addiction Research and Theory, 16*(2), 193–203.

Ford, J. D., Stockton, P., Kaltman, S., & Green, B. L. (2006). Disorders of extreme stress (DESNOS) symptoms are associated with type and severity of interpersonal trauma exposure in a sample of healthy young women. *Journal of Interpersonal Violence, 21*(11), 1399–1416.

Ford, J. D., Wasser, T., & Connor, D. F. (2011). Identifying and determining the symptom severity associated with polyvictimization among psychiatrically impaired children in the outpatient setting. *Child Maltreatment, 16*(3), 216–226.

Fox, N. A., & Levitt, L. A. (1995). *Violence Exposure Scale for Children—Revised (VEX-R)*. College Park, MD: Institute for Child Study, University of Maryland.

Freyd, J. J., DePrince, A. P., & Gleaves, D. H. (2007). The state of betrayal trauma theory: Reply to McNally—conceptual issues and future directions. *Memory, 15*(3), 295–311.

Grasso, D., Saunders, B., Williams, L. M., Hanson, R., Smith, D., & Fitzgerald, M. M. (2011). *Patterns of multiple victimization among maltreated children in Navy families.* Manuscript submitted for publication.

Hagenaars, M. A., Fisch, I., & van Minnen, A. (2011). The effect of trauma onset and frequency on PTSD-associated symptoms. *Journal of Affective Disorders, 132*(1–2), 192–199.

Hawkins, S. S., & Radcliffe, J. (2006). Current measures of PTSD for children and adolescents. *Journal of Pediatric Psychology, 31*(4), 420–430.

Herman, J. L. (1992). Complex PTSD: A syndrome in survivors of prolonged and repeated trauma. *Journal of Traumatic Stress, 5*(3), 377–391.

Hobfoll, S. E. (1989). Conservation of resources: A new attempt at conceptualizing stress. *American Psychologist, 44*(3), 513–524.

Hobfoll, S. E. (2001). The influence of culture, community, and the nested-self in the stress process: Advancing conservation of resources theory. *Applied Psychology: An International Review, 50*(3), 337–370.

Holt, M. K., Finkelhor, D., & Kantor, G. K. (2007). Multiple victimization experiences of urban elementary school students: Associations with psychosocial functioning and academic performance. *Child Abuse and Neglect, 31*(5), 503–515.

Kassam-Adams, N., Fleisher, C. L., & Winston, F. K. (2009). Acute stress disorder and posttraumatic stress disorder in parents of injured children. *Journal of Traumatic Stress, 22*(4), 294–302.

Kaufman, J., Jones, B., Stieglitz, E., Vitulano, L., & Mannarino, A. P. (1994). The use of multiple informants to assess children's maltreatment experiences. *Journal of Family Violence, 9*(3), 227–248.

Kim, B. N., Kim, J. W., Kim, H. W., Shin, M. S., Cho, S. C., Choi, N. H., et al. (2009). A 6–month follow-up study of posttraumatic stress and anxiety/depressive symptoms in Korean children after direct or indirect exposure to a single incident of trauma. *Journal of Clinical Psychiatry, 70*(8), 1148–1154.

Luthra, R., Abramovitz, R., Greenberg, R., Schoor, A., Newcorn, J., Schmeidler, J., et al. (2009). Relationship between type of trauma exposure and posttraumatic stress disorder among urban children and adolescents. *Journal of Interpersonal Violence, 24*(11), 1919–1927.

McEwen, B. S. (2000). The neurobiology of stress: From serendipity to clinical relevance. *Brain Research, 886*(1–2), 172–189.

Pynoos, R. S., Steinberg, A. M., & Piacentini, J. C. (1999). A developmental psychopathology model of childhood traumatic stress and intersection with anxiety disorders. *Biological Psychiatry, 46*(11), 1542–1554.

Saunders, B. E. (2003). Understanding children exposed to violence: Toward an integration of overlapping fields. *Journal of Interpersonal Violence, 18*(4), 356–376.

Scott-Storey, K. (2011). Cumulative abuse: Do things add up? An evaluation of the conceptualization, operationalization, and methodological approaches in the study of the phenomenon of cumulative abuse. *Trauma, Violence, and Abuse, 12*(3), 135–150.

Skelton, K., Ressler, K. J., Norrholm, S. D., Jovanovic, T., & Bradley-Davino, B. (2011). PTSD and gene variants: New pathways and new thinking. *Neuropharmacology, 62*(2), 628–637.

Stover, C. S., & Berkowitz, S. (2005). Assessing violence exposure and trauma symptoms in young children: A critical review of measures. *Journal of Traumatic Stress, 18*(6), 707–717.

Strand, V. C., Sarmiento, T. L., & Pasquale, L. E. (2005). Assessment and screening tools for trauma in children and adolescents: A review. *Trauma, Violence, and Abuse, 6*(1), 55–78.

Straus, M. A., Hamby, S.L., Boney-McCoy, S., & Sugarman, D.B. (1996). The Revised Conflict Tactics Scales (CTS2): Development and preliminary psychometric data. *Journal of Family Issues, 17,* 283–316.

Turner, H. A., Finkelhor, D., & Ormrod, R. (2010). Poly-victimization in a national sample of children and youth. *American Journal of Preventive Medicine, 38*(3), 323–330.

Turner, R. J., & Lloyd, D. A. (1995). Lifetime traumas and mental health: The significance of cumulative adversity. *Journal of Health and Social Behavior, 36,* 360–376.

van der Kolk, B. A. (2005). Developmental trauma disorder. *Psychiatric Annals, 35*(5), 401–408.

Walter, K. H., Horsey, K. J., Palmieri, P. A., & Hobfoll, S. E. (2010). The role of protective self-cognitions in the relationship between childhood trauma and later resource loss. *Journal of Traumatic Stress, 23*(2), 264–273.

CHAPTER 6

The Translational Evidence Base

Ruth R. DeRosa
Lisa Amaya-Jackson
Christopher M. Layne

Given the dramatic rise in the number of evidence-based treatments (EBTs) in child mental health (Kazdin, 2011), it has become increasingly difficult for clinicians and agencies with finite resources to select a "core" or common set of evidence-based interventions to adopt into everyday practice. Timely comments from Chorpita and his colleagues (2011) underscore this trend: "In our recent efforts to examine how to choose a set of EBTs to fit an organization's service population, we discovered that simply selecting a set of no more than a dozen treatments from among all EBTs for children yields more than 67 sextillion possibilities" (p. 493). Within the child trauma field, data from randomized controlled trials (RCTs) are becoming increasingly available, and studies to date include a range in age from toddlers and preschoolers (Lieberman, Ghosh Ippen, Van Horn, 2006; Scheeringa, Weems, Cohen, Amaya-Jackson, & Guthrie, 2011) to school-age children and adolescents in a variety of settings (e.g., Chaffin, Funderburk, Bard, Valle, & Gurwitch, 2011; Deblinger, Mannarino, Cohen, Runyon, & Steer, 2011; Ford, Steinberg, Hawke, Levine, & Zhang, 2012; Kolko, 2010; Layne et al., 2008; Najavits, Gallop, & Weiss, 2006). Although treatment options and best-practice recommendations regularly appear in the literature in ways that reflect the evolving evidence base (e.g., Ford & Cloitre, 2009; Dorsey, Briggs, & Woods, 2011), clinicians and agencies alike must nevertheless make consequential and challenging decisions regarding what and how to adopt, orient, train, implement, support, and sustain their efforts to provide clinical practice informed by both the latest research and skilled expertise.

The pioneer of the evidence-based practice (EBP) movement in medicine, David Sackett (Sackett, Rosenberg, Gray, Haynes, & Richardson, 1996), described EBP as "the judicious, explicit, and conscientious use of the evidence base to guide one's clinical practice" (p. 71). Clinicians must integrate the best available research evidence while using their clinical expertise and taking into consideration their patient's unique values and circumstances (Sackett et al., 1996). EBP requires systematic assessment, identification of specific goals, flexible and informed critical thinking, and implementation of the core components of treatment with ongoing evaluation of therapeutic progress. A central tenet of EBP—and perhaps the most intrinsically "human" element guiding its success—is critical thinking. *Critical thinking* (i.e., critical appraisal) refers to the ability and willingness to assess the evidence, to seek contradicting and confirming evidence, to monitor one's biases, and to make objective judgments based upon well-supported reasons (Profetto-McGrath, 2005). Indeed, adherence to an EBP requires (rather than precludes) that clinicians think and act judiciously while simultaneously utilizing the core components of the treatment.

Training in multiple treatments alone, however, is not synonymous with an EBP approach. Instead, EBP, as defined above, requires a learning culture with institutions partnering with therapists to foster a commitment to profession-long learning and development. In the treatment of complex, multiproblem, traumatized children and families, critical thinking is especially crucial as clinicians strive to provide the best care possible in an era in which guiding theory, proposed diagnostic criteria, and interventions are still in formative stages of development (see Chapters 14 and 18, this volume), and efforts to identify the "active ingredients" or mechanisms of therapeutic change are in a nascent stage (see Amaya-Jackson & DeRosa, 2007; Layne, 2011; Layne, Warren, Watson, & Shalev, 2007). As community-based clinicians work to integrate EBTs into practice, many discussions, controversies, papers, recommendations, and even new journals, such as *Implementation Science,* have emerged describing the challenges and barriers of adoption and implementation. Clinicians and clinical researchers alike have described the benefits of collaborative, comprehensive training and consultation in providing EBTs to community practices (Lyon, Stirman, Kerns & Bruns, 2011; Toth & Manly, 2011; Ebert, Amaya-Jackson, Markiewicz, Kisiel, & Fairbank, 2011). Not surprisingly, however, training workshops alone do not improve treatment outcome (Lopez, Osterberg, Jensen-Doss, & Rae, 2011). In addition to training methods, Ruzek and Rosen (2009) highlight other factors that can enhance the effective dissemination of EBTs for posttraumatic stress disorder (PTSD), including such clinician factors as competence, readiness to adopt a practice, and perceived attributes of the treatment; and organizational factors such as dissemination priorities, quality assurance programs, and ongoing training support. Until recently, much of the literature has taken primarily a deficit-based perspective, focusing on barriers such as therapist attitudes and motivation, organizational "buy-in" and resources, lack of treatment fidelity, and inadequate training/consultation (Jensen-Doss, Hawley, Lopez, & Osterberg, 2009; Asgary-Eden & Lee, 2011).

These challenges underscore the joint need for ongoing, evidence-based assessment of clients (e.g., Haynes, Smith, & Hunsley, 2011; Hunsley & Mash, 2008), and ongoing, evidence-based training and education of therapists in order to support treatment fidelity and success. As community-based clinicians, agencies, and statewide programs have begun to adopt EBTs (e.g., Ebert et al., 2011; Nakamura et al., 2011; Kauth, Sullivan, Cully, & Blevins, 2011; McHugh & Barlow, 2010), it has become clear that the science behind the "how" of treatment implementation is as important as the "what" (i.e., the specific treatment elements being implemented) (Becker & Stirman, 2011; Fixsen, Naoom, Blase, Friedman, & Wallace, 2005; Hoagwood, Burns, & Weisz, 2002). Of particular interest, in an in-depth qualitative examination of implementation that served as part of a larger RCT, titled Child System and Treatment Enhancement Projects or "Child STEPs," Palinkas et al. (2008) describe a conceptual model that may serve as a useful guide for enhancing training methods for the treatment of traumatized youth and families. An especially promising feature of the Palinkas et al. model is that, instead of focusing primarily on barriers, it describes components of the learning environment in EBT implementation that may play a role in the successful adoption of child and family interventions. We propose that the Palinkas et al. model may serve as a heuristic framework for conceptualizing key ingredients for enhancing current trauma training and critical thinking skills—which may, in turn, support more widespread, routine use of EBP approaches. Rather than focusing on barriers and risk factors for implementation problems, the Palinkas et al. (2008) model emphasizes what is working and which factors may facilitate success. Accordingly, in this chapter we adopt the Palinkas et al. (2008) model as a guiding framework to organize and systematically consider implications for training in trauma-focused treatments and for the application of an EBP approach to trauma work with children. For each factor proposed in the model, we describe pertinent developments in the literature that may be used to effectively harness these factors in the field of childhood traumatic stress treatment.

Overview of the Child STEPs Implementation Model

During a large, randomized clinical effectiveness trial for the treatment of childhood anxiety, depression, and conduct problems, Palinkas et al.

(2008) interviewed 60 clinicians at two different sites, reviewed minutes of therapy consultation teleconferences, and surveyed hundreds of hours of participant observations during the ongoing RCT. Analysis of clinicians' intentions to continue to use the treatment at the end of the study revealed three categories: (1) intends to faithfully continue to implement the treatment, (2) intends to engage in partial implementation of the treatment, or (3) intends to abandon EBTs in the study. The authors identified seven additional themes that they incorporated into a heuristic model to describe the associations among key variables and intentions to use the treatment long term (see Figure 6.1). The themes were organized into two categories, consisting of *preimplementation factors* and *short-term implementation factors*. We describe each set of factors in turn.

Preimplementation Factors

Palinkas et al. (2008) hypothesized that three themes that are present before treatment implementation begins contribute to the likelihood of long-term use by clinicians. These consist of (1) lag time between training and use, (2) clinician engagement, and (3) clinician–treatment fit. Not surprisingly, the longer the lag time between training and first client, the less likely clinicians were to report that they intended to continue to implement the treatment after the study. Clinician engagement factors include motivation, enthusiasm, and commitment to participating in the RCT project. *Clinician–treatment fit* refers to previous clinical experiences such as theoretical orientation and whether or not the clinician had worked with the treatment population before or had previous exposure to structured therapies.

Short-Term Implementation Factors

Palinkas et al. (2008) also identified four possible determinants of long-term use of the treatments during the first several months of implementing the treatment interventions. *Clinician's first impressions* refers to positive and negative beliefs and expectations after just starting the treatment (e.g., feeling that the protocol was too difficult for the client, too rigid, too simplistic for complex cases, too complex for parents to use, or they didn't have the time to cover the material in session). Clinician skill level or competence is also an important factor, as supervisors noted significant differences across therapists in their abilities to prepare for sessions and teach different skill sets. *Clinician–researcher adaptability* refers to (1) the degree to which therapists involved in the study were willing and able to be flexible and creative while adhering to the core components of the treatment, and (2) the degree to which the researchers were willing and able to translate across different therapy orientations and periodically adjust protocols within therapists' frameworks without abandoning the core treatment components. And finally, the most frequently cited positive factor was the relationship

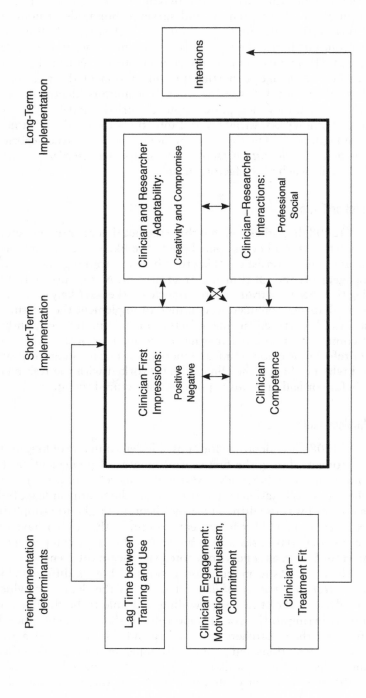

FIGURE 6.1. Child STEPs model of EBT implementation. From Palinkas et al. (2008). Copyright 2008 by the American Psychiatric Association. Reprinted with permission from *Psychiatric Services*.

between the clinicians and researchers. *Clinician–researcher interactions* refer to time spent engaging in supportive conversations during treatment consultations and in social interactions outside of consultation.

Examination of Implementation Factors

Clinician–Treatment Fit and Competence

The discussion of fit often refers to orientation: namely, does the orientation of the EBT match the clinician's orientation? However, in the area of child trauma, perhaps a more important question of fit is, Do the clinicians, regardless of orientation, have the foundational trauma-related conceptual knowledge and significant practice with trauma-informed clinical reasoning and judgment? Amaya-Jackson, representing the National Child Traumatic Stress Network (NCTSN), conducted a series of focus groups with experienced trauma clinicians with a variety of theoretical orientations from around the country who were using critical thinking skills in an EBP approach to thoughtfully tailor EBTs to best suit the needs of their clients while seeking to implement the core components of the treatments (Amaya-Jackson & DeRosa, 2007). The NCTSN trauma therapists, having implemented three or more EBTs in their agencies, came to the focus groups with different disciplinary perspectives from a variety of settings and worked with children of all ages. Based on the latest research and their clinical judgment and expertise, they came to a consensus during the discussions that EBTs were limited in their ability to address their complex trauma cases that present with multiple current stressors in combination with complex PTSD behaviors. They shared the approaches that they used to address complex cases without abandoning core components of EBTs or reverting to previous methods, uninformed by trauma theory and research, which they no longer felt were acceptable practices. The ability to do this requires knowledge of the complex sequelae of trauma, based on latest research, and critical thinking skills with clinical competence.

Examination of treatment implementation practices in the trauma field has just begun to emerge in the literature. Couineau and Forbes (2011) found that less experienced practitioners working with child sexual abuse were less likely to implement exposure techniques than the more experienced practitioners (defined as those with graduate degrees and more years of clinical experience) who were treating war veterans. The authors proposed an interaction between clinician experience and client type; however, this description does not provide a causal explanation outlining why the therapists made particular treatment choices. Specifically, were clinical judgments based on the behavior and treatment needs of their emotionally and behaviorally dysregulated clients as indicated by the extant complex trauma literature, or did their judgments reflect a significant lack of trauma-informed training? An in-depth assessment of these choices—for example, timing of exposure techniques—without rigid a priori assumptions is essential. With the confounding variables of clinical experience and treatment plan in this study, readers cannot draw definitive conclusions; however, the study does highlight the critical need for training in trauma theory, in the developmental impact of chronic stress, and in best-practice recommendations for complex trauma treatment.

Indeed, current evidence suggests that more trauma training is needed among practitioners in general. In a recent survey conducted by the American Psychological Association Practice Organization of over 200 practicing psychologists (Cook, Dinnen, Rehman, Bufka & Courtois, 2011), 64% expressed interest in receiving more specialized trauma training. Unfortunately, the majority of training programs for therapists and counselors in mental health fields do not provide trauma-specific training, despite the strong likelihood that they will encounter trauma survivors in their clinical practice (Cook et al., 2011; Courtois & Gold, 2009).

In order to address the gap and inconsistent standard in trauma training, the NCTSN has developed the Core Curriculum on Childhood Trauma (CCCT; Layne et al., 2011). This curriculum, intended to serve as a foundation for trauma-informed care, is useful to all clinicians from different disciplines before they receive more advanced clinical training and supervision in EBTs. Unlike traditional didactic models, the CCCT integrates problem-based learning (PBL) principles with in-depth case materials in a team-based learning environment. PBL is a routine part of many medical school programs and has been successfully incorporated into other social science curricula (Schlett et al., 2010). Based on adult active learning principles, the CCCT exposes participants to detailed "real-world" traumatic case material to enhance experiential knowledge and clinical reasoning skills. A key feature of this training is its goal of integrating knowledge acquisition with knowledge application or skill, providing repeated practice in critical thinking skills in guided small-group or team-based forums. Students of PBL approaches have been found to retain knowledge for much longer periods of time, make more accurate diagnoses, demonstrate more effective clinical problem-solving strategies, and score higher on measures of teamwork, interpersonal skills, and self-reflective abilities (Distelhorst, Dawson, Robbs, & Barrows, 2005; Schlett et al., 2010).

The conceptual foundation for the CCCT consists of three theoretical domains: (1) concepts for understanding the traumatic experience (e.g., "Traumatic events are inherently complex and consist of different traumatic moments that are encoded at multiple levels in the brain and body"); (2) concepts for understanding the consequences of trauma exposure and its aftermath (e.g., "Responses to trauma are rooted in neurobiology and involve the stress responses system and key brain structures"); and (3) guiding principles for intervention with trauma-exposed children and families (e.g., "Working with trauma-exposed youth and families can evoke distress in providers that makes it more difficult for them to provide good care")

(Layne et al., 2011, p. 9). Building on information from the child maltreatment literature, content areas are drawn from the fields of psychology, human development and social ecology, developmental neurobiology, and developmental psychopathology (Layne et al., 2011).

CCCT-based training involves presenting participants with incremental bits of clinical data that gradually "flesh out" the case. With each successive chunk of information, learners are invited to (1) list important information (and thereby practice sorting pertinent details), (2) generate hunches and hypotheses (practice resisting assumptions and premature decisions), (3) identify learning needs (practice identifying areas in which they need more knowledge or skills), and (4) plan next steps (practice identifying missing information and how to test hypotheses). A pilot evaluation indicated that the CCCT was well received as gauged both by open-ended qualitative reports as well as significant pre–post increases in participants' perceived self-efficacy in applying the core concepts to their clinical work (Layne et al., 2011). Next steps for evaluating the CCCT include assessing changes in therapist performance and competency in clinical settings. By providing interactive learning with "real-life" case descriptions and scenarios, coupled with an opportunity to actively apply trauma-based principles and knowledge, this curriculum arguably could address not only clinician–treatment fit, as outlined in the Palinkas et al. (2008) model, but also has great promise to enhance the clinician competence factor (Amaya-Jackson, 2011).

Clinician Engagement and First Impressions

The *clinician engagement* and *first impressions* factors in the Palinkas et al. (2008) model refer to clinicians' motivation, attitudes, commitment, beliefs, and expectancies before and after their initial implementation of the treatment. How might trainers actively harness these factors in implementing a new treatment? The psychotherapy literature has just begun to address this question. To address expectancies and future motivation, training orientations may benefit from incorporating adult learning principles. For example, Steinfeld, Coffman, and Keyes (2009) report that during training and implementation of EBTs in a large multisite project, it took 2 years for therapists to routinely and comfortably use cognitive-behavioral therapy (CBT) skills throughout their practice. Joyce and Showers (2002) estimate that it takes 20–25 iterations of a newly learned behavior before professionals achieve consistent professional change. In addition, Lyon et al. (2011) point to research suggesting that while learning new skills, clinicians may actually experience a decrease in competency before surpassing their original performance level. This decrease, however temporary, has significant implications for morale and clinicians' first impressions of treatment implementation, especially if they expect that with supervision/consultation they will be proficient after seeing only a few clients over a

6-month period. The speed with which practitioners acquire proficiency in trauma treatment will also depend on the amount of previous trauma training, such as the foundation provided by the CCCT, because the relation between existing knowledge and learning any new skills is an important variable in the success or failure of trainings (see Lyon et al., 2011).

Varra, Hayes, Roget, and Fisher (2008) point out that learning a new treatment also brings psychological stress that can include a decrease in confidence, clinical uncertainty, and highlight a deficient skill set. Based on the premise that learning new EBTs is influenced by emotion and the beliefs and expectancies of success, Varra et al. (2008) designed a study to investigate the impact of increasing clinicians' willingness to implement an EBP by changing their relationship to thoughts and feelings about barriers to implementation. Specifically, the authors included a training component drawn from Acceptance and Commitment Therapy (Acceptance and Commitment Training [ACT]; Hayes et al., 2004) to "alter the impact of thoughts and emotions rather than to alter the content, frequency, or intensity of thoughts and emotions" (Varra et al., 2008, p. 450) about barriers to treatment implementation. Counselors in the ACT condition made significantly more referrals for pharmacotherapy at follow-up 3 months later and were more willing to use empirically supported psychotherapy, compared to counselors in the educational control condition.

The authors reported that, at post and follow-up, participants in the ACT group were more likely to describe barriers to treatment *and* less likely to believe them compared to the controls. In addition, counselors in the ACT reported greater psychological flexibility at post and 3-month follow-up compared to individuals in the control group. Analysis of mediators revealed that participants who reported more psychological flexibility were also more willing and more likely to refer to pharmacotherapy. Psychological flexibility here was defined as the ability to choose behaviors and be flexible in their actions *in spite of* difficult thoughts and feelings. Interestingly, Palinkas et al. (2008) quote a clinician with a seemingly similar viewpoint during their discussion of positive engagement and the stress of learning new techniques; "I am going to do their study whether it feels good or not. This is what I signed up for, and I'm going to do it!" (p. 742). This therapist appears to value honoring the commitment to the study. In a similar fashion, the ACT component also linked therapist values and behaviors so that explicit commitments were intimately tied with the therapist's purpose and meaning in his or her professional life. Linking purpose, meaning, and goals is also effective for building therapeutic alliances (Tryon & Winograd, 2011); thus, it is not surprising that strengthening such links would enhance clinician engagement and behavior change as well.

Clinician–Researcher Adaptability and Social Interactions

In their 2008 paper, Palinkas et al. describe the implementation of the Child STEPs program (See Figure 6.1), an RCT of treatments for children and adolescents. More recently, results of the Child STEPs program evaluation indicated that a modular treatment approach that allowed the practitioner to flexibly alter the sequence of the treatment components was associated with better treatment outcome (Weisz et al., 2012). In other words, clinicians who learned a modularized version of the treatment (consisting of the individualized tailoring of treatment components depending on each child's needs, strengths, and circumstances), compared to a traditional, structured, fixed-session manual, not only reported that they were more likely to use the treatment in the future, but also had better treatment outcomes compared to clinicians who administered either the traditional manualized treatment or treatment as usual (Weisz et al., 2012). An evaluation of the specific components implemented revealed that clinicians using the modularized treatment included 17% more "other" content compared to the standard EBT (7%), leading the authors to conclude that this factor may have allowed clinicians to address more problem areas. An interesting contrasting hypothesis is found in the proposition by Norcross and Lambert (2011), who draw on the psychotherapy outcome literature to propose that tailoring treatment to the client increases effectiveness not primarily due to the use of enhanced treatment techniques, but rather due to a synergistic confluence of therapeutic factors, including client factors (e.g., positive vs. adverse life events, social support), the therapeutic relationship (e.g., common therapeutic factors such as warmth and therapeutic alliance), treatment method, and positive expectancy.

Adaptability, as defined by Palinkas et al. (2008), was operationalized as a modularized approach that allowed therapists to select the sequencing of the treatment components depending on the needs of their clients. In addition, the authors described and measured the creative ways in which clinicians tailored the material to align with their orientation while still adhering to the treatment's core components. Palinkas and colleagues also described three essential factors in their success: the perceptions that the researchers were willing to (1) work to build a common language, (2) translate terms across orientations to facilitate identification of common goals or treatment targets, and (3) identify clinicians' strengths and effectively and flexibly defer or direct them depending on their rationale and the clinical circumstances.

These collaborative efforts may have also been enhanced by clinician–researcher social interactions. Palinkas et al. (2008) identify this theme—which included participation in social activities such as lunch, pot luck dinners, and discussions unrelated to the project—as the most frequently cited by study participants. Clinicians described occasionally discussing non-work-related issues, stressors, and clients outside the scope of the study. These findings point to the importance of meaningful interpersonal relationships between researchers, supervisors, and clinicians that transcend project-related concerns. Norcross and Lambert (2011) underscore the point that "treatment methods are relational acts" (p. 5), and by extension, we would argue, so also are the training methods employed to coach practitioners in psychotherapy treatments. Rather than passively relegating the meaning and effects of the training relationships to "common factors" or relationship factors that might come naturally, the Palinkas et al. model suggests that training would benefit from incorporating specific relationship-building practices both in and outside of the consultation time.

One could thus argue that researcher–clinician or trainer–trainee collaborative behaviors and interactions are also an important part of the science of training individuals in treatment methods and implementation success, just as the "common factors" have emerged as powerful predictors in psychotherapy research.

Conclusion

Although the exact course of future trauma treatment development and training is still unfolding, we nevertheless propose that an EBP approach to trauma work can assist our field in its journey while also providing maximum benefit to clinicians and the children and families they treat. Understanding the possible impact of trauma exposure and its aftermath; the potential emotional, cognitive, interpersonal, and biological consequences; the existing protective factors; foundational trauma theory; and the common principles that undergird effective psychotherapy—all are likely to enhance any EBT training. The literature we reviewed suggests that a curriculum such as the CCCT has the potential of actually increasing treatment adherence and effectiveness because it helps to clarify the aims and structure of the treatment design and the logic behind the selection of specific intervention objectives.

A central tenet of EBP is that our empirical and theoretical knowledge base is constantly evolving. Thus, the "best-practice" factors judged at a given time to be necessary for effective outcomes should not be assumed to rest solely on the shoulders of either treatment technique alone or the therapeutic alliance alone, nor should the "active ingredients" of effective treatment be considered to be known, fixed, and immutable. Rather, creating a culture that actively integrates learning on an ongoing basis as an essential feature of evidence-based "practice" (the verb), including regular exposures to (or critical appraisal of) reviews of the current trauma literature, coupled with ongoing systematic assessments of clients, has the potential to support critical thinking and thereby enhance clinical judgment and decisions (Amaya-Jackson, 2011; see also Haynes et al., 2011; Hunsley & Mash, 2008).

The application of "assessment-informed" critical thinking within a supportive and validating team context or peer supervision group (for the solo practitioner) cultivates a willingness to seek out and evaluate both confirming and contradictory hypotheses and information in ways that contribute to better outcomes and less therapist burnout (Craig & Sprang,

2010; Pross & Schweitzer, 2010). Such teams may also benefit from strategies, described previously in ACT (Varra et al., 2008), which support the ability to make informed choices and to act flexibly despite difficult emotions that often arise while facing multiple barriers to implementation and learning new techniques. Helping practitioners and administrators alike to identify personal value-based goals and commitments to learning and professional development may also enhance engagement and EBP behaviors.

Creating a collaborative culture that fosters interpersonal relationships over time across multiple training sessions and consultation meetings is also emerging as a key ingredient to success (e.g., Becker & Stirman, 2011; Fixsen et al., 2005; Cohen & Mannarino, 2008; Lyon et al., 2011). To be clear, our earlier description of the cross pollination of ideas and strategies, involving flexibility, adaptability, creativity, and collaboration, are not intended to imply that modifying core treatment components is necessarily efficacious or routinely advised. Rather, as Nock, Goldman, Wang, and Albano (2004) note, "because all potential modifications are not listed in the manual, there is [therefore] no need to discard the EBT in favor of using an unsupported approach" (p. 777). Similar to an EBP approach, these authors suggest the application of the scientific method with each case as informed by systematic data collection. The fact that multiple verbs are used in the literature to describe alterations in how treatments are implemented (e.g., *tailoring, adapting, modifying, extending, incorporating*) without clear and consistent accompanying definitions is perhaps both emblematic and a "milepost marker" of the continuing evolution of EBP in the mental health field. For example, we propose that *tailoring* may best refer to alterations in language, selecting specific activities, verifying the length, or resequencing one or more treatment components. *Modifying* may refer to more in-depth alterations to a treatment, such as rewriting or adding material to the implementation manual, inserting or changing primary intervention objectives, and so forth, for a particular population, perhaps analogous to the "off-label" use of medication (Nock et al., 2004). Due to their more pervasive nature, such modifications clearly call for separate outcome evaluations within specific populations and settings—that is, to "assess along the way," as proposed by Amaya-Jackson and DeRosa (2007). Notably, *adapting* appears in the literature in ways that suggest its interchangeability with the above definitions and increase ambiguity in the literature. For example, the term *adaptability*, as defined by Palinkas et al. (2008), appears to refer to our above definition of *tailoring*. However, *modularized* by Weisz et al. (2012), or the term *adaptation* appear to include changes in the treatment that refer our definition of modification. Rigorous empirical evaluations, including "dismantling" designs for treatment elements that can be compartmentalized, such that they can be either included or omitted (e.g., prolonged exposure) and "mechanisms"-based designs, which examine potential mediators and moderators of therapeutic change over time, are critical (Layne, 2011).

Child and family trauma treatment is perhaps analogous to jazz music. Although jazz is a musical genre that offers, and indeed expects, individual expression, it does so within the context of a clearly defined chord progression that provides an underlying pattern, logical structure, and pulse that supply the backbone and driving force for each individual tune. So, too, clinicians may tailor treatments in accordance with individual clients' specific needs, strengths, circumstances, and informed wishes, based on principles of EBP that are "in sync" with the chord progression of core intervention. Talented musicians and clinicians alike must couple theory with practical application, be dedicated to lifelong learning and professional development, and collaborate and share in sync with colleagues and consumers—be they clients, audience members, community partners, or policy makers. We hope that such structured and clinical creativity, guided by sound clinical theory, evidence-based assessment, wise clinical judgment, and an evolving evidence base will foster enduring professional excellence and performance.

References

Amaya-Jackson, A., & DeRosa, R. R. (2007). Treatment considerations for clinicians in applying evidence-based practice to complex presentations in child trauma. *Journal of Traumatic Stress, 20*(4), 379–390.

Amaya-Jackson, L. (2011, November). *Challenges and opportunities in training a trauma-informed MH workforce in using the NCTSN core curriculum on childhood trauma to create "gold standard" training for evidence-based students and new practitioners* (C. Layne, Chair). Paper presented at the annual meeting of the International Society for Traumatic Stress Studies, Baltimore.

Asgary-Eden, V., & Lee, C. M. (2011). So now we've picked an evidence-based program, what's next?: Perspectives of services providers and administrators. *Professional Psychology: Research and Practice, 42*(2), 169–175.

Becker, K. D., & Stirman, S. W. (2011). The science of training in evidence-based treatments in the context of implementation programs: Current status and prospects for the future. *Administration Policy in Mental Health, 38*, 217–222.

Chaffin, M., Funderburk, B., Bard, D., Valle, L. A., & Gurwitch, R. (2011). A combined motivation and parent–child interaction therapy package reduces child welfare recidivism in a randomized dismantling field trial. *Journal of Counseling and Clinical Psychology, 79*(1), 84–95.

Chorpita, B. F., Rotheram-Borus, M. J., Daleiden, E. L., Bernstein, A., Cromley, T., Swendeman, D., et al. (2011). The old solutions are the new problem: How do we better use what we already know about reducing the burden of mental Illness? *Perspectives on Psychological Scinece, 6*(5), 493–497.

Cohen, J. A., & Mannarino, A. P. (2008). Disseminating and implementing trauma-focused CBT in community settings. *Trauma, Violence, and Abuse, 9*(4), 214–226.

Cook, J. M., Dinnen, S., Rehman, O., Bufka, L., & Courtois, C. (2011). Responses of a sample of practicing psychologists to questions about clinical work with trauma and interest in specialized training. *Psychological Trauma: Theory, Research, Practice and Policy, 3*(3), 253–257.

Courtois, C. A., & Gold, S. N. (2009). The need for inclusion of psychological trauma in the professional curriculum: A call to action. *Psychological Trauma: Theory, Research, Practice and Policy, 1*, 3–23.

Craig, C. D., & Sprang, G. (2010). Compassion satisfaction, compassion fatigue, and burnout in trauma treatment therapists. *Anxiety, Stress, and Coping, 23*(3), 319–339.

Deblinger, E., Mannarino, A. P., Cohen, J. A., Runyon, M.K., & Steer, R. A. (2011). Trauma-focused cognitive behavioral therapy for children: Impact of trauma narrative and treatment length. *Depression and Anxiety, 38*(1), 67–75.

Distelhorst, L. H., Dawson, E., Robbs, R. S., & Barrows, H. S. (2005). Problem-based learning outcomes: The glass half-full. *Academic Medicine, 80*, 294–299.

Dorsey, S., Briggs, E. C., & Woods, B. A. (2011). Cognitive-behavioral treatment for posttraumatic stress disorder in children and adolescents. *Child and Adolescent Psychiatric Clinics of America, 20*, 255–269.

Ebert, L., Amaya-Jackson, L., Markiewicz, J., Kisiel, C., & Fairbank, J. (2011). Use of the breakthrough series collaborative to support broad and sustained use of evidence-based trauma treatment for children in community practice settings. *Administration and Policy in Mental Health and Mental Health Services Research, 23*, 1–13.

Fixsen, D., Naoom, S. F., Blase, D. A., Friedman, R. M., & Wallace, F. (2005). *Implementation research: A synthesis of the literature.* Tampa: University of South Florida. Available online at *http://nirn.fmhi.usf.edu/resources/publications/Monograph/index.cfm.*

Ford, J. D., & Cloitre, M. (2009). Best practices in psychotherapy for children and adolescents. In C. A. Courtois & J. D. Ford (Eds.), *Treating complex traumatic stress disorders: An evidence-based guide* (pp. 59–81). New York: Guilford Press.

Ford, J. D., Steinberg, K. L., Hawke, J., Levine, J., & Zhang, W. (2012). Randomized trial comparison of emotion regulation and relational psychotherapies for PTSD with girls involved in delinquency. *Journal of Clinical Child and Adolescent Psychology, 41*(1), 27–37.

Hayes, S. C., Bissett, R., Roget, N., Padilla, M., Kohlenberg, B. S., & Fisher, G. (2004). The impact of acceptance and commitment training and multicultural training on the stigmatizing attitudes and professional burnout of substance abuse counselors. *Behavior Therapy, 35*, 821–836.

Haynes, S. N., Smith, G. T., & Hunsley, J. D. (2011). *Scientific foundations of clinical assessment.* London: Routledge.

Hoagwood, K., Burns, B. J., & Weisz, J. R. (2002). A profitable conjunction: From science to service in children's mental health. In B.J. Burns & K. Hoagwood (Eds.), *Community treatment for youth: Evidence-based interventions for severe emotional and behavioral disorders* (pp. 327–338). New York: Oxford University Press.

Hunsley, J., & Mash, E. J. (Eds.). (2008). *Guide to assessments that work.* New York: Oxford University Press.

Jensen-Doss, A., Hawley, K. M., Lopez, M., & Osterberg, L. D. (2009). Using evidence-based treatments: The experiences of youth providers working under a mandate. *Professional Psychology: Research and Practice, 40*(4), 417–424.

Joyce, B., & Showers, B. (2002). *Student achievement through staff development* (3rd ed.). Alexandria, VA: Association for Supervision and Curriculum Development.

Kauth, M. R., Sullivan, G., Cully, J., & Blevins, D. (2011). Facilitating practice changes in mental health clinics: A guide for implementation development in health care systems. *Psychological Services, 8*(1), 36–47.

Kazdin, A. E. (2011). Evidence-based treatment research: Advances, limitations, and next steps. *American Psychologist, 66*(8), 685–698.

Kolko, D. J. (2010, August). *Dissemination and implementation of AF-CBT in community settings: Initial findings from a RCT.* Paper presented at the annual meeting of the American Psychological Association, San Diego, CA.

Layne, C. M. (2011). Developing interventions for trauma-exposed children: A comment on progress to date. *Archives of Pediatric Adolescent Medicine, 165*(1), 89–90.

Layne, C. M., Ghosh Ippen, C., Strand, V., Stuber, M., Abramovitz, R., Reyes, G., et al. (2011). Curriculum on childhood trauma: A tool for training a trauma-informed workforce. *Psychological Trauma: Theory, Research, Practice, and Policy, 3*(3), 243–252.

Layne, C. M., Saltzman, W. R., Poppleton, L., Burlingame, G. M., Pasalic, A., Durakovic, E., et al. (2008). Effectiveness of a school-based group psychotherapy program for war-exposed adolescents: A randomized controlled trial. *Journal of the American Academy of Child and Adolescent Psychiatry, 47*(9), 1048–1062.

Layne, C. M., Warren, J. S., Watson, P. J., & Shalev, A. Y. (2007). Risk, vulnerability, resistance, and resilience: Toward an integrative conceptualization of posttraumatic adaptation. In M. J. Friedman, T. M. Keane, & P. A Resick (Eds.), *Handbook of PTSD: Science and practice* (pp. 497–520). New York: Guilford Press.

Lieberman, A. F., Ghosh Ippen, C., & Van Horn, P. (2006). Child–parent psychotherapy: 6-month follow-up of a randomized controlled trial. *Journal of the American Academy of Child and Adolescent Psychiatry, 45*(8), 913–918.

Lopez, M., Osterberg, L. D., Jensen-Doss, A., & Rae, W. A. (2011). Effects of workshop training for providers under mandated use of evidence-based practice. *Administrative Policy in Mental Health, 38*, 301–312.

Lyon, A. R., Stirman, S. W., Kerns, S. E., & Bruns, E. J. (2011). Developing the mental health workforce: Review and application of training approaches from multiple disciplines. *Administration and Policy in Mental Health and Mental Health Services Research, 38*(4), 238–253.

McHugh, R. K., & Barlow, D. H. (2010). The dissemination and implementation of evidence-based psychological treatments. *American Psychologist, 65*(2), 73–84.

Najavits, L. M., Gallop, R. J., & Weiss, R. D. (2006). Seeking safety therapy for adolescent girls with PTSD and substance use disorder: A randomized controlled trial. *Journal of Behavioral Health Services and Research, 33*(4), 453–463.

Nakamura, B., Chorpita, B. F., Hirsch, M., Daleiden, E., Slavin, L., Amundson, M. J., et al. (2011). Large-scale implementation of evidence-based treatments for children 10 years later: Hawaii's evidence-based services initiative in children's mental health. *Clinical Psychology: Science and Practice, 18*(1), 24–35.

Nock, M. K., Goldman, J. L., Wang, Y., & Albano, A. M. (2004). From science to practice: The flexible use of evidence-based treatments in clinical settings. *Journal of the American Academy of Child and Adolescent Psychiatry, 43*(6), 777–780.

Norcross, J. C., & Lambert, M. J. (2011). Evidence-based therapy. In J. C. Norcross (Ed.), *Psychotherapy relationships that work* (2nd ed., pp. 2–24). New York: Oxford University Press.

Palinkas, L. A., Schoenwald, S. K., Hoagwood, K., Landsverk, J., Chorpita, B. F., & Weisz, J. R. (2008). An ethnographic study of implementation of evidence-based treatments in child mental health: First steps. *Psychiatric Services, 59*(7), 738–746.

Profetto-McGrath, J. (2005). Critical thinking and evidence based practice. *Journal of Professional Nursing, 21*(6), 364–371.

Pross, C., & Schweitzer, S. (2010). The culture of organizations dealing with trauma: Sources of work-related stress and conflict. *Traumatology, 16*(4), 97–108.

Ruzek, J. I., & Rosen, R. C. (2009). Disseminating evidence-based treatments for PTSD in organizational settings: A high priority focus area. *Behaviour Research and Therapy, 47*, 980–989.

Sackett, D. L., Rosenberg, W. M., Gray, J. A., Haynes, R. B., & Richardson, W. S. (1996). Evidence-based medicine: What it is and what it isn't. *British Medical Journal, 312*, 71–72.

Scheeringa, M. S., Weems, C. F., Cohen, J. A., Amaya-Jackson, L., & Guthrie, D. (2011). Trauma-focused cognitive-behavioral therapy for posttraumatic stress disorder in three through six year old children: A randomized clinical trial. *Journal of Child Psychology and Psychiatry, 52*(8), 853–860.

Schlett, C. L., Doll, H., Dahmen, J., Polacsek, O., Federkeil, G., Fischer, M. R., et al. (2010). Job requirements compared to medical school education: Difference between graduates from problem-based learning and conventional curricula. *BMC Medical Education, 10*, 1–8.

Steinfeld, B. I., Coffman, S. J., & Keyes, J. A. (2009). Implementation of an evidence-based practice in clinical setting: What happens when you get there? *Professional Psychology: Research and Practice, 40*(4), 410–416.

Toth, S. L., & Manly, J. T. (2011). Bridging research and practice: Challenges and successes in implementing evidence-based preventive intervention strategies for child maltreatment. *Child Abuse and Neglect, 35*, 633–636.

Tryon, G. S., & Winograd, G. (2011). Goal consensus and collaboration. In J. C. Norcross (Ed.), *Psychotherapy relationships that work* (2nd ed,, pp. 153–167). New York: Oxford University Press.

Varra, A. A., Hayes, S. C., Roget, N., & Fisher, G. (2008). A randomized control trial examining the effect of acceptance and commitment training on clinician willingness to use evidence based pharmacotherapy. *Journal of Consulting and Clinical Psychology, 76*(3), 449–458.

Weisz, J. R., Chorpita, B. F., Palinkas, L. A., Schoenwald, S. K., Miranda, J., Bearman, S. K., et al. (2012). Testing standard and modular designs for psychotherapy treating depression, anxiety, and conduct problems in youth: A randomized effectiveness trial. *Archives of General Psychiatry, 69*, 274–282.

CHAPTER 7

Clinical Assessment and Diagnosis

Julian D. Ford
Kathleen Nader
Kenneth E. Fletcher

Clinical assessment of children and adolescents who have, or may have, complex trauma histories requires a number of special considerations over and above the standard technical, ethical, and relational requirements for pediatric mental health assessment. This chapter provides an overview of these considerations for clinicians when assessing child/adolescent clients' complex trauma histories, posttraumatic stress disorder (PTSD) symptoms, and the forms of dysregulation (i.e., emotional, somatic, cognitive, behavioral, relational, self) that are sequelae of complex trauma exposure (see Ford & Cloitre, 2009). First we describe an integrative framework for childhood trauma assessment and diagnosis.

Developmental Trauma Disorder: Complex Traumatic Stress Disorder in Childhood

Based on decades of scientific and clinical study, it has become clear that children who are victimized by abuse or prolonged exposure to violence, *and* whose primary relationship(s) with adult caregivers are disrupted, destroyed, or lost as a direct or indirect result, tend to suffer from protracted and difficult-to-remediate problems in several domains of *self-regulation* (Ford, 2010). Developmental trauma disorder (DTD) was formulated by expert clinicians to describe the self-regulation deficits based on their clinical observations and clients' personal descriptions of the difficulties they were experiencing, as well as the scientific evidence base (van der Kolk, 2005). Revisions over a 5-year period led to the development of a criterion set and semistructured interview (Ford and Developmental Trauma Disorder Work Group, 2011) that is being validated in an international field trial study, which is anticipated to be completed at approximately the same time as this book's publication (Ford is the study's principal investigator and can be contacted for more information about the study; *jford@uchc.edu*).

The DTD Structured Interview (DTD-SI Version 8.0) assesses seven criteria representing complex trauma exposure (i.e., interpersonal victimization and disruption[s] of relationships with primary caregiver[s]), three types of dysregulation (i.e., affective/somatic; cognitive/behavioral, and self/interpersonal), posttraumatic spectrum symptoms (i.e., PTSD intrusive reexperiencing *and* active avoidance symptoms), a duration of at least 6 months, and at least moderate to severe (i.e., Children's Global Assessment Scale [CGAS] ≤ 51) functional impairment. The 15 symptoms assessed by the DTD-SI correspond to a new formulation of DTD (see Figure 7.1), adapted from van der Kolk's (2005) proposal based on an empirical deconstruction of posttraumatic dysregulation into its affective/bodily, attentional/behavioral, and self/relational components (Ford, 2005).

Clinical and Ethical Considerations in Complex Trauma Assessment with Children and Adolescents

Children and adolescents who have experienced complex traumas are highly resilient, despite the fact that they also suffer complex problems with self-regulation as a major consequence. In order to establish a genuine working alliance as a foundation for assessment with these youth, the clinician must strike a delicate balance between validating their strengths and recognizing and accommodating their vulnerabilities. What may appear superficially to be oppositionality and defiance may be primarily a defensive/reactive aggressiveness (Ford, Fraleigh, & Connor, 2010) that should be documented in the assessment but not confused with proactive aggression. Or what may appear to be a morbid preoccupation with self-harm and death may be primarily an attempt to make sense of, and cope, with overwhelming anxiety and dysphoria associated with betrayal (see Schore, Chapter 1, this volume), abandonment or loss (see Lanius et al., Chapters 2, and Kaehler, Chapter 4, this volume), and the cumulative impact of a

A. Exposure: Experienced/witnessed multiple or prolonged adverse events for at least a year.

   A.1. Direct experience or witnessing of repeated and severe episodes of interpersonal violence;

   A.2. Significant disruptions of protective caregiving due to repeated changes in primary caregiver; repeated separation from the primary caregiver; or exposure to severe and persistent emotional abuse

B. Affective and Physiological Dysregulation. Impaired developmental competencies related to affect or arousal regulation, generally and during life transitions.

   B.1. Inability to modulate or tolerate extreme affect states (e.g., fear, anger, shame, grief), including prolonged and extreme tantrums, or immobilization

   B.2. Inability to modulate, tolerate, or recover from extreme bodily states

   B.4. Impaired capacity to describe emotions or bodily states

C. Attentional and Behavioral Dysregulation: The child exhibits impaired developmental competencies for attentional or behavioral responses to threats.

   C.1. Attention-bias toward or away from potential threats

   C.2. Impaired capacity for self-protection, including extreme risk-taking or thrill-seeking

   C.3. Maladaptive attempts at self-soothing

   C.4. Habitual (intentional or automatic) or reactive self-harm

   C.5. Inability to initiate or sustain goal-directed behavior

D. Self and Relational Dysregulation. The child's developmental competencies in personal identity and involvement in relationships are impaired.

   D.1. Persistent extreme negative perception of and emotional reaction to self, including (a) self-loathing, and (b) viewing self as damaged, helpless, ineffective, or defective.

   D.2. Compensatory adultified (precocious) attempts to take on the role of caregiver/protector for own caregiver(s) and difficulty tolerating reunion with caregivers after separation

   D.3. Extreme persistent distrust, defiance, or lack of reciprocal behavior in close relationships

   D.4. Reactive physical or verbal aggression toward peers, caregivers, or other adults

   D.5. Inappropriate (excessive or promiscuous) seeking of intimate contact (including sexual or physical intimacy), or excessive reliance on peers or adults for safety and reassurance

   D.6. Impaired capacity to regulate empathic arousal: (a) lacks empathy for, or intolerant of, expressions of distress of others, or (b) excessive responsiveness to the distress of others

   E.   At least one PTSD intrusive re-experiencing symptom and one active avoidance symptom

   F.   Duration at least 6 months

   G.   Impairment: ≤ 51 on the Children's Global Assessment Scale

FIGURE 7.1. DTD Structured Interview criteria and sample items. Excerpted from Ford and Developmental Trauma Disorder Work Group (2011).

B.1a. *Extreme Negative Affect States*

Do you ever get so upset or emotional that you blow up, or shut down totally (can't think), or feel totally overwhelmed or like you'll never feel okay again?
☐ **Yes** *(Continue)* ☐ **No** *(Skip to B.1b.)*

If Yes: How old were you when this first happened? ____ Did this happen in the past 6 months? **Yes No**

When this happens, do you feel (note all applicable): ____ Scared ____ Mad ____ Sad ____ Frustrated ____ Guilty ____ Ashamed ____ Disgusted ____Unhappy ____ Hopeless ____ Embarrassed ____ Resentful ____ Other: _____

What happens when you feel that upset or emotional? _____

How often does/did this happen? ____ Almost every day ____ 2 or 3 times a week ____ Less than once a week

☐ **Not Present** *(Skip to B.1b.) Developmentally normative expressions of negative affect/distress*

☐ **Subthreshold** *(Skip to B.1b.) Experiences occasional transient episodes of moderate distress*

☐ **Threshold** *Experiences frequent or ongoing states of negative affect/distress of severe intensity*

☐ **Severe** ____ *Loss of conscious awareness* ____ *Loss of body functions* ____ *Dissociative shifts in self-state*

B.1b. *Impaired Recovery from Extreme Negative Affect States*

Sometimes when you are upset or emotional does it take a long time to calm down and feel okay again?

If Yes: How old were you when this first happened? ____ Did this happen in the past 6 months? **Yes No**

When this happens, do you feel (note all applicable): ____ Scared ____ Mad ____ Sad ____ Frustrated ____ Guilty ____ Ashamed ____ Disgusted ____ Unhappy ____ Hopeless ____ Embarrassed ____ Resentful ____ Other: _____

What do you do to try to feel okay again? _____

How often does/did this happen? ____ Almost every day ____ 2 or 3 times a week ____ Less than once a week

☐ **Not Present** *(Skip to B.2.) Developmentally normative transient difficulties recovering from distress*

☐ **Subthreshold** *(Skip to B.2.) Occasionally requires help to fully recover from persistent distress*

☐ **Threshold** *Frequently or consistently cannot recover from persistent distress despite substantial help*

☐ **Severe** *Extreme negative affect:* ____ *Is continuously Present* ____ *Cyclically returns* ____ *Escalates over time*

B.1a. *Extreme Negative Affect States*

Does your child ever get so upset or emotional that s/he blows up, or shuts down totally (can't think), or feels totally overwhelmed or like s/he'll never feel okay again?

B.1b. *Impaired Recovery from Extreme Negative Affect States*

Sometimes when your child feels upset or emotional does it take her/him a long time to calm down and feel okay again?

FIGURE 7.1 *(continued)*

life characterized by recurrent psychological trauma that leads, in turn, to a sense of hopelessness and a foreshortened future (see Alexander, Chapter 3, this volume).

A frequent concern about screening/assessment for potentially disturbing issues in childhood, such as trauma history, aggression, self-harm, and suicidality, is that this process could endanger children by destabilizing them and precipitating crises. It is crucial that these sensitive topics be addressed in a manner that does not directly or indirectly coerce or pressure children or adolescents to disclose or acknowledge information that they do not want, or feel able, to divulge. It also is essential to immediately and calmly follow up on disclosures with support and services that enhance the child's sense of safety and personal control, including involving persons in the child's family or support system in a manner that reassures the child and ensures appropriate ongoing monitoring and assistance with coping. Evidence from a randomized controlled trial of screening for suicidality found no iatrogenic effects following screening for suicidal ideation or attempts with high-risk (i.e., depressed, substance-abusing, prior suicide attempts) youth (Gould et al., 2005). Screened youth were *less,* not more, suicidal or depressed after the screening. A field study of legally detained youth who were screened for trauma history, PTSD, suicidality, and substance abuse risk also found no instances of deterioration or crises (Ford, Hartman, Hawke, & Chapman, 2008). Moreover, trauma history and symptom screening led to the initiation of trauma-informed services in juvenile detention centers throughout an entire state that have been shown to be associated with reduced violent incidents and disciplinary sanctions (Ford & Hawke, 2012).

The generic goals of screening (i.e., to identify children and adolescents in need of services/supports) and assessment (i.e., to identify problems and strengths/resources that are the targets for, and markers of, treatment outcome/prevention) must be tailored to fit the unique circumstances and needs of those with histories of complex trauma (Courtois & Ford, 2013; see Figure 7.2). The core goal of treatment—*enhancing actual and perceived safety and resilience by enhancing the ability to self-regulate in the affective, somatic, cognitive, behavioral, and self/identity domains*—provides a context for screening and assessment. From this perspective, it is crucial to screen or assess for a wide range of potential traumatic events that may have threatened the child's safety and compromised the child's development and ability to self-regulate (see Table 7.1 for a list of validated child/adolescent trauma history screening and assessment measures). In addition, it is imperative to screen/assess not only past but also current or potential future retraumatization *and* posttraumatic reenactments. The latter are not added exposures to traumatic stressors, but instead are current contexts or events that activate posttraumatic intrusive memories, avoidance, emotional numbing, or hyperarousal (e.g., situations, people, or activities that are reminders of abuse).

Goals for Treatment/Prevention with Children with Complex Trauma Histories

A. **Safety: Recognize and Prevent Trauma and Reenactments**

B. **Affect Dysegulation: Enhance Ability to Manage Extreme Arousal States**

C. **Somatic Dysregulation: Repair the Mind–Body Split**

D. **Cognitive Dysregulation: Enhance Self-Determination and Autonomy**

E. **Behavioral Dysregulation: Enhance Personal Control and Self-Efficacy**

F. **Relational Dysregulation: Enhance Attachment Security**

G. **Self Dysregulation: Enhance Sense of Self and Personal Identity**

H. **Resilience: Maintain Functioning and Overcome Comorbidities**

Specific Objectives

Screening and assessment with children with histories of complex trauma should identify the problems and strengths that, respectively, reduce or enhance, a youth's ability to:

1. Anticipate and recognize reenactments of traumatic events and develop self-protection/self-enhancement skills to prevent retraumatization/revictimization of self or others

2. Develop and/or restore emotion regulation, that is, the ability to access and identify emotions (especially core emotions and affective schemas such as shame, horror, self-loathing, exploitation, and betrayal) and the capacity for and tolerance of emotional expression (emotion regulation) as a means of self-development

3. Acquire or regain capacities for bodily self-awareness and arousal regulation that have been split off or compartmentalized in the form of somatoform dissociation

4. Develop or regain cognitive and behavioral regulatory capacities to prevent or reduce the severity/frequency of dissociation, addiction, self-harm, impulsivity, compulsion, and aggression toward self and others (including sexual behavior problems)

5. Experience relational safety and attunement in family, peer, and treatment relationships as a "secure base" from which to develop or regain secure inner working models

6. Shift self-concept from permanently damaged to resiliently recovering from injury and from helpless/ineffective to pursuing autonomous self-determination

FIGURE 7.2. Complex trauma-specific goals and objectives to guide screening and assessment. Adapted from Courtois and Ford (2013, Ch. 4, pp. 88–90). Copyright 2013 by The Guilford Press. Adapted by permission.

Further, screening/assessment should address the full range of self-regulatory competencies and problems. Youth with complex trauma histories are very vulnerable to profound emotion dysregulation, including persistent severe negative emotion states (e.g., shame, rumination, catastrophizing) and difficulties in modulating (e.g., alexithymia, explosive anger, inconsolable sadness and grief) and recovering from distress. These problems often include (or for young children, predominantly take the form of) difficulty with bodily functioning and problems in learning, memory,

TABLE 7.1. Complex Trauma History Screening Instruments

Measure	Population	Description
Childhood Trauma Questionnaire Short Form (Bernstein et al., 2003; *www.psychcorp.com*)	Ages 12–17 years; psychiatric patients and community sample[a, b, c]	28-item self-report questionnaire, subscales (Emotional, Physical, Sexual Abuse; Emotional, Physical Neglect), and validity scale (minimization/denial)
Dimensions of Stressor Exposure (DOSE; Fletcher, 1996; *Kenneth.Fletcher@ umassmed.edu)*	Ages 8–18 years; psychiatric and community samples[c]	50-item clinician-administered scale (26 items characterize each stressful event; 24 items specific to sexual abuse)
Traumatic Experiences Screening Instrument (TESI; Daviss et al., 2000; Ford et al., 2000, 2008; *www.ncptsd.org*)	Ages 6–17 years; psychiatric patients, emergency patients, and juvenile-justice–involved youth[a, b] Ages 3–17 years[c]	15- to 24-item clinician-administered (ages 3–17) or child self-report (ages 11–17) measure of direct or witnessed exposure to noninterpersonal (accident, illness, disaster, loss) or interpersonal (abuse, neglect, family/community violence) traumatic victimization; probes for age(s) of onset, recency, risk factors, and Criterion A2 peritraumatic distress
UCLA Post Traumatic Stress Disorder Reaction Index (PTSD-RI; Steinberg et al., 2004; *ASteinberg@mednet. ucla.edu)*	Ages 7–17 years; psychiatric, school, child protection, medical, and community populations[b, c]	13 self- or parent-rated items answered yes–no (disaster, accident, medical trauma, assault, loss, abuse): "VERY SCARY, DANGEROUS OR VIOLENT things that sometimes happen to children. These are times where someone was HURT VERY BADLY OR KILLED, or could have been."

[a]Normed; [b]validated; [c]field tested.

and behavior (e.g., impulsivity, aggression, withdrawal). Complex trauma often begins with adversities or deficiencies in a child's relational "base" (i.e., caregiver, family, peer, school, and community support systems) that create an attitude of confusion, distrust, withdrawal, or hostility that can become a pervasive expectancy of exploitation, abandonment, betrayal, or maltreatment. This negative attitude, in turn, can create a vicious cycle undermining the youth's subsequent relationships (e.g., via disorganized working models, limited empathy; detachment/loneliness) and self-concept (e.g., via guilt, shame, self-doubt, or self-loathing), which further undermine all other regulatory capacities.

Assessing Dysregulation in Children and Adolescents Who Have Complex Trauma Histories

There is no gold standard screening or assessment measure for complex posttraumatic dysregulation in children and adolescents. However, the clinician and researcher can select from a variety of validated and field-tested (and in some cases, norm-based) measures that assess caregiver- or self-rated dysregulation in children and adolescents (Table 7.2). Most of these instruments are designed for screening rather than definitive assessment, but they can be used in conjunction with detailed clinical or research interviewing to provide a multimeasure (and ideally, multiperspective [including caregiver views, as well as, or for, young children, in lieu of] self-report and interviewer behavioral observations) assessment of dysregulation across the domains that are potentially impaired as a result of exposure to complex trauma.

It also is important to address differential diagnosis in both clinical and research assessment of children with complex trauma histories. Symptoms reflecting dysregulation may be better accounted for by psychiatric conditions that are prevalent among traumatized children but that do not necessarily result from trauma exposure (although often exacerbated by complex trauma). Relevant psychiatric disorders include the full range of affective, anxiety, behavioral, psychotic, somatoform, and developmental disorders of childhood and adolescence. Validated and widely used semistructured interviews for child/adolescent psychiatric disorders include the Child and Adolescent Psychiatric Assessment (CAPA; Angold & Costello, 2000) and the preschool version (PAPA; Egger et al., 2006), the Kiddie Schedule for Affective Disorders and Schizophrenia (K-SADS; Kaufman, Birmaher, Brent, Rao, & Ryan, 1996), and the Missouri Assessment of Genetics Interview for Children (MAGIC; Reich & Todd, 2002). As depicted in Table 7.3, the diagnoses addressed include some of the types of dysregulation associated with complex trauma exposure. The CAPA and PAPA specifically assess self-depreciation, self-hatred, inhibition, and feeling unloved.

In addition to interviews, self-report (usually for children ages 8 years and older) and parent or teacher rating assessment measures may provide additional multi-informant data that cover a wider range of the dysregulation symptoms than diagnostic interviews (Table 7.3). The Child Behavior Checklist (CBCL; Achenbach & Ruffle, 2000) and Behavior Assessment System for Children/Behavioral and Emotional Screening System (BASC/BESS; Dowdy et al., 2011) are normed and validated self- and parent/teacher-report questionnaires that also screen/assess a wider range of symptoms related to dysregulation than diagnostic interviews. A "dysregulation profile" (DRP) was developed empirically to identify children with a form of

TABLE 7.2. Psychometric Screening Measures Assessing Child/Adolescent Dysregulation

Measure	Population	Description
	Emotion dysregulation	
Children's Alexithymia Measure (Way et al., 2010)	Ages 5–17 years; in mental health services with trauma histories[b, c]	14-item caregiver-rated reliable and validated single-factor measure of difficulty putting words into feelings and avoiding disclosure of feelings
Symptoms of Traumatic Stress—Child Version (SOTS-C; Ford et al., 2013)	Ages 5–17 years; in psychiatric or juvenile justice services[b, c]	Clinician rating (7-point severity scale) of affective dysregulation (discharge, intolerance, confusion), excluding depression/psychosis
Behavior Rating Inventory of Executive Function (BRIEF; Goia et al., 2002; Isquith et al., 2004; LeJeune et al., 2010)	Ages 6–17 years (BRIEF and short-form BRIEF) and 2–5 years (BRIEF-P)[a, b, c]	86-item parent or teacher rating scale (24-item short form): BRIEF Emotional Regulation factor (Emotional Control, Shift scales); BRIEF-P Inhibitory Control factor
Child and Adolescent Functional Assessment Scale® (CAFAS®; Hodges, 2005; www.cafas.com)	Ages 6–17 years; in mental health services[a, b, c]	Clinician/record review ratings (4-point scale: *none, mild, moderate, severe*) of mood/emotion regulation problems
Emotion Awareness Questionnaire (EAQ; Rieffe et al., 2007)	Ages 8–14 years; in mental health services and school students[b, c]	25-item self-report (3-point rating scale) with reliable/validated subscales: Differentiation (7 items), Communication (5 items), Bodily Symptoms (6 items), Awareness of Others' Emotions (7 items)
Trait Emotional Intelligence Questionnaire (TEIQue; Petrides, 2009; Mavroveli et al., 2007, 2008)	Ages 8–12 years (child form) and 13–17 years (short form) school students[b, c]	30- (short-form) and 83-item (child form) self-report (7-point Likert ratings) measure that reliably/validly assesses 15 emotional intelligence factors
Alexithymia Questionnaire for Children (Rieffe et al., 2006)	Ages 9–16 years; school students[b, c]	20-item self-report (3-point rating scale) with reliable/factor-derived subscales measuring problems identifying, describing, externalizing emotions
Management of Shame State (Ahmed, 2001)	Ages 9 years and older; in justice system[b, c]	2 scenario-based self-rated 5-item factor scales for shame acknowledgment and displacement
Cognitive Emotion Regulation Questionnaire (CERQ; Garnefski et al., 2007, 2009; Amone-P'Olak et al., 2007; Tortella-Feliu et al., 2010)	Ages 9–11 years; school students (CERQ-K), and 12–18 years, students, medical patients, and war survivors (CERQ)[a, b, c]	36-item self-report (5-point rating scale) with reliable/validated subscales: Self-Blame; Other-Blame; Acceptance; Planning; Positive Refocusing; Rumination; Positive Reappraisal; Putting into Perspective; Catastrophizing

Abbreviated Dysregulation Scale (Mezzich et al., 2001; Pardini et al., 2003)	Ages 10–early 20 years; in community, substance abuse, juvenile justice samples[b]	10-item reliable/validated self-report subscale assessing difficulty with recovery from emotional distress

Somatic dysregulation

Symptoms of Traumatic Stress—Child Version (SOTS-C; Ford et al., 2013)	Ages 5–17 years; in psychiatric or juvenile justice services[b, c]	Clinician rating (7-point severity scale) of somatic dysregulation
Children's Somatization Inventory (CSI-C; Vila et al., 2009; Walker et al., 2009)	Ages 11–16 years; students and pediatric patients[a, b, c]	35-item reliable/validated self- or parent-rating scale (24-item short-form); three factors: Pain/Weakness, Gastrointestinal, Pseudoneurological
Somatic Complaint List (SCL; Jellesma et al., 2007; Rieffe et al., 2006)	Ages 9–16 years; school students and medical patients[b, c]	8- to 11-item self-report (5-point scale: *almost never* to *quite often*) of bodily discomfort or illness

Cognitive dysregulation

Symptoms of Traumatic Stress—Child Version (SOTS-C; Ford et al., 2013)	Ages 5–17 years; in psychiatric or juvenile justice services[b, c]	Clinician rating (7-point severity scale) of pathological dissociation
Behavior Rating Inventory of Executive Function (Goia et al., 2002; Isquith et al., 2004; LeJeune et al., 2010)	Ages 6–17 years (BRIEF and short-form BRIEF); 2–5 years (BRIEF-P)[a, b, c]	86-item parent or teacher rating scale (24-item short-form): Behavior Regulation factor (Inhibit, Self-Monitor scales), Metacognition factor (Working Memory, Initiate, Plan/Organize, Organization of Materials, Task–Monitor scales)
Child and Adolescent Functional Assessment Scale® (CAFAS®; Hodges, 2005; www.cafas.com)	Ages 6–17 years; in mental health services[a, b, c]	Clinician/record review rating (4-point scale: *none, mild, moderate, severe*) of Thinking Problems
Trauma Symptom Checklist for Children (TSCC; Briere, 1996)	Ages 6–17 years; in schools, health care, mental health services[a, b, c]	5-item factor-analysis-derived Dissociation sub-scale (daydreaming, detachment, derealization, depersonalization)
Adolescent Dissociative Experiences Scale (ADES; Armstrong et al., 1997; Farrington et al., 2001; Keck et al., 2004)	Ages 11–16 years; in the community and in psychiatric services[b, c]	20-item reliable/validated self-report (0–11 scale or 6-point Likert scale); one factor for absorption, depersonalization, amnesia, passive influence
Children's Cognitive Styles Questionnaire (CCSQ; Mezulis et al., 2006, 2011)	Ages 11–15 years; students[b, c]	20-item validated/reliable self-report, 4 negative scenarios rated for internality, stability, globality, self-inference, and expected outcomes. (*continued*)

TABLE 7.2. (*continued*)

Measure	Population	Description
Attentional Control Scale (Derryberry & Reed, 2002)	Ages 17–22 years; students[b, c]	20-item self-report scale assessing ability to focus or shift attention efficiently under stress

Behavioral self-regulation and dysregulation

Measure	Population	Description
Symptoms of Traumatic Stress—Child Version (SOTS-C; Ford et al., 2013)	Ages 5–17 years; in psychiatric or juvenile justice services[b, c]	Clinician rating (7-point severity scale) of impulsive aggression, self-harm, and risk taking
Child and Adolescent Needs and Strengths Mental Health Version (CANS-MH; Lyons, 1999; *www.nctsnet.org/sites/ default/files/assets/pdfs/ measures/CANS-MH. pdf*)	Ages 2–20 years; in mental health services[b, c]	Clinician/record review ratings (4-point scale: *none, mild, moderate, severe*): danger to others, runaway, sexually abusive, peer affiliations, crime/delinquency, attention deficit/ impulse control, oppositional behavior, antisocial behavior, substance abuse
Child and Adolescent Functional Assessment Scale® (CAFAS®; Hodges, 2005; *www.cafas.com*)	Ages 6–17 years; in mental health services[a, b, c]	Clinician/record review ratings (4-point scale: *none, mild, moderate, severe*) of Delinquency, Aggression, Self-Harm, Substance use
Children's Impact of Traumatic Events Scale–R (CITES-R; Wolfe et al., 1991; Crouch et al., 1999)	Ages 8–16 years[b]	Subscales (Sexual Activity, Eroticism) validated in relation to the Trauma Symptom Checklist for Children
Scale for Suicidal Ideation (Steer, Kumar, & Beck, 1993)	Ages 12–17 years; psychiatric inpatients[b, c]	Self-report measure of active–passive suicidality and specific plans for suicide
Suicidal Ideation Questionnaire (SIQ; Reynolds, 1987; Chapman & Ford, 2008; Huth-Bocks et al., 2007; Vitiello et al., 2009)	Ages 12–18 years; community, juvenile justice, and psychiatric samples[a, b, c]	15- (SIQ Jr.; ages 12–15) and 30-item (SIQ; ages 16–18) self-report measure assessing active and passive suicidal thoughts and intentions
Deliberate Self-Harm Inventory (DSHI; Gratz et al., 2002; Latimer et al., 2009)	Ages 17–30 years; students[a, b, c]	9-item self-report of nonsuicidal self-harm (e.g., cutting, burning, carving, bone breaking, biting, head banging); cutoff of 5+ for moderate risk

Relational functioning/working models/empathy

Measure	Population	Description
Strange Situation (Ainsworth et al., 1978; Main & Cassidy, 1988; Moss et al., 2009; Rosen & Burke, 2009)	Ages 1–7 years[b, c]	Clinic-based behavior observation procedure with 3- to 45-minute structured episodes of separation and reuniting with a caregiver

Attachment Q-sort (Vaughn & Waters, 1990)	Ages 1–5 years[b, c]	In-home naturalistic interaction observations and interviews with mothers
Southampton Test of Empathy for Preschoolers (STEP; Howe et al., 2008)	Preschoolers[b, c]	8 videotaped vignettes of children elicit reactions selected by choosing a facial expression (angry, happy, sad, or fearful); scored for understanding and sharing of others' emotion
Symptoms of Traumatic Stress—Child Version (SOTS-C; Ford et al., 2013)	Ages 5–17 years; in psychiatric or juvenile justice services	Clinician rating (7-point severity scale) of disorganized attachment and sexualization
MacArthur Story–Stem Battery (Minnis et al., 2006; Robinson et al., 2000)	Ages 7–9 years	10 story stems completed by child with a puppet family; coded for competition, sharing, jealousy, empathy, conflict resolution/escalation, aggression, affiliation, affection, compliance, opposition, blame, reconciliation, and dishonesty
Attachment Security Scale (Kerns et al., 2000; Weimer et al., 2004)	Ages 9 years– adolescence[b, c]	Self-report of secure, ambivalent, or avoidant attachment with primary caregiver(s)
Adolescent Attachment Interview (Miga et al., 2010); Adult Attachment Interview (Allen et al., 2004); Family Attachment Interview (FAI) (Scharfe, 2002)	Ages 13 years– adulthood[b, c]	Semistructured interviews coded for secure, preoccupied, dismissing, ambivalent, or avoidant attachment working models related to primary caregiver(s)
Children's Impact of Traumatic Events Scale–R (CITES-R; Wolfe et al., 1991; Crouch et al., 1999)	Ages 8–16 years[b, c]	Subscales (Negative Reactions by Others, Social Support) validated in relation to the Trauma Symptom Checklist for Children
Inventory of Parent and Peer Attachment (IPPA; Armsden & Greenberg, 1987; Sternberg et al., 2005); People in My Life (PIML; Ridenour et al., 2006)	Ages 10–13 years (PIML), 13–18 years (IPPA); youth in community and at-risk or psychiatric samples[b, c]	25-item self-report questionnaires assessing mutual trust, quality of communication, and anger/alienation with mother, father, and peers
UCLA Loneliness Scale—Revised (Russell, Peplau, & Cutrona, 1980; Mahon, 1995)	Ages 12 years– adulthood[b, c]	20-item self-report scale measures feelings of loneliness in interpersonal relationships
Interpersonal Reactivity Index (Davis, 1983)	Ages 17 years–early adult students[b, c]	28-item self-report scale assesses four dimensions of empathy (7 items each, 5-point scale): fantasy, perspective-taking, concern, sympathy

(continued)

TABLE 7.2. (*continued*)

Measure	Population	Description
	Self-dysregulation	
Perceived Competence Scales for Children (Harter, 1982; Harter & Pike, 1984)	Ages 4 years–adult[b, c]	35–63 items (7-items per subscale) *Ages 4–7:* pictorial scales for Cognitive, Physical Appearance, Physical Competence, Peer Acceptance, Behavioral Conduct. *Children:* Scholastic/Athletic Competence, Physical Appearance, Peer Acceptance, Behavioral Conduct, Global Self-Worth. *Adolescent:* adds Close Friendships, Romantic Relationships, Job Competence
Expectations Test (ET; Gully, 2003)	Ages 4–16 years[b, c]	16 ambiguous photographs elicit answers to (1) feelings, (2) expected outcomes, and (3) control. Responses classified as (1) negative—*sexual abuse, physical harm, separation, other*; (2) neutral; (3) positive; (4) unknown
Child Attribution and Reaction Survey (Ferguson et al., 1999)	Ages 5–12 years[b]	8 age-appropriate scenarios validated to elicit shame or guilt reactions
Symptoms of Traumatic Stress—Child Version (SOTS-C; Ford et al., 2013)	Ages 5–17 years; in psychiatric or juvenile justice services[b, c]	Clinician rating (7-point severity scale) of beliefs: (1) self as permanently damaged or harmful; (2) world as permanently dangerous or harmful
Children's Interpretations of Interpersonal Distress/Conflict (Zahn-Waxler et al., 1990)	Ages 7–17 years[b, c]	4 stories with photographs; responses coded for remorse, self-punishment, reparation, apology, and blameworthiness
Piers–Harris Children's Self-Concept Scale–2 (Piers & Herzberg, 2002)	Ages 7–18 years[a, b, c]	6 scales (Behavioral, Intellectual/School Status, Physical Attributes, Freedom from Anxiety, Popularity, Happiness, and Satisfaction) and 2 validity (inconsistency, bias) scales
Situation-Specific Shame Questions (Feiring et al., 2002)	Ages 7 years and older; sexually abused children/youths[b, c]	4 items assessing sexual-abuse-related beliefs of self as transparently guilty, ostracized, singled-out, and dirty
Tennessee Self-Concept Scale–2 (Fitts & Warren, 1996)	Ages 7–14 years and 13–adult community and psychiatric populations[a, b, c]	6 factor-analytic scales (Academic, Family, Moral, Personal, Physical, Social) and 5 validity scales; 20-item short-form

(*continued*)

Self-Esteem Inventory (Coopersmith, 1989)	Ages 8–13 years[a, b, c]	32-item youth self-report of self as competent, successful, significant, and worthy in general, with peers, and at school, with a validity (response distortion) scale
Test of Self-Conscious Affect (Tangney & Dearing, 2002)	Ages 8–17 years[b, c]	Semistructured scenarios elicit developmentally relevant responses validated for children and adolescents
State Shame and Guilt Scale (SSGS; Tangney & Dearing, 2002)	Ages 12–17 years[b, c]	15-item self-rating scale of in-the-moment feelings of shame, guilt, and pride
Relational Self-Concept Scale (Schott & Bellin, 2001)	Ages 13–16 years[a, b, c]	6-factor-analytic scales (School Competence, Academic Performance, Actual–Ideal Peer–Parent Acceptance, Physical)
Trauma-Related Guilt Inventory (TRGI; Kubany et al., 1996)	Ages 15 years–adult[b, c]	32-items with 3 scales: Global Guilt, Distress, and Guilt Cognitions (responsibility, wrongdoing, justification)
Personal Feelings Questionnaire–2 (PFQ2; Harder & Zalma, 1990)	Ages 16 years and older[a, b, c]	A 10-item Shame subscale and a six-item Guilt subscale, validated in relation to 11 scales with college freshmen

[a]Normed; [b]validated; [c]field tested.

bipolar disorder, but recent studies have shown that children with this profile are at risk for many of the problems associated with complex trauma exposure (e.g., substance abuse, suicidality; Holtmann et al., 2011). More recent findings indicate that a CBCL profile originally assessing PTSD symptoms may better serve as a short-form of the DRP than to identify children at risk for PTSD (Althoff, Ayer, Rettew, & Hudziak, 2011).

Four omnibus self-report questionnaires with factor-analysis-derived subscales provide the broadest coverage of the types of dysregulation associated with complex trauma history. The Trauma Symptom Checklist for Children (TSCC; Briere, 1996) has subscales for anger, sexual concerns, anxiety, depression, dissociation, and posttraumatic stress. The Children's Impact of Traumatic Events Scale—Revised (CITES-R; Wolfe, Gentile, Michienzi, Sas, & Wolfe, 1991) has subscales for self-blame/guilt, others' negative reactions, vulnerability, dangerous world, sexual activity, eroticism, and PTSD symptom features (Crouch, Smith, Ezzell, & Saunders, 1999). The Children's Responses to Trauma Inventory (CRTI; Alisic & Kleber, 2010) similarly has subscales for the PTSD symptom clusters and one for "other" posttraumatic reactions (e.g., crying, guilt, somatic distress, regression, recklessness, fears). Finally, the Minnesota Multiphasic Personality

TABLE 7.3. DTD Features Assessed by Broadband Assessment Measures

Domain	PAPA/ CAPA	MAGIC	K-SADS	CBCL	BASC	MMPI-A	DTD-SI
Emotion dysregulation							
Persistent negative affect	X	X	X	X	X	X	X
Cannot recover from negative affect				X			X
Alexithymia						X	X
Somatic dysregulation							
Somatic preoccupation	X	X	X	X	X	X	X
Somatoform dissociation							X
Cognitive dysregulation							
Attention bias to threat						X	X
Psychoform dissociation							X
Behavioral dysregulation							
Self-harm/risky behavior				X	X	X	X
Impulsivity	X	X	X	X	X	X	X
Anger/aggression	X	X	X	X	X	X	X
Relational dysregulation							
Isolation/withdrawal					X	X	X
Deficit in empathy						X	X
Disorganized attachment							X
Problematic sexuality				X			X
Self-dysregulation							
Shame (self as damaged)	X					X	X
Vulnerability (self as victim)	X					X	X

Inventory for Adolescents (MMPI-A; Veltri et al., 2009) has numerous clinical/content subscales assessing facets of dysregulation (Table 7.3).

Assessing PTSD in Children and Adolescents Who Have Complex Trauma Histories

PTSD symptoms often are manifested and reported differently by children and adolescents than adults. As a result, adaptations in the PTSD criteria for children appear in the new version of the American Psychiatric Association's *Diagnostic and Statistical Manual of Mental Disorders* (DSM-5; American Psychiatric Association, 2013). Principally, these changes involve allowing dissociative flashbacks to include "trauma-specific reenactment . . . in play" and reducing the number of symptoms required in the "negative alterations cognitions and mood" and "alterations in arousal and reactivity" criteria for a PTSD diagnosis from three symptoms to two—based on clinical and research observations that children (especially younger than school age) tend to be impaired by fewer and more global symptoms than older individuals.

For all ages, DSM-5 separates what was Criterion C (avoidance and emotional numbing) into two criteria: (1) active avoidance and (2) emotional distress in reaction to trauma memories or reminders. This is important because children/youth with complex trauma histories may tend to deny active avoidance while acknowledging "negative alterations in cognitions and mood" that include new symptoms: "persistent and exaggerated negative expectations about one's self, others, or the world (e.g., 'I am bad,' 'no one can be trusted,' 'I have lost my soul forever,' . . . 'the world is completely dangerous')"; "persistent distorted blame of self or others about the cause or consequences of the traumatic event(s)"; and "pervasive negative emotional state—for example, fear, horror, anger, guilt, or shame." The hyperarousal criterion for PTSD also includes "aggressive behavior" and "reckless or self-destructive behavior," which are forms of behavioral dysregulation that often follow exposure to complex trauma.

Anticipating the need for clinical screening of not only classic (DSM-IV) but also the more complex trauma-relevant symptoms in DSM-5 and in the DTD syndrome, a brief clinician rating scale for PTSD (and DTD; see below) symptoms has been developed and field-tested for reliability and validity with children and adolescents (ages 5–17 years) in psychiatric treatment or the juvenile justice system: the Symptoms of Traumatic Stress Scale for Children—Revised (SOTS-C-R; Ford, Opler, Muenzenmaier, Shelley, & Grennan, 2013). This scale has single items assessing intrusive reexperiencing, avoidance, emotional numbing, and hyperarousal symptoms. Symptom ratings are made on a 7-point scale with specific operational definitions for *not present, normal range, mild, moderate, moderate–severe, severe,* and *extreme.*

Assessing Resilience in Children and Adolescents Who Have Complex Trauma Histories

Resilience to exposure to traumatic stressors can take a number of forms (Layne et al., 2008), but when complex trauma occurs it most often involves retaining or regaining adequate functioning by coping with or managing, rather than maintaining complete imperviousness to, traumatic stress reactions (Cook et al., 2005). Resilience is enhanced by personal (e.g., optimism, problem-solving skills, mindfulness; Joseph & Wood, 2010) and relational or environmental (e.g., social support, socioeconomic status) strengths and resources (Walter, Horsey, Palmieri, & Hobfoll, 2010).

A 25-item posttraumatic resilience scale has been developed for adults, the Connor–Davidson Resilience Scale (CDRS; Connor & Davidson, 2003), and recently shown to have evidence of reliability and structural and convergent validity with a large sample of Chinese youth (ages 11–23 years) following a severe earthquake (Yu et al., 2011). The CDRS yields a total score that reflects several aspects of self-efficacy, with three items (one for social support, two for spiritual faith) that load weakly on the total score. A longer but relatively brief self-report measure, the 54-item (4-point Likert scale) Behavioral and Emotional Rating Scale (BERS; Epstein, Ryser, & Pearson, 2002; *www.proed.com*) has five factor-analysis-based subscales—interpersonal strengths, family involvement, intrapersonal strengths, school functioning, and affective strengths—and a total score. Validated brief measures that specifically assess children's and adolescents' optimism and self-efficacy include the 24-item Perceived Control Scale for Children (PCSC; Weisz, Southam-Gerow,& McCarty, 2001), the 6-item Children's Hope Scale (Snyder et al., 1997), and the 10-item subscale of the Abbreviated Dysregulation Inventory for Cognitive Self-Regulation (Mezzich, Tarter, Giancola, & Kirisci, 2001).

Resilience following complex trauma is enhanced by emotional, cognitive, and behavioral self-regulation (Cook et al., 2005). Items potentially reflecting these types of self-regulation are interspersed throughout the BERS subscales. The ability to tolerate or alter the intensity, valence, or meaning of distressing emotions and thoughts has been assessed by self-report with sixth and seventh graders with the 20-item Secondary Control Scale for Children (SCSC; Weisz, Francis, & Bearman, 2010) and with 12- to 17-year-olds with the 30-item Expectancies for Negative Mood Regulation scale (NMR; Ford, Steinberg, Hawke, Levine, & Zhang, 2012). The rationale for "secondary control" as a distinct form of self-regulation is that it involves the ability to "influence the personal psychological impact of objective conditions on oneself, by adjusting oneself to fit those conditions" (Weisz et al., 2010, p. 885).

The Child and Adolescent Functional Assessment Scale® (CAFAS®; Hodges, 2005) and Child and Adolescent Needs and Strengths scale (CANS; Lyons et al., 1999) enable trained raters to quantify children's strengths and resources within the home, community, school, and legal domains based upon interview or records review. The CAFAS assesses adaptive functioning and family/social support. The CANS elicits detailed ratings on physical health, school achievement, intellectual development, school behavior, school attendance, sexual development, family/caregiver strengths (supervision, involvement, knowledge, organization, residential stability, resources, safety), and the child's strengths (interpersonal, relationship permanence, education, vocation, well-being, optimism, spiritual/religious, talents, interests, inclusion). For children with clinically significant intellectual or behavioral impairment, measures of more basic adaptive functioning should be used. For example, the Vineland Adaptive Functioning Scale–II (Sparrow, Cicchetti, & Balla, 2006) is a normed and validated semistructured clinical interview with caregivers assessing infants', children's, or adolescents' communication, daily living skills, socialization, and motor skills (up to age 6 years, only), as well as an overall measure of adaptive functioning and a maladaptive behavior index rating.

More detailed information on strengths in the interpersonal domain can be obtained using the Social Adjustment Interview for Children and Adolescents (SAICA; John, Gammon, Prusoff, & Warner, 1987; Kliewer & Sullivan, 2008). This self- or parent-report measure was validated with several community and clinical populations to assess 6- to 18-year-olds' social functioning and problems. Subscales include school (academic and social), "spare-time activities," peer relationships and "heterosexual adjustment," and family (home and sibling) relationships.

Two briefer indices of functioning are the single-rating CGAS (Shaffer et al., 1983)—a clinician/interviewer rating with detailed anchors for each 10-point interval on a 100-point scale, normed and validated for children ages 4–16 years old—and the Columbia Impairment Scale (CIS; Bird et al., 1993)—a 13-item parent-rated or youth self-report assessment that provides a single numerical score based upon all domains of function. Note that PTSD semistructured interviews such as the Clinician Administered PTSD Scale—Children and Adolescents (CAPS-CA) (Nader et al., 1996), and multisymptom structured and semistructured interviews for children and adolescents such as the CAPA/PAPA, MAGIC, and K-SADS/PL, obtain a global interviewer rating of functioning in the home/family, with peers, and in school or extracurricular activities. The CITES-R also includes subscales assessing social support and empowerment (Wolfe et al., 1991).

Conclusion

Although the forms of childhood dysregulation associated with exposure to complex trauma are not codified in DSM-5 as DTD, clinicians and researchers have an array of instruments with which to screen and assess complex trauma exposure and its sequelae. These measures should be used cautiously to develop and test clinical and research hypotheses following the quality parameters described by Egger (2009, p. 559): "(1) multiple sessions, (2) multiple informants, (3) a multidisciplinary approach, (4) a multicultural perspective, (5) multiple modes of assessment, and (6) a multiaxial diagnostic formulation and treatment plan." Bottom line: Complex trauma and its sequelae require correspondingly complex assessment.

References

Achenbach, T. M., & Ruffle, T. M. (2000). The Child Behavior Checklist and related forms for assessing behavioral/emotional problems and competencies. *Pediatric Review, 21*, 265–271.

Ahmed, E. (2001). Shame management: Regulating bullying. In E. Ahmed, N. Harris, J. Braithwaite, & V. Braithwaite (Eds.), *Shame management through reintegration* (pp. 211–314). Cambridge, UK: Cambridge University Press.

Ainsworth, M. D., Blehar, M. C., Waters, E., & Wall, S. (1978). *Patterns of attachment: A psychological study of the strange situation.* Hillsdale, NJ: Erlbaum.

Alisic, E., & Kleber, R. J. (2010). Measuring posttraumatic stress reactions in children. *Journal of Child and Adolescent Trauma, 3,* 192–204.

Allen, J. P., McElhaney, K. B., Kuperminc, G. P., & Jodl, K. M. (2004). Stability and change in attachment security across adolescence. *Child Development, 75*(6), 1792–1805.

Althoff, R. R., Ayer, L. A., Rettew, D. C., & Hudziak, J. J. (2011). Assessment of dysregulated children using the Child Behavior Checklist. *Psychological Assessment, 22*(3), 609–617.

American Psychiatric Association. (2013). *Diagnostic and statistical manual of mental disorders* (5th ed.). Arlington, VA: Author.

Amone-P'Olak, K., Garnefski, N., & Kraaij, V. (2007). Adolescents caught between fires: Cognitive emotion regulation in response to war experiences in Northern Uganda. *Journal of Adolescence, 30,* 655–669.

Angold, A., & Costello, E. J. (2000). The Child and Adolescent Psychiatric Assessment (CAPA). *Journal of the American Academy of Child and Adolescent Psychiatry, 39*(1), 39–48.

Armsden, G. C., & Greenberg, M. T. (1987). The Inventory of Parent and Peer Attachment: Individual differences and their relationship to psychological well-being in adolescence. *Journal of Youth and Adolescence, 16,* 427–453.

Armstrong, J. G., Putnam, F. W., Carlson, E. B., Libero, D. Z., & Smith, S. R. (1997). Development and validation of a measure of adolescent dissociation: the Adolescent Dissociative Experiences Scale. *Journal of Nervous and Mental Disease, 185*(8), 491–497.

Bernstein, D. P., Stein, J. A., Newcomb, M. D., Walker, E., Pogge, D., Ahluvalia, T., et al. (2003). Development and validation of a brief screening version of the Childhood Trauma Questionnaire. *Child Abuse and Neglect, 27*(2), 169–190.

Bird, H. R., Shaffer, D., Fisher, P., Gould, M. S., Staghezza B., Chen, J., et al. (1993). The Columbia Impairment Scale (CIS): Pilot findings on a measure of global impairment for children and adolescents. *International Journal of Methods in Psychiatric Research, 3,* 167–176.

Briere, J. (1996). *Trauma symptom checklist for children (TSCC): Professional manual.* Odessa, FL: Psychological Assessment Resources.

Chapman, J. F., & Ford, J. D. (2008). Relationships between suicide risk, traumatic experiences, and substance use among juvenile detainees. *Archives of Suicide Research, 12*(1), 50–61.

Connor, K. M., & Davidson, J. R. T. (2003). Development and validation of a new resilience scale. *Depression and Anxiety, 18,* 76–82.

Cook, A., Spinazzola, J., Ford, J. D., Lanktree, C., Blaustein, M., Cloitre, M., et al. (2005). Complex trauma in children and adolescents. *Psychiatric Annals, 35*(5), 390–398.

Coopersmith, S. (1989). *Coopersmith Self-Esteem Inventories.* Palo Alto, CA: Consulting Psychologists Press.

Courtois, C. A., & Ford, J. D. (2013). *Treatment of complex trauma: A sequenced, relationship-based approach.* New York: Guilford Press.

Crouch, J. L., Smith, D. W., Ezzell, C. E., & Saunders, B. E. (1999). Measuring reactions to sexual trauma among children: Comparing the Children's Impact of Traumatic Events Scale and the Trauma Symptom Checklist for Children. *Child Maltreatment, 4,* 255–263.

Davis, M. H. (1983). Measuring individual differences in empathy: Evidence for a multidimensional approach. *Journal of Personality and Social Psychology, 44,* 113–126.

Daviss, W. B., Mooney, D., Racusin, R., Ford, J. D., Fleischer, A., & McHugo, G. J. (2000). Predicting posttraumatic stress after hospitalization for pediatric injury.

[Print]. *Journal of the American Academy of Child and Adolescent Psychiatry,* *39*(5), 576–583.

Derryberry, D., & Reed, M. A. (2002). Anxiety-related attentional biases and their regulation by attentional control. *Journal of Abnormal Psychology, 111,* 225–236.

Dowdy, E., Twyford, J. M., Chin, J. K., Distefano, C. A., Kamphaus, R. W., & Mays, K. L. (2011). Factor structure of the BASC-2 Behavioral and Emotional Screening System Student Form. *Psychological Assessment, 23,* 379–387.

Egger, H. L. (2009). Psychiatric assessment of young children. *Child and Adolescent Psychiatric Clinics of North America, 18*(3), 559–580.

Egger, H. L., Erkanli, A., Keeler, G., Potts, E., Walter, B. K., & Angold, A. (2006). Test–retest reliability of the Preschool Age Psychiatric Assessment (PAPA). *Journal of the American Academy of Child and Adolescent Psychiatry, 45*(5), 538–549.

Epstein, M. H., Ryser, G., & Pearson, N. (2002). Standardization of the Behavioral and Emotional Rating Scale: Factor structure, reliability, and criterion validity. *Journal of Behavioral Health Science and Research, 29,* 208–216.

Farrington, A., Waller, G., Smerden, J., & Faupel, A. (2001). The Adolescent Dissociative Experiences Scale: Psychometric properties and difference in scores across age groups. *Journal of Nervous and Mental Disease, 189,* 722–727.

Feiring, C., Taska, L., & Lewis, M. (2002). Adjustment following sexual abuse discovery: The role of shame and attributional style. *Developmental Psychology, 38,* 79–92.

Ferguson, T. J., Stegge, H., Miller, E. R., & Olsen, M. E. (1999). Guilt, shame, and symptoms in children. *Developmental Psychology, 35*(2), 347–357.

Fitts, W. H., & Warren, W. L. (1996). *Tennessee Self-Concept Scale: Manual.* Los Angeles: Western Psychological Services.

Fletcher, K. (1996). Psychometric review of Dimensions of Stressful Events (DOSE) Ratings Scale. In B. H. Stamm (Ed.), *Measurement of stress, trauma, and adaptation* (pp. 144–151). Lutherville, MD: Sidran Press.

Ford, J. D. (2005). Treatment implications of altered neurobiology, affect regulation, and information processing following child maltreatment: *Psychiatric Annals, 35,* 410–419.

Ford, J. D. (2010). Conceptualizing complex posttraumatic stress syndromes in childhood and adolescence: Toward a developmental trauma disorder diagnosis. In V. Ardino (Ed.), *Post-traumatic syndromes in children and adolescents* (pp. 433–448). London: Wiley/Blackwell.

Ford, J. D., & Cloitre, M. (2009). Best practices in psychotherapy for children and adolescents. In C. A. Courtois & J. D. Ford (Eds.), *Treating complex traumatic stress disorders: An evidence-based guide* (pp. 59–81). New York: Guilford Press.

Ford, J. D., & Developmental Trauma Disorder Work Group. (2011). *Developmental Trauma Disorder Structured Interview (DTD-SI).* Farmington, CT: University of Connecticut Health Center. Available by contacting *jford@uchc.edu.*

Ford, J. D., Fraleigh, L. A., & Connor, D. F. (2010). Child abuse and aggression among psychiatrically impaired children. *Journal of Clinical Child and Adolescent Psychology, 39*(1), 25–34.

Ford, J. D., Hartman, J. K., Hawke, J., & Chapman, J. C. (2008). Traumatic victimization, posttraumatic stress disorder, suicidal ideation, and substance abuse risk among juvenile justice-involved youths. *Journal of Child and Adolescent Trauma, 1,* 75–92.

Ford, J. D., & Hawke, J. (2012). Trauma affect regulation psychoeducation group and milieu intervention outcomes in juvenile detention facilities. *Journal of Aggression, Maltreatment, and Trauma, 21*(4), 365–384.

Ford, J. D., Opler, L. A., Muenzenmaier, K., Shelley, A., & Grennan, M. (2013). *Symptoms of Traumatic Stress for Children (SOTS-C) clinician manual.* Toronto: Multi-Health Systems.

Ford, J. D., Racusin, R., Ellis, C. G., Daviss, W. B., Reiser, J., Fleischer, A., & Thomas,

J. (2000). Child maltreatment, other trauma exposure, and posttraumatic symptomatology among children with oppositional defiant and attention deficit hyperactivity disorders. *Child Maltreatment, 5*(3), 205–217.

Ford, J. D., Steinberg, K. L., Hawke, J., Levine, J., & Zhang, W. (2012). Randomized trial comparison of emotion regulation and relational psychotherapies for PTSD with girls involved in delinquency. *Journal of Clinical Child Adolescent Psychology, 41*(1), 27–37.

Garnefski, N., Koopman, H., Kraaij, V., & ten Cate, R. (2009). Cognitive emotion regulation strategies and psychological adjustment in adolescents with a chronic disease. *Journal of Adolescence, 32,* 449–454.

Garnefski, N., Rieffe, C., Jellesma, F., Meerum Terwogt, M., & Kraaij, V. (2007). Cognitive emotion regulation strategies and emotional problems in 9–11-year-old children: The development of an instrument. *European Child and Adolescent Psychiatry, 16,* 1–9.

Gioia, G. A., Isquith, P. K., Retzlaff, P. D., & Espy, K. A. (2002). Confirmatory factor analysis of the Behavior Rating Inventory of Executive Function (BRIEF) in a clinical sample. *Child Neuropsychology, 8,* 249–257.

Gould, M., Marrocco, F., Kleinman, M., Thomas, J., Mostkoff, K., Cote, J., et al. (2005). Evaluating iatrogenic risk of youth suicide screening programs: A randomized controlled trial. *Journal of the American Medical Association, 293*(13), 1635–1643.

Gratz, K. L., Conrad, S. D., & Roemer, L. (2002). Risk factors for deliberate self-harm among college students. *American Journal of Orthopsychiatry, 72*(1), 128–140.

Gully, K. (2003). *Expectations Test professional manual.* Salt Lake City, UT: Peak Ascent.

Harder, D. H., & Zalma, A. (1990). Two promising shame and guilt scales: A construct validity comparison. *Journal of Personality Assessment, 55,* 729–745.

Harter, S. (1982). The Perceived Competence Scale. *Child Development, 53,* 87–97.

Harter, S., & Pike, R. (1984). The pictorial scale of perceived competence and social acceptance for young children. *Child Development, 55,* 1969–1982.

Hodges, K. (2005). Child and Adolescent Functional Assessment Scale. In T. Grisso, G. Vincent, & D. Seagrave (Eds.), *Mental health screening and assessment in juvenile justice* (pp. 123–136). New York: Guilford Press.

Holtmann, M., Buchmann, A. F., Esser, G., Schmidt, M. H., Banaschewski, T., & Laucht, M. (2011). The Child Behavior Checklist—Dysregulation Profile predicts substance use, suicidality, and functional impairment. *Journal of Child Psychology and Psychiatry, 52*(2), 139–147.

Howe, A., Pitten Cate, I. M., Brown, A., & Hadwin, J. A. (2008). Empathy in preschool children: The development of the Southampton Test of Empathy for Preschoolers (STEP). *Psychological Assessment, 20,* 305–309.

Huth-Bocks, A.C., Kerr, D.C.R., Ivey, A.Z., Kramer, A.C., & King, C.A. (2007). Assessment of psychiatrically hospitalized suicidal adolescents. *Journal of the American Academy of Child and Adolescent Psychiatry, 46*(3), 387–395.

Isquith, P. K., Gioia, G. A., & Espy, K. A. (2004). Executive function in preschool children: Examination through everyday behavior. *Developmental Neuropsychology, 26,* 403–422.

Jellesma, F. C., Rieffe, C., & Terwogt, M. M. (2007). The Somatic Complaint List. *Journal of Psychosomatic Research, 63*(4), 399–401.

John, K., Gammon, G. D., Prusoff, B. A., & Warner, V. (1987). The Social Adjustment Inventory for Children and Adolescents (SAICA): Testing of a new semistructured interview. *Journal of Clinical Child and Adolescent Psychology, 26*(6), 898–911.

Joseph, S., & Wood, A. (2010). Assessment of positive functioning in clinical psychology: Theoretical and practical issues. *Clinical Psychology Review, 30*(7), 830–838.

Kaufman, J., Birmaher, B., Brent, D., Rao, U., & Ryan, N. (1996). Schedule for Affective

Disorders and Schizophrenia for School-Age Children—Present and Lifetime version (K-SADS-PL): Initial reliability and validity data. *Journal of Clinical Child and Adolescent Psychology, 36,* 980–988.

Keck Seeley, S. M., Perosa, S. L., & Perosa, L. M. (2004). A validation study of the Adolescent Dissociative Experiences Scale. *Child Abuse and Neglect, 28*(7), 755–769.

Kerns, K. A., Tomich, P. L., Aspelmeier, J., & Contreras, J. (2000). Attachment-based assessments of parent–child relationships in middle childhood. *Developmental Psychology, 36,* 614–626.

Kliewer, W., & Sullivan, T. N. (2008). Community violence exposure, threat appraisal, and adjustment in adolescents. *Journal of Clinical Child and Adolescent Psychology, 37*(4), 860–873.

Kubany, E., Haynes, S., Abueg, F., Manke, F., Brennan, J., & Stahura, C. (1996). Development and validation of the Trauma-Related Guilt Inventory. *Psychological Assessment, 8,* 428–444.

Latimer, S., Covic, T., Cumming, S. R., & Tennant, A. (2009). Psychometric analysis of the Self-Harm Inventory using Rasch modelling. *BMC Psychiatry, 9,* 53.

Layne, C., Beck, C., Rimmasch, H., Southwick, J., Moreno, M., & Hobfoll, S. (2008). Promoting 'resilient' posttraumatic adjustment in childhood and beyond. In D. Brom, R. Pat-Horenczyk & J. D. Ford (Eds.), *Treating traumatized children: Risk, resilience, and recovery* (pp. 13–47). London: Routledge.

LeJeune, B., Beebe, D., Noll, J., Kenealy, L., Isquith, P., & Gioia, G. (2010). Psychometric support for an abbreviated version of the Behavior Rating Inventory of Executive Function (BRIEF) Parent Form. *Child Neuropsychology, 16,* 182–201.

Lyons, J. S. (1999). *Child and adolescent needs and strengths (CANS-MH): An information integration tool for children and adolescents with mental health challenges.* Chicago: Praed Foundation.

Mahon, N. E., Yarcheski, T. J., & Yarcheski, A. (1995). Validation of the revised UCLA Loneliness Scale for adolescents. *Research in Nursing and Health, 18*(3), 263–270.

Main, M., & Cassidy, J. (1988). Categories of response to reunion with the parent at age six: Predictable from infant attachment classifications and stable over a 1-month period. *Developmental Psychology, 24,* 415–526.

Mavroveli, S., Petrides, K. V., Rieffe, C., & Bakker, F. (2007). Trait emotional intelligence, psychological well-being, and peer-rated social competence in adolescence. *British Journal of Developmental Psychology, 25,* 263–275.

Mavroveli, S., Petrides, K. V., Shove, C., & Whitehead, A. (2008). Investigation of the construct of trait emotional intelligence in children. *European Journal of Child and Adolescent Psychiatry, 17,* 516–526.

Mezulis, A. H., Funasaki, K., & Hyde, J. (2011). Negative cognitive style trajectories in the transition to adolescence. *Journal of Clinical Child and Adolescent Psychology, 40*(2), 318–331.

Mezulis, A. H., Hyde, J. S., & Abramson, L. Y. (2006). The developmental origins of cognitive vulnerability to depression. *Developmental Psychology, 42,* 1012–1025.

Mezzich, A., Tarter, R., Giancola, P., & Kirisci, L. (2001). The Dysregulation Inventory. *Journal of Child and Adolescent Substance Abuse, 10,* 35–43.

Miga, E. M., Hare, A., Allen, J. P., & Manning, N. (2010). The relation of insecure attachment, states of mind, and romantic attachment styles to adolescent aggression in romantic relationships. *Attachment and Human Development, 12*(5), 463–481.

Minnis, H., Millward, R., Sinclair, C., Kennedy, E., Greig, A., Towlson, K., et al. (2006). The Computerized MacArthur Story Stem Battery—a pilot study of a novel medium for assessing children's representations of relationships. *International Journal of Methods in Psychiatry Research, 15,* 207–214.

Moss, E., Bureau, J., Béliveau, M., Zdebik, M., & Lépine, S. (2009). Links between children's attachment behavior at early school-age, their attachment-related representations, and behavior problems in middle childhood. *International Journal of Behavioral Development, 33,* 155–166.

Nader, K., Newman, E., Weathers, F., Kaloupek, D., Kriegler, J., & Blake, D. (1996). *Clinician-Administered PTSD Scale for Children and Adolescents (CAPS-CA).* Los Angeles: Western Psychological Press.

Pardini, D. A., Lochman, J. E., & Frick, P. J. (2003). Callous/unemotional traits and social–cognitive processes in adjudicated youths. *Journal of the American Academy of Child and Adolescent Psychiatry, 42,* 364–371.

Petrides, K. V. (2009). *Technical manual for the Trait Emotional Intelligence Questionnaires (TEIQue).* London: London Psychometric Laboratory.

Piers, E. V., & Herzberg, D. S. (2002). *Piers–Harris Children's Self-Concept Scale: Manual* (2nd ed.). Los Angeles: Western Psychological Services.

Reich, W., & Todd, R. (2002). *Missouri Assessment of Genetics Interview for Children specifications manual.* St. Louis, MO: Washington University School of Medicine.

Reynolds, W.M. (1987). *Suicidal Ideation Questionnaire: Professional manual.* Odessa, FL: Psychological Assessment Resources.

Ridenour, T., Greenberg, M., & Cook, E. (2006). Structure and validity of People in My Life: A self-report measure of attachment in late childhood. *Journal of Youth and Adolescence, 35,* 1037–1053.

Rieffe, C., Meerum Terwogt, M., Petrides, K.V., Cowan, C., Miers, A.C., & Tolland A. (2007). Psychometric properties of the Emotion Awareness Questionnaire for children. *Personality and Individual Differences, 43,* 95–105.

Rieffe, C., Oosterveld, P., & Meerum Terwogt, M. (2006). An alexithymia questionnaire for children: Factorial and concurrent validation. *Personality and Individual Differences, 40,* 123–133.

Robinson, J., Herot, C., Haynes, P., & Mantz-Simmons, L. (2000). Children's story stem responses: A measure of program impact on developmental risks associated with dysfunctional parenting. *Child Abuse and Neglect, 24,* 99–110.

Rosen, K. S., & Burke, P. B. (1999). Multiple attachment relationships within families: Mothers and fathers with two young children. *Developmental Psychology, 35,* 436–444.

Russell, D., Peplau, L. A., & Cutrona, C. E. (1980). The revised UCLA Loneliness Scale. *Journal of Personality and Social Psychology, 39,* 472–480.

Scharfe, E. (2002). Reliability and validity of an interview assessment of attachment representations in a clinical sample of adolescents. *Journal of Adolescent Research, 17,* 532–551.

Schott, G. R., & Bellin, W. (2001). The relational self-concept scale: A context-specific self-report measure for adolescents. *Adolescence, 36*(141), 85–103.

Shaffer, D., Gould, M. S., Brasic, J., Ambrosini, P., Fisher, P., Bird, H., et al. (1983). A children's global assessment scale (CGAS). *Archives of General Psychiatry, 40*(11), 1228–1231.

Snyder, C. R., Hoza, B., Pelham, W. E., Rapoff, M., Ware, L., Danovsky, M., et al. (1997). The development and validation of the Children's Hope Scale. *Journal of Pediatric Psychology, 22*(3), 399–421.

Sparrow, S., Cicchetti, D., & Balla, D. (2006). *Vineland–II: Vineland Adaptive Behavior Scales: Teacher rating form manual* (2nd ed.). Circle Pines, MN: American Guidance Services.

Steer, R. A., Kumar, G., & Beck, A. T. (1993). Self-reported suicidal ideation in adolescent psychiatric inpatients. *Journal of Consulting and Clinical Psychology, 61*(6), 1096–1099.

Steinberg, A. M., Brymer, M. J., Decker, K. B., & Pynoos, R. S. (2004). The University of California at Los Angeles Post-Traumatic Stress Disorder Reaction Index. *Current Psychiatry Reports, 6*(2), 96–100.

Sternberg, K. J., Lamb, M. E., Guterman, E., Abbott, C. B., & Dawud-Noursi, S.

(2005). Adolescents' perceptions of attachments to their mothers and fathers in families with histories of domestic violence. *Child Abuse and Neglect, 29*(8), 853–869.

Tangney, J.P., & Dearing, R. L. (2002). *Shame and guilt.* New York: Guilford Press.

Tortella-Feliu, M., Balle, M., & Sese, A. (2010). Relationships between negative affectivity, emotion regulation, anxiety, and depressive symptoms in adolescents as examined through structural equation modeling. *Journal of Anxiety Disorders, 24*(7), 686–693.

van der Kolk, B. A. (2005). Developmental trauma disorder: Toward a rational diagnosis for children with complex trauma histories. *Psychiatric Annals, 35*(5), 401–408.

Vaughn, B. E., & Waters, E. (1990). Attachment behavior at home and in the laboratory: Q-sort observations and Strange Situation classifications of one-year-olds. *Child Development, 61,* 1965–1973.

Veltri, C. O., Graham, J. R., Sellbom, M., Ben-Porath, Y. S., Forbey, J. D., O'Connell, C., et al. (2009). Correlates of MMPI-A scales in acute psychiatric and forensic samples. *Journal of Personality Assessment, 91*(3), 288–300.

Vila, M., Kramer, T., Hickey, N., Dattani, M., Jefferis, H., Singh, M., et al. (2009). Assessment of somatic symptoms in British secondary school children using the Children's Somatization Inventory (CSI). *Journal of Pediatric Psychology, 34*(9), 989–998.

Vitiello, B., Silva, S. G., Rohde, P., Kratochvil, C. J., Kennard, B. D., Reinecke, M. A., et al. (2009). Suicidal events in the Treatment for Adolescents with Depression Study (TADS). *Journal of Clinical Psychiatry, 70*(5), 741–747.

Walker, L. S., Beck, J. E., Garber, J., & Lambert, W. (2009). Children's Somatization Inventory: Psychometric properties of the revised form. *Journal of Pediatric Psychology, 34,* 430–440.

Walter, K. H., Horsey, K. J., Palmieri, P. A., & Hobfoll, S. E. (2010). The role of protective self-cognitions in the relationship between childhood trauma and later resource loss. *Journal of Traumatic Stress, 23*(2), 264–273.

Way, I., Applegate, B., Cai, X., Franck, L., Black-Pond, C., Yelsma, P., et al. (2010). Children's Alexithymia Measure (CAM). *Journal of Child and Adolescent Trauma, 3*(4), 303–318.

Weimer, B. L., Kerns, K. A., & Oldenburg, C. (2004). Adolescents' interactions with a best friend: Associations with attachment style. *Journal of Experimental Child Psychology, 88,* 102–120.

Weisz, J. R., Francis, S. E., & Bearman, S. (2010). Assessing secondary control and its association with youth depression symptoms. *Journal of Abnormal Child Psychology, 38*(7), 883–893.

Weisz, J. R., Southam-Gerow, M. A., & McCarty, C. A. (2001). Control-related beliefs and depressive symptoms in clinic-referred children and adolescents: Developmental differences and model specificity. *Journal of Abnormal Psychology, 110*(1), 97–109.

Wolfe, V.V., Gentile, C., Michienzi, T., Sas, L., &Wolfe, D.A. (1991). The Children's Impact of Traumatic Events Scale. *Behavioral Assessment, 13,* 359–383.

Yu, X. N., Lau, J. T., Mak, W. W., Zhang, J., Lui, W. W., & Zhang, J. (2011). Factor structure and psychometric properties of the Connor–Davidson Resilience Scale among Chinese adolescents. *Comprehensive Psychiatry, 52*(2), 218–224.

Zahn-Waxler, C., Kochanska, G., Krupnick, J., & McNew, D. (1990). Patterns of guilt in children of depressed and well mothers. *Developmental Psychology, 26,* 51–59.

PART II

INDIVIDUAL PSYCHOTHERAPY MODELS

CHAPTER 8

Integrative Treatment of Complex Trauma

Cheryl Lanktree
John Briere

Since the advent of posttraumatic stress disorder (PTSD) as a psychiatric diagnosis (American Psychiatric Association, 1980), clinical understanding of trauma and its effects has tended to emphasize relatively circumscribed psychological reactions to a single, isolated event, such as a rape or motor vehicle accident. More recently, however, clinicians and researchers have identified what may be a more typical scenario, at least in clinical populations: generally described as *complex trauma*. Complex trauma involves a combination of early- and later-onset traumatic events, frequently including repetitive childhood sexual, physical, and/or psychological abuse, and, in many cases, caretaker neglect (Courtois & Ford, 2009; Cook et al., 2005). In addition, exposure to multiple traumas is often associated with lower socioeconomic status: those experiencing poverty, social marginalization, or homelessness are more likely than others to have undergone a variety of especially adverse events, including, for example, peer sexual and physical assault, community and gang-related violence, commercial sexual exploitation, and murder or injury of a family member or friend (Briere & Scott, 2012; Brown, 2009; Singer, Anglin, Song, & Lunghofer, 1995).

Together, the accumulation of multiple adverse and traumatizing events and, for some, the ongoing effects of negative social conditions can lead to a wide range of psychological outcomes in children and youth. These include anxiety, depression, cognitive distortions, posttraumatic stress, interpersonal problems, insecure attachment, revictimization, and, in the case of older children and adolescents, substance abuse, suicidality, and other dysfunctional or self-endangering behaviors (Cook et al., 2005; van der Kolk, 2005). Cumulative trauma also increases the likelihood of aggression, criminality, and subsequent incarceration or other forms of institutionalization (Grisso, Vincent, & Seagrave, 2005). Unfortunately, social discrimination and marginalization also may mean that that the traumatized person has reduced access to appropriate health, mental health, or social services (Perez & Fortuna, 2005), further compounding his or her psychosocial difficulties.

Given these complexities, treatment approaches for children and others that are limited to a single modality (e.g., exposure therapy, cognitive therapy, or psychiatric medication) may be insufficient—especially if the intervention is not adapted to the specific experiences, needs, and cultural matrix of the affected individual. A multimodal treatment strategy may be useful in such cases, especially one that takes into account not only the panoply of symptoms and problems that may accrue from complex trauma, but also the sociocultural environment in which the client is embedded.

In response to these various issues, *integrative treatment of complex trauma* (ITCT) was designed to provide a culturally informed, multicomponent approach to the treatment of complex trauma effects. It consists of two separate intervention packages: *ITCT for children* (ITCT-C; Lanktree & Briere, 2008) for those from 8 to 12 years old, and *ITCT for adolescents and young adults* (ITCT-A; Briere & Lanktree, 2008, 2011) for those from 12 to 21.

First developed at the Miller Children's Abuse and Violence Intervention Center (MCAVIC) in Long Beach, California, ITCT-C and ITCT-A were later expanded in collaboration with the Psychological Trauma Program of the University of Southern California (USC) Department of Psychiatry. Under the auspices of the National Child Traumatic Stress Network (NCTSN), and funded by the Substance Abuse and Mental Health Services Administration (SAMHSA), the ITCT treatment guides were adapted and revised from 2005 until 2009, with input from MCAVIC and USC staff, an expert panel on cultural issues, a community advisory council, and attendees from a nationwide NCTSN Learning Community on ITCT. The ITCT-A treatment guide has been further expanded to its current form (Briere & Lanktree, 2011).

Empirical Support for ITCT

A record review of 151 MCAVIC-USC clients (Lanktree et al., 2012) recently examined the effectiveness of ITCT in reducing Trauma Symptom

Checklist for Children (TSCC; Briere, 1996) scores in a culturally diverse, largely inner-city sample of children and adolescents. Most had experienced multiple types of trauma, typically some combination of childhood sexual or physical abuse, psychological maltreatment, emotional neglect, family violence, loss of a loved one, and community violence, often compounded by caretaker–child attachment issues. In addition, some were referred by local hospitals and clinics following a traumatic medical condition (e.g., AIDS), injury (e.g., gunshot wound), or invasive medical procedure (e.g., amputation). Due to SAMHSA funding requirements for treatment development and testing, but not randomized control studies, no wait list or alternative treatment comparison group was included in this study.

Most clients (67%) were in treatment for an average of 7 months (range = 3 months to more than a year), with longer treatment duration associated with more severe initial symptomatology. Clients' scores on each of the TSCC scales (*Anxiety, Depression, Anger, Posttraumatic Stress, Dissociation,* and *Sexual Concerns*) decreased an average of 41% from pre- to posttest ($p < .001$). There were no differences in treatment effectiveness in relation to gender, number of traumas, ethnicity, or whether the client received ITCT-C or ITCT-A. However, longer-term treatment was associated with greater symptom reduction, as per other research in this area (e.g., Lanktree & Briere, 1995).

Overview of ITCT

ITCT is an evidence-based, multicomponent therapy that integrates treatment principles from the complex trauma literature (Cook et al., 2005; Courtois & Ford, 2009), attachment theory (Bowlby, 1988), the self-trauma model (Briere, 2002), and components of trauma-focused cognitive-behavioral therapy (TF-CBT; Cohen, Mannarino, & Deblinger, 2006; see Chapter 10, this volume). It involves semistructured protocols and interventions that are customized to the specific issues and capacities of each client, since complex posttraumatic outcomes are notable for their variability across different individuals.

An important and relatively unique aspect of ITCT is its ongoing monitoring of treatment effects over time. Ideally, this involves initial and periodic psychometric and interview-based evaluation of the child's symptomatology in a number of different areas, as well as assessment of his or her socioeconomic status, culture, ongoing level of support systems and coping skills, family and caretaker relationships, attachment issues, and functional self capacities. The client's social and physical environments are considered as well for evidence of new stressors, changes in family financial and housing status, potential danger from revictimization, and exposure to community violence.

Assessments take place at intake and at 3-month intervals throughout treatment, and are coded and organized based on one of two versions of the *Assessment–Treatment Flowchart* (ATF): the ATF-C for use in ITCT-C, and the ATF-A for use in ITCT-A. Each ATF version allows the therapist to review therapy and environmentally related changes in symptomatology or psychosocial problems over time, based on repeatedly collected interviews, psychological tests, and information from other sources such as parents or teachers (Briere & Lanktree, 2011; see also *www.johnbriere.com* for ITCT forms and handouts). ATF domains, which are rated on a 1 ("Not currently a problem, do not treat") to 4 ("Most problematic, requires immediate attention") scale, include areas such as environmental safety, caretaker support, depression, anger, low self-esteem, posttraumatic stress, grief, attachment insecurity, suicidality, and self-injury, each of which may increase or decrease from one assessment period to the next (see the case example at the end of this chapter). Successful treatment, for example, might reduce the child's posttraumatic stress during assessment period 1, yet his or her self-injurious behavior might be unaffected or even increase for some reason (e.g., new stressors, peer relationship changes, or a new instance of abuse) during assessment period 2.

Based on information from the ATF, the therapist uses a *PROBLEMS-TO-COMPONENTS GRID* (PCG) to customize the client's treatment, applying the empirically supported components described later in this chapter. Most of those with complex posttraumatic outcomes will, by definition, have multiple targets for intervention requiring multiple treatment components, sometimes within the same session. Over time, these various interventions can be initiated or terminated, or intensified or reduced, as a function of changing ATF ratings. In this way, use of the ATF formally encourages "midcourse corrections," wherein the clinician may shift from, for example, therapeutic exposure to an increased focus on safety or affect regulation issues. Which, how, and when a given component is used will vary according to the immediate needs of the client and the relative importance of the treatment target, as indicated on the ATF.

Unlike many structured trauma treatment approaches, ITCT does not recommend a preestablished number of sessions for every client. Instead, therapy can range from several months to a year or more, with clients in the ITCT outcome study requiring an average of 7 months (Lanktree et al., 2012). Overall, the pace of treatment is guided by consideration of the "therapeutic window" (Briere, 2002), a concept that stresses the need to provide (1) therapeutic exposure, cognitive restructuring, and relational processing of trauma memories, and yet, at the same time, (2) careful attention to the treatment process so that it does not overwhelm the child's affect regulation capacities and lead to avoidance or retraumatization. This need for titrated exposure and processing may extend the total time required for treatment.

ITCT especially focuses on social and cultural issues. Attention is paid to the use of culturally appropriate treatment resources (e.g., play therapy toys and games, books, and psychoeducational materials), and the focus and context of treatment is adapted to the child's sociocultural milieu (Lanktree, 2008). Also taken into account are cultural phenomena that can assist the client's progress in therapy, including, for some, use of the extended family as a physical, psychological, and social support system.

ITCT-C and ITCT-A include most of the same treatment components, except that ITCT-C places a greater emphasis on expressive and play therapy modalities (including sand tray, games, and toy-based play), whereas ITCT-A devotes more attention to verbal psychotherapy and interventions to reduce impulsive, aggressive, or other tension-reduction behaviors. ITCT-C also focuses more on involving the family and key adults (e.g., teachers), since younger children are more dependent on caretakers than older adolescents and young adults. ITCT-C often includes more sessions with primary caretakers, as well as family and group therapy. Parent education classes are provided as needed, especially for caretakers struggling with proper responses to challenging or problematic child behaviors. Both versions of ITCT have been applied in outpatient child trauma clinics, public school settings, and in "alternative education" schools (Lanktree, 2008).

ITCT Treatment Components

Following completion of the ATF and consulting the PCG, the clinician applies the following specific ITCT components as needed.

Relationship Building and Support

A positive therapeutic relationship is crucial to the effectiveness of ITCT, as has been found for psychotherapy in general (Lambert & Barley, 2001). Although relationship building is considered one of the initial components in ITCT, the therapist may need to return to this component at other stages of treatment, especially when the client is addressing particularly difficult traumatic or relational material. Therapist behaviors and responses that increase the client's sense of safety include several ITCT subcomponents, especially *nonintrusiveness, visible positive regard, reliability and stability,* and *transparency*. Therapist behaviors that can enhance the client's sense of feeling understood and of being less alone include *attunement, empathy, acceptance, understanding,* and *curiosity* about the client's perspective and internal experience (Briere & Lanktree, 2011). The clinician is an active agent in therapy, especially in terms of communicating caring and positive regard, and encourages the client to express his or her thoughts and feelings throughout the therapy process.

ITCT emphasizes the management of countertransference, since a therapist's responses to his or her own memories and schemas can reduce the client's perceived level of safety in treatment, and can diminish the clinician's capacity to accurately diagnose and intervene. It is important that the therapist regularly monitor him- or herself during the therapy process; avoid dismissive, judgmental, or authoritarian behaviors; self-regulate emotions; and seek supervision and/or consultation whenever appropriate.

Safety Interventions

Childhood maltreatment and other relational traumas are associated with a greater likelihood of subsequent substance abuse, unsafe sexual practices, self-endangering behavior, aggression, and a greater risk of further victimization. ITCT interventions to enhance safety include (1) regular assessment and intervention of the client's danger to self (e.g., suicidality) and others (e.g., assaultiveness); (2) collaboration with child protection or law enforcement (including mandated reporting and assistance in making crime reports); (3) systems-level advocacy; (4) referral for additional mental health resources or medical treatment; and (5) in the case of ongoing child abuse, exploitation, or domestic violence, the development of "safety plans." In some cases, the therapist may need to refer the child or adolescent and his or her family to a homeless or domestic violence shelter. These interventions are often paramount in work with multitraumatized young people, and may be necessary repeatedly before and during significant trauma processing.

Psychoeducation

Children with histories of interpersonal violence often are victimized in the context of overwhelming emotion, narrowed or dissociated attention, and a relatively early stage of cognitive development. There may have been a lack of consistent, nurturing caretakers. Preverbal experiences may further contribute to fragmented, incomplete, or inaccurate explanations of traumatic events.

The psychoeducation component of ITCT allows the clinician to provide the client with information regarding the nature of trauma and its effects. Not only does this increase the child or adolescent's fund of accurate information, it can reduce feelings of isolation and of being different from others, validate feelings and perceptions, and facilitate cognitive processing of trauma. In younger or less verbal clients, psychoeducational materials can provide a concrete framework for discussion of topics such as sexual victimization, sexual development, and sexual identity issues that might otherwise feel too threatening. Although often presented early in therapy, carefully screened handouts, books, and other media (e.g., DVDs, YouTube files), and additional verbal information can be provided throughout the treatment process.

Affect Regulation Training

Above and beyond classic posttraumatic symptoms, children and adolescents with complex trauma histories often experience relatively uncontrollable emotional states that overwhelm existing affect regulation capacities. When this occurs, the client may compensate with avoidance strategies such as dissociation, substance abuse, and externalizing behavior (Briere, Hodges, & Godbout, 2010). High levels of avoidance, in turn, may interfere with psychological recovery by blocking the client's access to upsetting memories and feelings during treatment.

ITCT includes interventions that increase the client's affect regulation skills, in some cases before, as well as during, trauma memory processing (see Cloitre et al., 2010, for a discussion of this issue). These include *grounding, progressive relaxation, guided imagery, visualization, breath training, meditation* and *mindfulness training, emotion identification,* and *trigger identification/intervention* (described separately below). All are focused on increasing the child's overall capacity to tolerate and downregulate negative feeling states, thereby reducing the likelihood that he or she will be overwhelmed by activated emotions.

Cognitive Processing

Trauma-related cognitive disturbance is generally addressed in ITCT through detailed verbal or play-based exploration of the traumatic event and its surrounding circumstances. Whether in discussion or play, the child or adolescent has the opportunity to hear—or witness him- or herself engage in—verbalizations or behaviors that reflect assumptions and perceptions that were encoded at the time of the trauma but that do not make sense in the (currently safe and supportive) here and now. For example, a youth may hear herself describing an abusive event that happened earlier in her life (e.g., "I got punished a lot because I was a bad kid"), and have a chance to update her narrative with what, upon reflection, she now knows about herself ("I didn't really do anything that bad, and I really didn't deserve to be beat up"), the abuser (e.g., "She was drunk all the time"), and the abuse process in general (e.g., "It wasn't my fault" or "Dad was out of control"). Similarly, the younger child may enact through play or in a sand-tray activity a memory of domestic violence between his parents and describe what he now thinks was happening, why it happened, and what his role was (or was not) during the event. In these ways, the client and therapist work together to create a more accurate cognitive model of the trauma and to process its implications for how the client currently thinks and feels.

The client is also encouraged to develop a more coherent narrative of the traumatic event(s). As the traumatic event is repetitively discussed or acted out in play or drawings, in detail, and in a gradual manner according to the client's emotional and self capacities, a process sometimes referred to as *context reinstatement* may occur: Additional details of the trauma are recalled as the story of the trauma is recounted, such that the narrative becomes more complete and more internally consistent over time. The therapist may encourage the client to map out, on a piece of paper, traumatic and nontraumatic events on a *trauma time line,* beginning early in life and ending in the present, thereby supporting the development of a more sequential and organized narrative.

Trigger Identification and Intervention

Many of the difficulties that trauma-exposed children and adolescents experience arise when stimuli or situations in their immediate environment trigger upsetting memories and associated cognitions and emotions. When these thoughts and feelings are reexperienced, the individual may engage in tension reduction behaviors in order to reduce distress associated with these memories. For example, an adolescent is (or perceives him- or herself to be) insulted or rejected by a peer. This event triggers memories of parental maltreatment or abandonment, which, in turn, activate abuse-era feelings of low self-esteem and thoughts about "getting even." These thoughts and memories may then activate anger and motivate an action (e.g., aggression) that is out of proportion to the actual insult by the peer and more relevant to his childhood than his current situation.

The *trigger awareness and intervention* component teaches the client how to identify and address triggers in the environment, as well as those that arise internally through thoughts, emotions, and sensations. This component can facilitate a greater sense of control and better interpersonal functioning by helping the child or adolescent to identify and avoid or alter situations in which triggering might be likely—or, if triggering has occurred, to change or better manage his or her emotional and behavioral responses.

In ITCT-A, in particular, the client and therapist work together using a *trigger grid* (available in Briere & Lanktree, 2011, and at *www.johnbriere. com*). The goals of the trigger grid exercise are for the client to:

1. Learn about triggers, including their capacity to elicit reactions that make it seem like a traumatic event is happening, even though, in fact, it is not.
2. Identify specific instances during which he or she has been triggered in the past.
3. Determine what seem to be the major triggers in his or her life.
4. Explore the thoughts and feelings associated with each major trigger, so that triggering, as a phenomenon, becomes more obvious to him or her.
5. Develop problem-solving strategies to deescalate the situation, including (a) "time-outs" (e.g., removing oneself from the

interaction); (b) analyzing the triggering stimulus or situation until a greater understanding changes his or her perception of the event; (c) increasing immediate support systems; (d) engaging in positive self-talk, relaxation, or distraction; or (e) engaging in physical and creative activities as soon as possible after being triggered, such as writing, exercise, dance, music, or art.

Titrated Exposure

In addition to the components outlined above, ITCT includes *therapeutic exposure* (e.g., Berliner, 2005; Cohen et al., 2006). This component involves exposing the client, during therapy, to memories of a traumatic event until the associated emotional responses are desensitized or habituated and thus can no longer be activated. The version used in ITCT, *titrated exposure,* involves controlling this process so that the activated emotions do not exceed the client's affect regulation capacity and thus do not overwhelm him or her. It is important that exposure be applied only to the extent that the client can tolerate the associated emotional activation. The chronically overwhelmed and avoidant child or adolescent, for example, may not be able to process trauma memories in any significant way without feeling retraumatized. In such cases, the relational, cognitive, and affect regulation components of ITCT may be more immediately relevant.

THE THERAPEUTIC WINDOW

The therapeutic window represents the psychological midpoint between inadequate and overwhelming activation of trauma-related emotion during treatment; it is a hypothetical "place" where therapeutic interventions are thought to be most helpful (Briere, 2002). Interventions within the therapeutic window are neither so nonevocative that they provide inadequate memory processing and maintain avoidance, nor so intense that they become overwhelming and punish awareness. In other words, interventions that take the therapeutic window into account are those that trigger trauma memories (i.e., through therapeutic exposure) and promote processing, but do not overwhelm the client's internal protective systems and activate unwanted avoidance responses.

The exposure process and how it is titrated vary according to the age of the child. In ITCT-C, exposure may involve play therapy, sand-tray work, drawing, painting, or making clay figures. Titration in ITCT-C often occurs when the clinician selects certain toys, games, or sand-tray figures for the child to work with and then joins the child in the game or activity in such a way that he or she can comment, redirect, support, soothe, and engage the child in activities that activate trauma memories but do not overwhelm.

When expressive/art therapy is used in ITCT-C, the child may draw a picture or write a poem about how he or she felt before being abused or otherwise traumatized, as compared to how he or she felt afterward. The client can draw a self-portrait of when he or she was hurt, create a collage, or make a drawing of a person or place that, in some manner, encourages the expression and processing of trauma-related feelings. Other options can include kinetic family drawings (i.e., of the family doing something) or drawing a "snapshot" of the child's family, each of which can elicit the child's memories of, and feelings for, different family members. Children also can bring in photo albums or pictures of themselves at different ages, as well as those of family members. Pictures are often quite evocative in terms of triggering traumatic memories, and thus may be effectively used as a form of therapeutic exposure. They also may trigger additional, more remote or avoided memories, which can then be processed as well.

In the case of ITCT-A, titrated exposure is done in a manner more similar to work with adults. Here exposure often involves conversations with the adolescent about trauma experiences, during which the therapist guides the process via questions, comments, and gentle instructions that allow the client to remember and express at a level of intensity that does not exceed the therapeutic window. Because adolescents in general, let alone those who are traumatized, often struggle with affect regulation as they encounter new developmental stimuli, titration by the therapist may be needed on a moment-to-moment basis. The clinician may encourage discussion of one topic, but not yet a more distressing one, ask about certain events and feelings but not others, support and verbally soothe at moments of greater stress, or even temporarily distract or redirect the youth away from a specific memory or mental state. At another moment, however, when the youth is more stable and has more access to affect regulation skills, previously avoided traumatic material can be revisited or introduced, albeit with care.

Relational Processing

The client's attachment history is central to the development of complex trauma and is integral to ITCT. One of the earliest impacts of abuse and neglect is thought to be on the child's internal representations of self and others, inferred from how he or she is treated by his or her caretakers. These early inferences about self and others often occur in the caretaker–child attachment process and form a generalized set of expectations, beliefs, and assumptions (see Chapters 1–3, this volume). In the case of abuse or neglect, these attachment schemas are likely to be especially negative, and may result in the child or youth behaving in ways that disrupt or prevent the development of healthy interpersonal relationships with others.

Attachment relationships can be improved and become more secure as the client–therapist relationship develops. This relationship serves several functions, including fostering a sense of empathic attunement in the child, providing support and validation, training in interpersonal skills, and the activation and processing of trauma-related relational schemas and associated negative emotional states (Briere & Scott, 2012; Kinsler, Courtois, & Frankel, 2009).

Regarding this last point, the therapeutic relationship is a powerful source of interpersonal triggers. The youth's increasing attachment to the therapist can activate implicit (i.e., nonverbal, sensory, experiential) memories of attachment experiences in childhood. For many clients, these early attachment memories include considerable abuse or neglect, which may be reexperienced in the form of maltreatment-related thoughts, feelings, and perceptions during the treatment process. These largely implicit "relational flashbacks" are often misperceived by the client as feelings and information about the current therapist–client relationship (see Briere & Scott, 2012, for more on these "source attribution errors"). Once activated and expressed, such cognitions and emotions can be discussed and processed in the context of the safety, soothing, and support associated with a positive therapeutic relationship.

As in the processing of simpler traumatic memories, the therapeutic processing of relational/attachment-level memories and their associations can be seen as involving the following (Briere, 2002):

- *Exposure:* The child or adolescent encounters stimuli in the therapeutic relationship (e.g., the clinician's caring and focus on the child's well-being) that, by virtue of their basic nurturing qualities, trigger attachment responses, including, somewhat paradoxically, implicit memories of early interpersonal abuse or neglect.
- *Activation:* As a result of therapeutic exposure, the young person experiences emotions and thoughts that occurred at the time of the relational trauma or attachment disruption and attributes them to the current (therapeutic) relationship.
- *Disparity:* Although the youth thinks and feels as if maltreatment, neglect, or abandonment is either happening or is about to happen, in reality the session is safe, and the therapist is not abusive, rejecting, or otherwise dangerous.
- *Counterconditioning:* As the therapeutic relationship triggers early memories of abuse or neglect, the child also experiences positive emotional states (e.g., love, interpersonal warmth) associated with growing attachment to the therapist. The presence of these positive emotional experiences at the same time as negative memories are elicited potentially counterconditions these memories over time, ultimately reducing their capacity to produce distress.
- *Desensitization:* The child's or adolescent's repeated exposure to relational trauma memories, triggered by his or her connection with the therapist, in combination with the reliable nonreinforcement and counterconditioning of his or her negative expectation and feelings

by the therapeutic relationship, leads to a disruption of the learned connection between relatedness and danger.

Although attachment activation and processing probably occur in similar ways for children and adolescents, clearly there are differences, as reflected in ITCT-C and ITCT-A. Perhaps most significantly, although the therapist may encourage the adolescent to form a bond with him or her that can trigger relational cognitions and affects, more caution is warranted in work with younger children. This is because the child's greater psychobiological drive to seek out primary attachments may cause him or her to become strongly engaged with, and dependent on, the clinician, only to experience attachment loss when the therapy ends and the relationship terminates. ITCT-C therefore encourages some level of attachment, but focuses more on improving the parent–child attachment connection primarily by working with the parent(s) or caretaker(s) to increase the quality of his or her relationship with the child, as noted in the later section on caretaker interventions. This is not always easy; the parent may have attachment issues of his or her own and/or may have other psychiatric, social, or relational difficulties that interfere with his or her capacity to be empathically attuned to, and supportive of, the child. In contrast, the therapist may be a much more compelling attachment target for the child, even though this connection is inevitably short-lived. This balance between providing positive connections for the child and allowing some level of therapeutic attachment activation—and yet not replacing the parent or caretaker in the primary attachment role—is one of the challenges of working with traumatized and/or neglected children.

Interventions for Identity Issues

Less described in many child or adolescent therapies, but still important, is the child or youth's capacity to access a stable internal sense of self, so that he or she can self-soothe at times of stress, perceive entitlement to personal well-being, discern boundaries, address appropriate needs, and experience self-efficacy. Yet, abused and neglected children often suffer from inadequate mirroring and attunement from their primary caregivers that limit their self and identity development. As suggested by recent neurobiological research (see Schore, Chapter 1, this volume) and the related attachment perspective, the need to dissociate or otherwise avoid trauma-related distress early in life may block the child's awareness of his or her internal state at the very time that a sense of self develops in children (Briere & Lanktree, 2011). Further, the hypervigilance needed by the endangered child in order to ensure survival may mean that much of his or her attention is directed outward—a process that detracts from internal awareness and is likely to result in decreased self-knowledge. ITCT seeks to reverse these processes in several ways.

PROVIDING RELATIONAL SAFETY

Introspection and self-exploration, which are thought to increase internal awareness, can occur only when the external environment does not require vigilance but instead provides mirroring and support. For this reason, the ITCT therapist especially endeavors to provide psychological safety and security in the session, both by providing a nonauthoritarian and supportive environment and by carefully avoiding criticism, rejection, judgment, or punitive responses.

SUPPORTING SELF-VALIDITY

The ITCT therapist should strive to visibly accept the child or adolescent's needs as intrinsically valid. Although his or her behavior may be problematic in some instances—for example, involving self-endangerment or aggression toward others—the client's underlying right to be happy and to meet his or her needs is reinforced by the therapist as entirely appropriate. As therapy facilitates increasing self-exploration and self-reference, the client may be able to gain a greater sense of identity, including greater self-knowledge and perceived self-worth.

SUPPORTING SELF-ACTUALIZATION VERSUS SOCIALLY BASED DEVALUATION

It also may be important to encourage discussion of the older child's or adolescent's beliefs, experiences, and perceptions regarding gender, cultural background, sexual orientation, and other sociocultural issues as they apply to him or her. Such interchanges ideally support the client's self-determination and self-acceptance and potentially negate cultural stereotyping or discrimination. Ultimately, the therapist's consistent and ongoing support for introspection, self-exploration, and self-identification allows the traumatized child or adolescent to develop a more articulated and accessible internal sense of self, beyond symptom resolution.

Family Therapy

Family therapy is conducted in ITCT when the client is not overwhelmed with posttraumatic symptoms and his or her caretaker(s) have the potential to be supportive. Primary foci for family therapy are *effective communication, appropriate caretaking* (including safety and protection of the child and age-appropriate expectations), *affect management, boundaries* and *roles,* and *attachment/relationship issues,* as well as *parental empathy, support, and emotional attunement.*

The ITCT family therapy module is loosely structured and provides guidance for sessions that can be conducted on a weekly or biweekly basis, following a course of individual therapy or in conjunction with individual therapy and collateral sessions. As with individual therapy in ITCT, the specific needs of the family are evaluated to determine the course and duration of treatment. When possible, all members of the family are included, with the exception of those who have been sexually abusive, physically dangerous, or are not currently able to contribute positively to the therapeutic process. Comprising a minimum of six sessions, this ITCT module includes assessment of family functioning and setting the goals of family therapy, facilitation of effective communication and expression of feelings, discussion of roles and boundaries, exploration of trauma exposures, enhancement of family relationships, and further trauma processing. During ongoing family therapy, additional issues may also need to be addressed, including cultural factors that contribute to identity and communication issues, the need to broaden the family's social network, and issues arising from foster placements.

Interventions with Caretakers

Whenever possible, ITCT involves the child or adolescent's parents or caretakers in treatment. Interventions are focused on increasing the youth's access to familial support, healthy attachments, and a positive parenting environment. It is also important to provide an opportunity for parents/caretakers to become aware of their reactions to their child's trauma, as well as their own histories of trauma, loss, and attachment issues. Collateral sessions with caretakers involve some combination of support, parent skills development, psychoeducation on abuse and the child/adolescent's response to it, and general developmental issues. Caretaker groups generally are held for 12 weeks and address issues associated with child maltreatment, the dynamics of abuse and abusers, parenting issues and strategies, coping skills and self-care, families of origin, trauma narratives, gender and cultural identity issues, attachment relationships, and intimacy/sexuality.

Group Sessions

ITCT group therapy modules include caretaker groups (parent education, skills development, and support), sexual abuse groups that complement or follow individual therapy, and group therapy sessions focused on other trauma, such as community violence, parental substance abuse, and/or domestic violence. As described in Briere and Lanktree (2011) these latter groups usually take place over 8–12 weeks and can be conducted in school or clinic settings.

An Example of ITCT Components in a Hypothetical Case

The following case is adapted from material presented in Briere and Lanktree (2011). Trauma histories and clinical presentations have been combined across multiple individuals, and the client's demographics have been altered. This is an example only; it is not meant to represent the average response to ITCT.

Athena is a 15-year-old Asian-Hispanic American female, referred for ITCT-A by her school counselor following an incident of drunkenness and suicidal threats at school. She was removed from her biological mother's care at age 6, after disclosing ongoing physical abuse and neglect, and was subsequently adopted by a European American couple. Athena had visitations with her biological mother on a monthly basis until age 9, later reporting that these times were chaotic and involved angry, verbal tirades and physical violence. Contact with her biological mother now occurs by phone only, given the chaotic nature of their relationship and her mother's continuing potential for abuse.

At intake, Athena reported chronic depression, low self-esteem, weight problems, and interpersonal conflicts, as well as long-term abuse of cold medication, alcohol, and marijuana. She acknowledged that substance use was more likely to occur when she was in the presence of older male friends and has led to several unprotected sexual encounters.

Following the intake interview, psychometric assessment, and collateral data collection, Athena was rated on the ATF-A as having a number of treatment targets. Her progress can be seen in reduced ratings at 3 and 6 months (see Figure 8.1).

After consulting the PCG, Athena's therapist began with an initial focus on establishing a positive therapeutic relationship. Because Athena's primary abusive figure was her biological mother, she had significant problems forming a trusting relationship with her female therapist. However, over a period of months she was able to be more open and disclosing in treatment and began to respond to the clinician as a benign, even helpful, person. Her therapist also worked with Athena on safety issues, including suicidality, substance abuse, and ways she might reduce her sexual behavior, or at least make it safer in terms of disease and pregnancy risk, and taught Athena the breathing exercise described in Briere and Lanktree (2011). Although she was willing to problem solve around sexual risk, she stated that her substance abuse was necessary for her ongoing functioning. Because her adoptive parents were attuned and supportive in their relationship with Athena, no caretaker or family therapy interventions were initiated at the beginning of treatment. However, they were periodically involved in therapy sessions, and ultimately in family therapy, focused primarily on reinforcing support and attachment connections and on facilitating better communication with Athena regarding her history and current concerns.

Athena spent considerable time in treatment recounting abuse experiences and "fights" she had experienced with her biological mother, although typically framing her maltreatment as deserved consequences for bad behavior. She also discussed conflicts and what appeared to be several coerced sexual experiences with peers while intoxicated. As per her abuse experiences, however, these were recounted as normal events or things

Client Name: *Athena*

Priority ranking (circle one for each symptom):

  1 = Not currently a problem: No treatment currently necessary
  2 = Problematic, but not an immediate treatment priority: Treat at lower intensity
  3 = Problematic, a current treatment priority: Treat at higher intensity
  4 = Most problematic, requires immediate attention
  (S) = Suspected, requires further investigation

Assessment period

Intake

Date:	7/12/11	10/22/11	1/15/12	_____
Problem area	Tx priority	Tx priority	Tx priority	Tx priority
1. Safety—environmental	1 2 **③** 4 (S)	**①** 2 3 4 (S)	**①** 2 3 4 (S)	1 2 3 4 (S)
2. Caretaker support issues	**①** 2 3 4 (S)	**①** 2 3 4 (S)	**①** 2 3 4 (S)	1 2 3 4 (S)
3. Anxiety	1 **②** 3 4 (S)	1 **②** 3 4 (S)	1 **②** 3 4 (S)	1 2 3 4 (S)
4. Depression	1 2 **③** 4 (S)	1 2 **③** 4 (S)	1 **②** 3 4 (S)	1 2 3 4 (S)
5. Anger/aggression	**①** 2 3 4 (S)	1 **②** 3 4 (S)	**①** 2 3 4 (S)	1 2 3 4 (S)
6. Low self-esteem	1 2 3 **④** (S)	1 2 **③** 4 (S)	1 **②** 3 4 (S)	1 2 3 4 (S)
7. Posttraumatic stress	**①** 2 3 4 (S)	1 2 **③** 4 (S)	1 **②** 3 4 (S)	1 2 3 4 (S)
8. Attachment insecurity	1 2 **③** 4 (S)	1 **②** 3 4 (S)	1 **②** 3 4 (S)	1 2 3 4 (S)
9. Identity issues	1 2 **③** 4 (S)	1 **②** 3 4 (S)	1 **②** 3 4 (S)	1 2 3 4 (S)
10. Relationship problems	1 2 **③** 4 (S)	1 **②** 3 4 (S)	1 2 **③** 4 (S)	1 2 3 4 (S)
11. Suicidality	1 2 **③** 4 (S)	**①** 2 3 4 (S)	**①** 2 3 4 (S)	1 2 3 4 (S)
12. Safety—risky behaviors	1 2 3 **④** (S)	1 **②** 3 4 (S)	**①** 2 3 4 (S)	1 2 3 4 (S)
13. Dissociation	**①** 2 3 4 (S)	**①** 2 3 4 (S)	**①** 2 3 4 (S)	1 2 3 4 (S)
14. Substance abuse	1 2 3 **④** (S)	1 2 3 **④** (S)	1 2 **③** 4 (S)	1 2 3 4 (S)
15. Grief	**①** 2 3 4 (S)	**①** 2 3 4 (S)	1 **②** 3 4 (S)	1 2 3 4 (S)
16. Sexual concerns and/or dysfunctional behaviors	1 2 **③** 4 (S)	**①** 2 3 4 (S)	1 2 **③** 4 (S)	1 2 3 4 (S)
17. Self-mutilation	**①** 2 3 4 (S)	**①** 2 3 4 (S)	**①** 2 3 4 (S)	1 2 3 4 (S)
18. Other:	1 2 3 4 (S)	1 2 3 4 (S)	1 2 3 4 (S)	1 2 3 4 (S)
19. Other:	1 2 3 4 (S)	1 2 3 4 (S)	1 2 3 4 (S)	1 2 3 4 (S)

FIGURE 8.1. Completed ATF-A for Athena.

she had precipitated. Although generally dismissive of the impact of these traumas, Athena eventually admitted to recent nightmares of being sexual assaulted. The clinician was supportive of Athena's trauma disclosures and communicated caring and concern when appropriate. At the same time, however, she avoided expressing agreement with Athena's belief that she had caused or deserved physical, sexual, or psychological maltreatment.

By assessment period 2 (12 weeks), Athena reported a reduction in sexual risk taking, generally by avoiding males with whom she had previously "partied." This also reduced her experience of relational conflict, since she was no longer subject to the emotional chaos associated with this behavior. Although the therapist doubted that merely avoiding males was a lasting solution, she was encouraged that Athena's current environment was physically safer. Athena also reported a decrease in depression and an increase in self-esteem, seemingly due to her growing attachment to the therapist, and a slightly increased sense of hope for her future. She denied any suicidal thoughts, plans, or impulses. She disclosed, however, that she was a bit more irritable with her adoptive mother and more likely to become angry over small things in general. This was normalized by the therapist as potential evidence that she was getting more in touch with her feelings, "because, actually, you've got things that you have a right to be mad about."

In the next 3 months, the clinician introduced the cognitive processing component of ITCT-A. Athena began to formally explore her negative views of herself and their probable basis in her birth mother's psychological and physical maltreatment of her. Early in this process, she defended her biological mother to the therapist, although the clinician was not, in fact, criticizing Athena's birth mother—instead affording her the opportunity to "go back" and recall what had happened when she was young, how she interpreted it then, and what she thought about it now. During this cognitive component, Athena frequently became emotionally upset and required help with grounding and doing the breathing exercise. Also introduced was the trigger identification and intervention component of ITCT-A, although this was initially difficult because Athena was unable to identify triggered emotional and cognitive responses as such. Eventually, however, she began to embrace this component, especially in terms of the increased behavioral control it afforded her. She began a healthier relationship with a boy she met at school, although this was associated with a greater awareness of being triggered in close relationships.

As shown in the third column of Figure 8.1, Athena continued to improve by the end of 6 months, with decreased ATF ratings on depression, anger, low self-esteem, risky behaviors, posttraumatic stress, and, surprisingly (given her refusal to discuss this issue), substance abuse. She continued to rate higher on relationship problems, substance abuse, and sexual concerns.

Athena remains in therapy, and her therapist expects that she will require a number of additional sessions. She is now more directly undergoing titrated exposure, focused primarily on her physical and psychological abuse history, but also on her prior sexual maltreatment by peers. The combination of her new relationship and growing attachment to her therapist appears to be stimulating more issues around attachment and abandonment. In addition, as she becomes less emotionally avoidant, she is verbalizing more distress about her life, past and present. Nevertheless, Athena reports these changes as evidence of continuing improvement.

Conclusion

ITCT is a multiversion, multicomponent treatment approach to the problems and symptoms experienced by traumatized children and youth. Although relatively structured, it can be adapted to the specific developmental level, symptoms, capacities, and cultural milieu of each client, and is not limited to a specific number of sessions. Repeated assessment is stressed in this model, allowing for "midcourse corrections" as the child's symptoms and problems change over time. Although the components of ITCT include cognitive, behavioral, and affect regulation interventions, a core focus is the therapeutic relationship and the remediation of attachment-level difficulties. Preliminary treatment outcome data indicate substantial effects of this treatment package on a sample of socially marginalized, multitraumatized children and adolescents.

References

American Psychiatric Association. (1980). *Diagnostic and statistical manual of mental disorders* (3rd ed.). Washington, DC: Author.

Berliner, L. (2005). The results of randomized clinical trials move the field forward. *Child Abuse and Neglect, 29,* 103–105.

Bowlby, J. (1988). *A secure base: Parent–child attachment and healthy human development.* New York: Basic Books.

Briere, J. (1996). *Trauma Symptom Checklist for Children (TSCC).* Odessa, FL: Psychological Assessment Resources.

Briere, J. (2002). Treating adult survivors of severe childhood abuse and neglect: Further development of an integrative model. In J. E. B. Meyers et al. (Eds.), *The APSAC handbook on child maltreatment* (2nd ed., pp. 175–202). Newbury Park, CA: Sage.

Briere, J., Hodges, M., & Godbout, N. (2010). Traumatic stress, affect dysregulation, and dysfunctional avoidance: A structural equation model. *Journal of Traumatic Stress, 23,* 767–774.

Briere, J., & Lanktree, C.B. (2008). *Integrative treatment of complex trauma for adolescents (ITCT-A): A guide for the treatment of multiply-traumatized youth.* Long Beach, CA: MCAVIC-USC, National Child Traumatic Stress Network, U.S. Department of Substance Abuse and Mental Health Services Administration.

Briere, J., & Lanktree, C. B. (2011). *Treating complex trauma in adolescents and young adults.* Los Angeles, CA: Sage.

Briere, J., & Scott, C. (2012). *Principles of trauma therapy: A guide to symptoms, evaluation, and treatment* (2nd ed.). Thousand Oaks, CA: Sage.

Brown, L. S. (2009). *Cultural competence in trauma therapy: Beyond the flashback.* Washington, DC: American Psychological Association.

Cloitre, M., Stovall-McClough, K. C., Nooner, K., Zorba, P., Cherry, S., Jackson, C. L., et al. (2010). Treatment for PTSD related to childhood abuse: A randomized controlled trial. *American Journal of Psychiatry, 167,* 915–924.

Cohen, J. A., Mannarino, A., & Deblinger, E. (2006). *Treating trauma and traumatic grief in children and adolescents.* New York: Guilford Press.

Cook, A., Spinazzola, J., Ford, J., Lanktree, C., Blaustein, M., Cloitre, M., et al. (2005). Complex trauma in children and adolescents. *Psychiatric Annals, 35,* 390–398.

Courtois, C. A., & Ford, J. D. (Eds.). (2009). *Treating complex traumatic stress disorders: An evidence-based guide.* New York: Guilford Press.

Ford, J. D., & Cloitre, M. (2009). Best practices in psychotherapy for children and adolescents. In C. A. Courtois & J. D. Ford (Eds.), *Treating complex traumatic stress disorders: An evidence-based guide* (pp. 59–81). New York: Guilford Press.

Grisso, Y., Vincent, G., & Seagrave, D. (Eds.). (2005). *Handbook of mental health screening and assessment for juvenile justice.* New York: Guilford Press.

Kinsler, P. J., Courtois, C. A., & Frankel, A. S. (2009). Therapeutic alliance and risk management. In C. A. Courtois & J. D. Ford (Eds.), *Treating complex traumatic stress disorders: An evidence-based guide* (pp. 183–201). New York: Guilford Press.

Lambert, M. J., & Barley, D. E. (2001). Research summary on the therapeutic relationship and psychotherapy outcome. *Psychotherapy, 38,* 357–361.

Lanktree, C. B. (2008, August). *Cultural adaptations to complex trauma treatment with children and adolescents.* Paper presented at the annual meeting of the American Psychological Association, Boston, MA.

Lanktree, C. B., & Briere, J. (1995). Outcome of therapy for sexually abused children: A repeated measures study. *Child Abuse & Neglect, 19,* 1145–1155.

Lanktree, C. B., & Briere, J. (2008). *Integrative treatment of complex trauma for children (ITCT-C): A guide for the treatment of multiply-traumatized children aged eight to twelve years.* Long Beach, CA: MCAVIC-USC, National Child Traumatic Stress Network, U.S. Department of Substance Abuse and Mental Health Services Administration.

Lanktree, C. B., Briere, J., Godbout, N., Hodges, M., Chen, K., Trimm, L., et al. (2012). Treating multi-traumatized, socially-marginalized children: Results of a naturalistic treatment outcome study. *Journal of Aggression, Maltreatment and Trauma, 21,* 813–828.

Perez, M. C., & Fortuna, L. (2005). Psychosocial stressors, psychiatric diagnoses and utilization of mental health services. *Journal of Immigrant and Refugee Services, 3,* 107–124.

Singer, M. I., Anglin, T. M., Song, L. Y., & Lunghofer, L. (1995). Adolescents' exposure to violence and associated symptoms of psychological trauma. *Journal of the American Medical Association, 273,* 477–482.

van der Kolk, B. A. (2005). Developmental trauma disorder: Toward a rational diagnosis for children with complex trauma histories. *Psychiatric Annals, 35,* 401–408.

CHAPTER 9

Dissociation-Focused Therapy

Sandra Wieland
Joyanna Silberg

Dissociation often emerges as a physiologically based coping mechanism when a primary caregiver is grossly inconsistent and unavailable to an infant or young child and when other traumas occur during development (Putnam, 1997). Repeated or chronic traumas—being faced with abandonment/neglect, chaos, inconsistency, and direct sexual, physical, and/or emotional abuse—make it necessary for children to protect themselves. Dissociation is a psychophysiological process that can protect children facing overwhelming emotions, body sensations, and/or knowledge of those experiences by enabling them to split off and separate these reactions from conscious awareness (see Schore, Chapter 1, this volume). This splitting-off process, however, can lead to an unstable and unreliable sense of self, of the world, or of others that, over time, can lead to fragmentation of the child's identity.

The current chapter discusses the various levels of dissociation that may occur in children who have experienced developmental and other forms of trauma and their dissociative symptoms. We trace the development of awareness of dissociation within the mental health community and describe the process of dissociation in terms of neurological and other conceptual frameworks. We explain why, when treating traumatized children, it is important to apply a therapeutic approach that identifies dissociation and gradually ameliorates entrenched dissociative patterns. A case study of a child with a dissociative disorder is used to illustrate these concepts.

Levels and Symptoms of Dissociation

Normative dissociation, such as getting absorbed in a video game or driving to work without being aware of the route taken, is a common phenomenon in both children and adults. Dissociation is quite different and less normative, however, when it is used to escape awareness of feelings and sensations associated with traumatic experiences, events, exposures, and environments. Originally, it may occur spontaneously in children as a psychophysiological response to repeated circumstances of fear, threat, and insecurity. Over time and in the face of ongoing danger, its use may become automatic, nonvoluntary, and progressive. Although its use is initially protective, it can become problematic and pathological when overgeneralized and applied outside of its original context, when it becomes automatic in response to cues associated with the unresolved trauma, and when it extends into adulthood. Although the sensations, feelings, knowledge, and learned behaviors resulting from overwhelming events may be blocked from conscious awareness, they are encoded neurologically and somatosensorily (Schore, 2003; van der Kolk, 2005). When an infant/child is traumatized and does not receive needed attention and consistent caring, soothing, and response, he or she must find other ways to cope and to self-soothe. Over time and while under ongoing states of duress without protection from harm, the traumatized child develops separated-off segments of memory, knowledge, emotion, or patterns of relating that are internalized (van der Hart, Nijenhuis, & Steele, 2006). The self may no longer be "whole," and the dissociated memories and sensations may be perceived as not being under the control of the conscious and executive self (for more detailed description of dissociative states, see Wieland, 2011a; Silberg, 2013; Silberg & Dallam, 2009; van der Hart et al., 2006).

Mild Dissociation

When a child is experiencing a mild level of dissociation (a blocking of awareness of what is going on around him or her), other people may notice that he or she is "spacing out." This child may show extreme reactivity (high upset or total withdrawal) without any of the "in-between" states associated with normal emotional shifts. The child in such a state is often unable to identify his or her own environment, emotions, or body sensations. At other times, the child may experience strong emotions as taking over and may perceive that he or she has little ability to control behavior, particularly when angry. The child may have some elaborated imaginary friends who are used as protection and soothing in times of stress, but the child knows these are imaginary. The child may struggle with remembering recent or past events or school-related information, but can generally access needed information with prompting. The child is aware when frightening events are happening or have happened, and is generally aware of what he or she is doing and feeling.

Moderate Dissociation

From the outside, moderate dissociation in a child may look quite similar to mild dissociation—diffuse "spaciness," inattention, and difficulty naming feelings and sensations, on one hand, and overreaction on the other—to what appear to be innocuous situations. The child's reactions are incongruous; they do not fit the situation. The child may swing quickly between feeling states, for example, between excitement and hopefulness at one extreme and extreme discouragement or hopelessness at the other. The child may feel disconnected from the outside world—for example, feeling outside of an event watching it happen (depersonalization), or inside the event but perceiving it to be unreal (derealization). Depersonalization and derealization usually occur initially in response to a frightening or terrifying experience or event but then continue to occur in situations similar in some way to the original circumstance. The child with moderate dissociation may also report imaginary friends who are perceived as having lives of their own.

Extreme Dissociation

A child with extreme dissociation may have experiences of self as divided between different states or identifies that hold separate information, emotions, physical sensations, or experiences. There may be baby-like states that provide a sense of respite for the older child through regression. There may be frightened self-states in which the child remembers a trauma and is easily triggered into fear and terror responses, or angry self-states, during which the child lashes out and that often serve a defensive or protective function. The child may feel divided among several parts of self that experienced trauma at different ages—some at his or her present age and even, for some children, an older part that developed to cope with difficult situations and to parent and soothe the child "from the inside." These children with extreme dissociation often have significant memory gaps and difficulties (amnesia) for recent and past behaviors. If the child reports imaginary friends, he or she may perceive them as real and as sharing or taking over control of his or her feelings and behavior.

From the outside, the child's eye gaze, facial expression, voice tone, body position, way of interacting, and developmental level may shift so dramatically that the parent or teacher perceives a completely "different child." The child may become unresponsive to current surroundings for a period of time, ranging from several seconds to minutes to hours. At other times, the shifts are subtler and the parent or teacher is simply left with a sense that the child is not functioning normally or is highly labile or excessively moody. It may take little by way of triggering to set off responses of shutdown or overreactivity in this child, who may also demonstrate radically different interests, food preferences, skills, or levels of attachment at different times and in different states of self. There may be physical problems related to different areas of the body—pain, movement, lack of control—for which there are no medical causes or reasons and which may come and go (i.e., in the form of somatoform dissociation; Nijenhuis, 2009). Subjectively, these children may experience sudden shifts in internal experiencing, including hallucinatory symptoms such as hearing or being aware of different voices in the head. Some children may talk aloud to themselves using different voices and use different names for themselves. At different times they may insist that others use these different names. Additionally, the child may be amnesic, in a global or in more circumscribed ways, including for awareness of positive as well as distressing relationships and experiences.

Per criteria included in the DSM-5, when the child (or later the adult) retains awareness of other states or ways of feeling or being, he or she is likely to meet criteria for the diagnosis of other specified dissociative disorder (American Psychiatric Association, 2013). When the child or adult in one identity state is amnesic for experiences in other states and one or more states emerge to take executive control of the self, the child then meets criteria for the diagnosis of dissociative identity disorder (DID; American Psychiatric Association, 2013). The child may or may not give specific names or other defining attributes (age, gender, feelings) to these dissociated identity states in either diagnosis.

Children with trauma-based dissociative symptoms often present similarly to children with other childhood disorders, in ways that can make differential diagnosis difficult. For example, the dazed looks and problems with attention and focus may be confused with the symptoms of attention-deficit disorder (ADD), or the child's dramatically shifting states and moods may resemble bipolar disorder. An out-of-context angry response to mild requests may look like bipolar disorder, oppositional defiant disorder, or conduct disorder. In fact, dissociative disorders may co-occur with each of these other disorders. It is essential in situations of comorbidity that dissociation be recognized, since the dissociation requires its own treatment—one that is specific and direct.

Recognition of Child Dissociation and the Need for Specific Therapeutic Interventions

Although the case of an 11-year-old child with extreme dissociation was described by Despine in 1840 (see McKeown & Fine, 2008), it was not until the 1980s that clinicians and researchers began to address this phenomenon of dissociation in children. Kluft (1984) hypothesized that dissociation in adults was a function of childhood trauma and would, therefore, have originated in childhood. Kluft also identified dissociation in some of the children of his adult patients and went on to successfully treat them using hypnosis, as he did with his adult patients (Kluft, 1984). In the late 1980s and 1990s, additional cases were reported in the literature (see review by Silberg & Dallam, 2009). Diagnostic measures—including the Child Dissociative Checklist (Peterson & Putnam, 1994), Children's Dissociative Experience Scale (Stolbach, 1997), Adolescent Dissociative Experiences Scale (Armstrong, Putnam, Carlson, Libero, & Smith, 1997), and the Adolescent Multidimensional Inventory for Dissociation (Ruths, Silberg, Dell, & Jenkins, 2002)—were developed for clinical practice and research. In 2004, dissociation was included in the guidelines for the treatment of child abuse released by the National Crime Victims Research and Treatment Center (Saunders, Berliner, & Hansen, 2004). More detailed guidelines for assessment and treatment of dissociative symptoms in children were released by the International Society for the Study of Trauma and Dissociation in 2004 (www.ISST-D.org). Developmental trauma disorder (van der Kolk, 2005), proposed for inclusion in the American Psychiatric Association's fifth revision of the *Diagnostic and Statistical Manual of Mental Disorders,* but ultimately excluded from it, includes dissociative symptoms as one of the common outcomes for children exposed to chronic attachment and other forms of interpersonal trauma.

Research demonstrates that dissociative symptoms are common in a broad range of adolescents in both clinical and nonclinical populations, including in delinquent youth (Carrion & Steiner, 2000), psychiatric inpatients (Brunner, Parzer, Schuld, & Resch, 2000), and girls with eating disorders (Farrington et al., 2002). Dissociative symptoms have been found to be strongly associated with sexual abuse (Trickett, Noll, & Putnam, 2011) and to be related to sequelae of chronic medical trauma and treatment, particularly when a painful procedure is employed and parents are involved in its implementation (Diseth, 2006). Child dissociation also has been found to be related to histories of disorganized attachment with primary caregivers, especially when early attachment problems, associated with chronic abuse and lack of caregiver response and protection, lead to ongoing fear and terror in the family (Ogawa, Sroufe, Weinfield, Carlson, & Egeland, 1997; see also Schore, Chapter 1, and Alexander, Chapter 3, this volume).

Understanding the way a traumatized child who dissociates may process information is a necessary first step toward developing a therapeutic approach. Deficits in right-brain cortical integration of sensory information are related to the development of dissociation and may leave the traumatized infant/child without an integrated sense of self (see Schore, Chapter 1, and Lanius et al., Chapter 2, this volume) and altered awareness of pain and visceral sensations (Bremner, 2009; Lanius, Bluhm, & Lanius, 2007; de Kloet & Rinne, 2007). Such neurobiological alterations are consistent with findings from research on early childhood interpersonal trauma and disorganized attachment (Schore, Chapter 1, and Alexander, Chapter 3, this volume). Liotti (2009) describes the shifting behaviors of the mother figure (comforting, needing comfort, hurtful–frightening, hurt–frightened), which place the child in the opposing positions of being comforted, having to comfort, being hurt or frightened, and creating hurt or fright. These shifting relational stances characteristic of disorganized attachment can lead to the fragmented information processing and self-fragmentation seen in dissociative children. Similarly, Putnam (1997) described how traumatized children may not develop integrated behavioral states that occur as a consequence of healthy development. Instead, these children show discrete (rather than continuous) behavioral states—sometimes from the time of infancy—that connote fragmented experience and information processing. These observations are consistent with the structural model of dissociation (van der Hart et al., 2006): When trauma is repetitive and severe, fundamental divisions of the self may occur that make it increasingly difficult for the child to maintain personal integration or integrated awareness of self or others.

Similarly, but with a focus on the integrative role of emotion in information processing and adjustment, Silberg (2013) proposes that overwhelming affect during early life trauma disrupts the development of the psychobiological affect regulation system. In order to eliminate what is overwhelming, the traumatized child seeks to avoid arousal and affect. With continued trauma, these avoidance responses become triggered by the many stimuli that serve as trauma reminders. Disssociative responses are understood as the initiation of automatic avoidance processes of behavior, identity, and affect that take over functioning without the child's central awareness in response to reminders of trauma (Silberg, 2013).

Dissociation-Focused Therapy as Integral in Treatment of Complex Traumatic Stress

A sequenced model of treatment, usually organized in three stages, has been suggested for complex trauma resolution in both children and adults, involving phases of (1) safety, stabilization, and strengthening; (2) trauma processing; and (3) reconnecting with the world (Herman, 1992). Such sequencing has recently received support from a survey of a cohort of identified experts in the treatment of complex and more standard forms of PTSD in adults, (Courtois, Ford, & Cloitre, 2011), a finding that is applicable to the treatment of children and adolescents. The importance of the identification and treatment of dissociation in each stage is increasingly recognized. Without attention to dissociation, treatment may be beneficial but will not be complete, all too often leaving the child (and later the adult) with unresolved split-off emotions sensations, behaviors, thoughts, or states of awareness (Silberg, 2013). When children or teens are not treated for disso-ciation, they are more vulnerable to further dissociation, particularly, when faced with traumatic reminders or other difficult events and experiences in the future. Traumatized and dissociative children may not be able to fully experience the therapist, the therapeutic interaction, or themselves as a par-ticipant in therapy due to their ongoing fragmentation. This too makes it imperative to identify and treat dissociative processes.

Stage 1 Treatment

Stage 1 of trauma treatment starts with assuring that the child is living in conditions of safety with relatively secure attachment relationships, and with helping the child develop an internalized sense of safety as well. Over time, the information about present safety needs to be passed to all parts of the self when the child is highly dissociated (see Silberg, 2013; Wieland, 2011a). At this stage the therapist might engage the child in drawing, play, or conversation that begins to elicit and assess his or her use of dissocia-tion and the extent of the dissociative process. For example, the child can be asked to draw a self-portrait wherein conflicting parts of the mind are illustrated, or the child can be assessed in play and conversation for evi-dence of dissociation.

Education about dissociation for both the child and the parent needs to occur early in the first stage of treatment (Silberg, 1996). For children, dolls or toys with multiple parts, and for adolescents, diagrams as well as draw-ings, can be used as a therapist explains how children use dissociation as a means of self-protection when frightened or hurt. During the educational process, the therapist can describe the dissociated parts of the self using child-friendly language, such as "your feelings talking to you" or "your reminder voice about bad things that happened" (Silberg, 2013). The therapist offers information about the "internal wisdom" of dissociation as a means of self-protection in times of danger but also emphasizes that dissociation can create problems in daily life when the feelings or states "pop out" and take over out of context and out of the individual's control. This begins discussion about a primary goal of treatment, which is to lessen the use of dissociation, and sets the stage for collaborative work throughout the therapy.

The therapist and child, hopefully with the assistance of the parent or other caretaker, can start to identify those aspects of the child's feelings or self that relate to past traumatic events, and recognize when they emerge in the present and seem to take over. For the child with DID, attention should be given to when a particular part came into being, what label or name the child has for the part, and its function within the child's self-regulatory and self-protection system. The theme right from the beginning of therapy is *not* that dissociated feelings or parts are bad or should be eliminated or avoided but that the child needs to recognize and thank them for the help they gave during the time of trauma, listen to the feelings or distress they express or hold, and give them a new role (as helpful feelings or parts of the child's self) within the safe (or safer) world in which the child is presently living. The therapist helps the child move toward increased self-awareness by asking him or her to "listen inside," draw pictures, or write or talk to other parts of the self that have been identified and thus to accept them.

As the child, parent, and therapist identify when and how these parts of self or dissociative states developed and now emerge, they can start to identify the situations or feelings that trigger and elicit each particular state. Thus, a critical part of this first stage of therapy is the identification of triggers and then helping the child learn to separate a trigger associated with past traumatic event (e.g., an abuser raising his voice) from an event in the present that has similar elements (e.g., a teacher raising her voice). The differentiation of past from present and of danger from safety is emphasized and reinforced throughout the treatment. Throughout, the therapist needs to remember that, with the dissociative child, he or she may not be accessing, in treatment, the part(s) that experienced the trauma. It is only when those hidden parts of the child that feel and react to the trauma of the past, perceive that "now" is different, that the child can begin to feel truly safe. The therapist can invite the child to dialogue with dissociated states or express dissociated feelings, perhaps using drawings, play objects, or imagery, about the "now" world. The bilateral stimulation in eye movement desensitization and reprocessing (EMDR) may be used with this work to support the internal conversations (Gomez, 2013; see also Wesselmann & Shapiro, Chapter 11, this volume).

Another important aspect of the first stage of therapy is stabilization—of both the child's internal reactivity and of the chaotic aspects of his or her world. Various methods can be used to help the child learn to identify his or her emotions and regulate overreactivity or dissociative shutdown. For example, the child can learn to breathe slowly and to use breath to counter reactivity. He or she can learn to shift awareness by using exercises such as standing on one foot, rolling on a gym ball, or wrapping up in a blanket. The therapist can inquire (e.g., "I wonder . . . ") how this feels for the scared or the angry part of the child, and what he or she is feeling physically and emotionally. Shifting the child's attention to a dissociated part of the self or feeling helps the child to develop a more integrated central awareness (e.g., "What I am feeling that I hadn't noticed"). Those experiences, together with activities such as playing music and moving to different rhythms, can enhance the child's emotion regulation capacities (see Perry & Dobson, Chapter 13, this volume).

As these activities are conducted with one or both parents (or other caregiver), attachment bonds can be strengthened—a very important part of stabilization and the reinforcement of safety. Encouraging parents to hold and rock or gently massage their child, to talk about feelings and body sensations, to find opportunities to feed him or her and to increase eye gazing between them can increase the child's attachment security while simultaneously developing the skills needed for emotion regulation. Particularly important is helping parents become attuned to the child's experience and to maintain their attunement as they interact with the child (Hughes, 2009). Although parents are encouraged to understand their child's impaired self-awareness and defensive use of dissociation, they also are encouraged to help their child take responsibility for age-appropriate actions, even if the child believes that those actions were controlled by another part of self. They can empathize with the child over the dilemma of being forced to take responsibility for something he or she doesn't recall or didn't feel he or she could control, and how frustrating that must be. This kind of support and help in establishing a position of integrated awareness and responsibility can simultaneously reduce the child's distress and sense of helplessness and encourage association and awareness, thus reducing dissociation. Behavioral programs can be used to reinforce access to memory of behaviors carried out by dissociated part(s). Silberg (2013) discusses a clinical case in which a child earns access to an honors-level program at school for remembering the destructive behavior he engaged in at home, for which he had become anmesic due to dissociation. The child's internal integration was facilitated by highlighting awareness of his destructive behavior even when he was not in his angry destructive state.

Stage 1 therapy also includes helping a child learn to get out of dissociative shutdown states that may be evoked by traumatic triggers within and outside of the treatment setting. Some children may become unresponsive (eyes closed, shallow or rhythmic breathing, rocking) and have difficulty being aroused when in these states. Since these states may be a form of altered consciousness and self-hypnosis, the therapist can use gentle hypnotic imagery to suggest moving into safety and then awakening, ready to handle feelings in a new way. The therapist helps the child and family to identify the events or feelings (triggers) that precede the onset of these states in order for them to learn and practice new methods for handling feelings or solving what has seemed to the child to be irreconcilable conflicts or unacceptable emotions. They also are assisted in learning grounding skills to use with the child.

For many parents, the concept of dissociation is difficult to understand and accept. They may view their child as defiant, disobedient, unmotivated, selfish, unintelligent, or strange. Unfortunately, these labels or related diagnoses (e.g., oppositional defiant disorder, attention-deficit/hyperactivity disorder, bipolar disorder, or some other disorder) may have been used by other professionals. Attuning to the parents' desperation and anger may be the hardest part of the therapist's work with the child. Indeed, many of the parents (whether birth, foster, or adoptive) of children who dissociate may also be dissociative. As the therapist works with the parents, the therapist can discuss the parents' experiences that are similar to those of their child's, especially with regard to unresolved trauma and loss. The therapist also can stress the importance of parents addressing their own issues and, at times, help parents to make the decision to seek their own therapy.

Although the family is usually the primary and most important system in which a child functions, he or she is in contact with other systems as well, such as school, church, community programs, or protective services. The therapist can play an important role in helping key members in other systems understand dissociation. Explaining the dynamics of dissociation and providing suggestions for important adults in the child's life can help to stabilize the child's world and increase his or her sense of safety (Yehuda, 2011). Providing education on dissociation to protective service workers means that children will experience more appropriate support from case or investigative workers because the workers will better understand how dissociation can block a child's ability to disclose abuse or to maintain personal continuity (Waters, 2007; see also Bloom, Chapter 15, this volume).

Stage 2

There is no clear line between Stage 1 (safety) and Stage 2 (trauma processing) in this treatment, particularly when working with children. During the first stage of work, as triggers are identified and processed, there often is reference to the time of trauma and how the present is different from the past. As nightmares, intrusive thoughts, or flashbacks occur and are worked on through artwork, play, imagery, or conversation, bits of trauma are being processed. The strengthening of attachment relationships both in therapy and in the family helps promote the child's self-regulation skills, allowing trauma processing to begin. The revisiting of trauma may temporarily destabilize the child—something all parties should know ahead of time. A return to Stage 1 work, with its emphasis on safety, stabilization, and strengthening, may be necessary and should be expected and not seen as a treatment failure.

Regardless of the therapist's approach to trauma treatment, attention to the dissociated feelings, sensations, cognitions, experiences and/or self-states of the child is essential for the child to reconnect with all aspects of the self. Dissociation-focused therapy can be integrated with any approach for processing trauma with children. For some children, trauma scenarios emerge within play, art, or their conversation, and the therapist can begin with gentle reflection or inquiry to encourage connection to the trauma-related and dissociated emotions, body sensations, or internalizations (Silberg, 2013; Wieland, 1998, 2011a). For others, therapist-introduced activities such as metaphorical play activities (Marks, 2011), hypnotic-type interventions (Grimmick, 2011), time-line narratives (Wieland, 2011b), storytelling, and "listening inside" (Silberg, 2011) can help the child process and become less phobic of all aspects of the trauma. EMDR bilateral stimulation can be used during these activities (Gomez, 2013; Marks, 2011; Wieland, 2011b).

Moments of dissociation are likely to occur during trauma processing.

The child might deny the impact of the trauma ("I really didn't mind what happened"), show a glazed or suddenly angry or scared look, or display a sudden body shift or voice tone change. Each of these manifestations needs to be recognized by the therapist and acknowledged in order for that dissociated feeling state to be included within the therapeutic interaction. The therapist's acknowledgment of all feelings helps the child welcome contradictions or inconsistencies in him- or herself.

Therapists without a clear understanding of dissociation are likely to respond to those moments of dissociation by immediately grounding the child back to the present. This grounding may be appropriate if there is a possibility of anyone getting hurt or the child becoming overwhelmed. However, if there is no such danger, the child's dissociation can be used within the therapy. For example, the therapist can state: "I noticed a really scared look come in just briefly. What does that part of you want us to know or need from us now? What can you tell that part of you?" Whether through play, art, movement, or discussion, the therapist can gently guide the child toward facing and reconnecting memories, emotions, body sensations, and/or behaviors that have been disconnected from the child's central awareness. Simply regrounding the child in the present may paradoxically serve to reinforce dissociative strategies, rather than allowing the integration of dissociated experiences.

Although attending to dissociated feelings and self-states in therapy can be useful and productive, the child needs to learn that it is not a good idea to purposefully switch to other self-states as a means of avoiding or coping. For example, when anger is too overwhelming or appears at inappropriate times (e.g., during school, at the end of a therapy session), a therapist can assist the child to become grounded in the present (e.g., "Look at your hands—they are the hands of a 12-year-old, not a 2-year-old"; "Place your feet on the floor and push down with all the strength of a 12-year-old and feel yourself here in this room now"). Then it is important to provide a link to this emotion or self-state (e.g., "Let the frightened you, the 2-year-old you, know that we can look at that fright a little bit at a time [at our next session]—we will connect with this feeling, this part of you, again and listen carefully to all that needs to be said"; "Can the 12-year-old part of you look out through your eyes now and help you adjust to what you need to do now?").

Whereas explicit memories can often be addressed directly, implicit memories, encoded in somatosensory form during the early years of life as the result of relational and other forms of trauma, are often only partially accessible to conscious awareness. They may surface metaphorically through nightmares, repetitive or unusual play patterns, or art. They may be at the base of the child's fears or seemingly innocuous questions. They may be expressed through behaviors that are destructive toward self or others, that are developmentally inappropriate, or that are overcontrolling. Therapists need to be alert and sensitive to trauma indications in each of these areas. Making gentle inquiry into, and linkages between what the child does express—albeit nonverbally—and the early trauma is important. For example, the therapist might say: "I notice that you're holding the girl doll upside down over the edge of the doll house, and it reminds me of the time your mother told me about when she saw your father holding you as a baby over the railing of the balcony. What would that have been like for the 'little you?'" By highlighting the past in this way within a safe supportive setting, the therapist is able to help the child experience not only the trauma but also the feelings, sensations, and internalizations from the trauma and the realization that the trauma is in the past and has been survived. During all of this work, and particularly if and when new destructive behaviors emerge, the therapist needs to be alert to feelings or self-states that may still be hidden and that have not yet been revealed in therapy (Waters & Silberg, 1996). Gentle inquiry (see Marks, 2011; Silberg, 2011, 2013) can be used to evoke and support these dissociated states and facilitate safe forms of expression either verbally or nonverbally within the session.

Stage 3

Herman (1992) referred to the third stage of trauma therapy as "reconnecting with the world." In dissociation-oriented treatment, this stage is often referred to as "integration and moving on." Reconnection of the child with his or her dissociated states occurs bit by bit throughout the first two stages of therapy. Most children experience what is known as "spontaneous integration"—that is, parts of the self merge to the point where they are no longer perceived or experienced as separate. For children with more extreme dissociation, integration metaphors (e.g., ingredients mix together to make a delicious cake; soccer players work together to form a strong team) or rituals (e.g., all parts holding hands and walking toward and into each other) can be used to strengthen and reinforce the concept of integration (Waters & Silberg, 1996). As in the earlier stages of therapy, the dissociation-informed therapist is alert for, and comments on, any instances of disconnection that occur. The therapist talks with the child and parent about times in the future when the child may again experience dissociation and ways the parent can assist the child in dealing with threatening experiences without disconnecting self or aspects of the experience from his or her central awareness.

Working Clinically with a Child with Extreme Dissociation: The Case of Henri

Henri, a 6-year-old Haitian boy adopted into a Canadian family with two children (a girl of 9 and a boy of 6), strode into the therapist's (SW) office with a very "take-charge" attitude. His adoptive mom had briefly explained his history in a Haitian orphanage that included malnutrition, physical and sexual abuse, witnessing adults and children being killed, all capped off by the 2010 earthquake. Over his years in the orphanage, he had been visited from time to time by his birth parents, who had placed him there at 20 months of age due to their poverty. His adoptive mom explained that over the past year in Canada, Henri had often and suddenly become very angry and aggressive, making threats such as cutting off his brother's head. In contrast, when he was scared, he curled up and cried like an infant. At some points, he hit his head on hard objects and at others he closed down and would not talk to anyone. Although he stated that he wanted friends, he was often quite intimidating when with other children. These changes in behavior, the extreme levels of dangerous and frightened behavior, and the observed regression suggested dissociation. The adoptive parents completed the Child Dissociative Checklist (Peterson & Putnam, 1994), and the score of 20 was highly consistent with a dissociative disorder. His completion of the projective house–tree–person test (Buck, 1970) suggested that Henri had little sense of family and experienced contradictions within his world. For a house he drew the therapist's office building, for a tree he drew an apple tree that was "healthy" but that had no apples drawn on it, and for people he drew children who were "super-happy" but had no friends.

Following an assessment session, the first series of interventions included psychoeducation and preparing the child and family for the treatment. SW talked with both Henri and his parents about dissociation and how children use it to protect themselves when in conditions of threat and danger. SW explained that although certainly a part of Henri knew that he was safe in Canada, there were probably many parts of him that he had split off in order to survive past experiences, and those parts, because they were connected to the past, would not automatically know about the safety of the present. SW emphasized how both she and the parents would need to work together to help all the parts of Henri realize that he was now safe. SW also talked about how Henri's internal system—his brain and his body—would not have had enough calming and soothing experiences during those years in Haiti and how he might need more of the holding, rocking, and rhythmic and feeding activities of the sort they had given to their other children when they were young—while cautioning that these needed to be done in ways that were comfortable and acceptable to 6-year-old Henri. Such explanations help parents learn about dissociation and also emphasize how important their role is in the therapeutic process and in reversing the automatic use of dissociation.

The next goal was to work on stabilizing Henri's behavior throughout the day. As Henri created a volcano in the sand tray, his mother discussed his agitation at bedtime when he talks about his bad memories of Haiti. SW suggested they find another time of day for Henri to talk about them and for Mom to create a box (either real or imaginary) with a lock, into which Henri could put his disclosed memories. As Mom locked the box, she could remind Henri of his present-day safety in Canada and ask him to tell "the part of him that lived through the bad memories in Haiti" that he is now safe in a new family and new country. Then for bedtime, SW suggested that Mom create a song about Henri coming to Canada and doing safe things with his new family. SW also suggested engaging in some rhythmic activity after locking the box and utilizing a body massage at bedtime to help settle Henri.

These early interventions did not cause much change in Henri's "nasty" behavior at home. Henri continued being particularly nasty to his mother whenever she said "no" to something he wanted, telling her she was not keeping him safe and putting her down in front of others. SW suggested that whenever possible, Mom should sit with Henri after such behavior— first stating his name and her name and that he was safe with her; then naming his anger at her and wondering if the anger was because she was not there when he'd had to go to the orphanage, an unsafe and scary place, and that she wishes she had been able to bring him to Canada then. She should emphasize that he is now safe and that even the "angry him" is safe. Mom was particularly concerned that Henri's nasty and threatening behavior happened whenever she said "no" to him and that he was try-ing to manipulate her to get his own way. SW explained that, because of past trauma, Henri's nervous system was in continual high arousal and he was on "high alert." Most children get upset or frustrated (i.e., their stress arousal system goes up but stays within a manageable range) when their requests or demands are refused. For Henri, already in high arousal, the upset would put him over the top of the manageable range and out of control. The "out-of-control" feeling probably was a trigger for old experi-ences and resulting dissociation to the point of switching to another state. SW suggested that before she refuses requests or disciplines him for nega-tive behavior, Mom should talk to him quietly to remind him where he is and that he is safe. Calming and grounding need to happen *prior to* discussion of the event. Whatever regular consequences the parents use to curb negative behavior should then be used to communicate to Henri that he is responsible for all his behavior in the present, even behavior that he cannot remember engaging in (possibly due to dissociative amnesia). In this way, he is encouraged and reinforced in learning that all parts of him are responsible for his behavior.

Attuning to the child's anger is an important part of connecting with him or her. Once again the emphasis is that all parts of Henri are accept-able, as are all of his emotions. Because children who dissociate often "erupt" when they are made to do something they do not want to do, parents often experience them as manipulative—and, indeed, they seem manipulative. Explaining how trauma creates a state of hyperarousal and reactivity within the child's nervous system can help the parent understand what's going on and to feel less threatened or manipulated by the child.

The next important step is to help Henri recognize that he can accept and be grateful to the many parts of himself and to start exploring the angry, hateful feelings he has been expressing. A few sessions later, Mom brought in a picture Henri had drawn of himself with two sets of eyes, one set that loved Mom, and another set ("the inside eyes") that hated her. SW asked when he'd noticed the "hating Mom feeling," and he said when she tells him "no" or tells him to go take a bath or do things he does not want to do. SW noted how important that "hating feeling" was—how that feeling had helped him hate (and not take in) the bad things that had happened to him in Haiti. SW suggested that Henri and Mom could thank the "hating part" for helping Henri during his time in Haiti. Then SW asked if the "hating part" knew that he was safe now. Henri started talking about seeing people getting beaten and killed when he was in Haiti. SW thanked him for telling her about that. Although Henri had moved into trauma processing here, SW did not feel that enough work had been done on Stage 1 safety and stabilization to move further into that area.

SW continued psychoeducation with Henri and his parents about accepting his "angry parts" and feelings. When he came in and picked up the foam bat and started hitting the large gym ball (SW had explained to him previously that the bat could be used for expressing anger in a safe way), SW asked if he had been angry during the week. Henri replied, "No." When SW asked Mom, she told about his banging doors and also banging his head against the wall. When SW asked Henri if he remembered those incidents, he nodded but she noted that he was staring with a blank look in his eyes. SW picked up a play tree trunk that has six small animals inside it and noted that people are like the tree trunk with many different feelings or parts inside (Any toy or doll with multiple parts can be helpful when explaining dissociation to children). When frightening things happen, feelings like fear and anger can get so large that they cannot be kept inside, so they get shoved out when it is not safe to express them. Doing so makes it hard because the anger is "on its own" and doesn't have the "thinking part" to help it. SW asked Henri which animal would be the angry part of him; he pulled out the tiger. SW asked what that part would say. Henri did not reply but Mom mentioned that he talked everyday about killing people and that his threats scare the other children in their family. At this point Henri was lying on his stomach over the gym ball. SW gently moved the ball back and forth and said: "So much happened in Haiti, so much killing happened in Haiti. What happened there was really scary but those things don't happen here in Canada. Can you tell the 'angry Henri' and the 'little scared Henri' that those things don't happen here, now?" SW then suggested that Mom and Henri thank the "angry Henri" for helping him survive in Haiti and that perhaps the "angry Henri" could have a new job now, rather than that of threatening to hurt people. The movement of the ball helped provide calming for Henri's physiological system, thus helping Henri connect to what was being said.

The next week, Mom reported that displays of anger and talk of killing had receded as they thanked the angry part of Henri. She and Henri, however, had not been able to come up with a new job for the angry part. Mom explained that she had told the children that Dad's mother was very sick, and she had asked them not to talk to him about it. Henri had immediately gone to his dad and talked to him about Grandma, all the time with a grin on his face. SW asked Henri what this was like for him, having Grandma so sick—she wondered if he was feeling sad like he'd felt when he lost his birth family and angry that he might lose someone else. Henri picked up the trunk with animals. SW noted that lots of different feelings would have come up in him and asked which would be the angry feelings (Henri pulled out the tiger) and the sad feelings (Henri pulled out the raccoon). Henri then picked up the crocodile puppet and used the crocodile to ask Mom why he did not have front teeth. SW noticed the crocodile asking questions and wondered if the angry part's new job could be to ask questions. Finding a new job for negative feeling parts allows the child to integrate that part rather than trying to control or get rid of it. When working with young children, their play often tells us what will be useful. With older children, asking them for their ideas is helpful.

Henri's behavior improved considerably during the following weeks. Mom reported that he was asking lots of questions. Dad came to the session with Henri and talked about Henri not taking responsibility for his negative behavior. When his brother would ask Henri to stop teasing and chasing him, Henri would insist that he was just playing and deny doing anything wrong. Henri clearly remembered this behavior, so it did not appear to be dissociative—possibly it involved a lack of understanding on his part. More likely, Henri had wanted people to stop doing what they were doing to him in Haiti, but no one had stopped. SW set up a game of ball between Henri and Dad and had Henri call out "stop" from time to time. Dad would immediately stop. SW asked them to continue this game at home because it allowed Henri to experience being noticed, heard, and responded to. The game helped him experience power in a positive way, which in turn reduced the sense of helplessness he'd felt previously. When working with children who dissociate, it is important to remember that all negative behavior is not a result of dissociation. Learning alternative and healthier behaviors and developing empathy for self and others are important parts of the therapy.

In a later session, when Henri was creating objects out of plasticine, SW asked him what he was making. Henri showed her a ball with a face on it, saying that it was he. SW asked about the marks on the other side, and he said that was the robot. Henri explained that the robot took over his body when Mom said he couldn't do something, and that it was the robot who teased his brother. SW noted, "Yes, different parts, but just like they are both on the ball, they are both you, and you are responsible for whatever any part of you does." Two weeks later, Mom said that Henri was not teasing as much but was demanding things in a very nasty voice. SW asked about the plasticine ball. Henri found it, but the face part could not be seen. Henri redid the face as SW talked about how all the parts could work together to not be nasty. Henri said, "It is like a team," and he and SW talked about how players on a team need to work together to win a game.

In time, Henri's behavior settled considerably—enough to begin more direct processing of the trauma. Although bits of the trauma had come up during the first stage of therapy as Henri talked about memories and nightmares, considerable abuse and detail had not been disclosed or discussed. Mom and SW met to review what was known about Henri's past. SW then created a story of Henri's early years: early months in a caring family but without enough food, being left at the orphanage, undergoing sexual and physical abuse at the orphanage, being burned with cigarettes and hit with sticks, witnessing a child getting killed, experiencing the earthquake, being taken away and put onto a plane, and finally being met by strange people speaking a strange language who were to become his new family. For each trauma segment in the story, SW outlined the feelings, thoughts, and physical sensations that Henri would likely have experienced (adaptation of the story time line used by Lovett, 2005). After processing each trauma segment, SW included a positive element (e.g., his body still being healthy, not being killed). Since it was not possible (or advisable) to review the whole story in one session, it was important to give Henri a sense of survival, safety, and hope at the end of each session. SW would read the story of the negative experiences, adding the likely feelings, thoughts, and sensations. After each segment, SW would then ask Henri to play out what happened in the sand tray, draw a picture of it, or imagine it to encourage exposure to and processing of the experience. Mom, as Henri's safe person, would then read about the positive elements.

The next week, SW started the session by reading the story about when Henri was left at the orphanage and his witnessing a baby getting seriously hurt on his very first night there. As SW read about fear and thoughts that something bad might happen to him, Henri's mouth curled up. SW validated that his fear in the present was coming up from what had happened to him back then. SW mentioned the frozen body feelings that he likely would have had, and Henri stood very still. After SW, and then Mom, finished reading their parts, SW asked Henri what he would like tell the "little him" through drawing, using the puppets, or using the figures in the sand tray about what had happened. Henri stood completely still at the sand tray and did not answer. SW opened the cupboards with the miniatures; she took out a little child figure but Henri reached in and took out the baby figure. He then chose soldiers with guns and lined them up on the edge of the sand tray. "They're shooting! The baby's running!" SW noted to Henri that there was no plane among the miniatures and that one was needed to take the baby to Canada—whereupon Henri reached into the cupboard, took out the dragon, and, placing the baby on the dragon's back, flew the dragon to Mom, who took the baby in her hands and told the soldiers they could not come to Canada.

Henri then took out the superman figure and put him in the sand tray while saying that he was dirty and then cleaning him off. SW asked the superman figure to tell the baby that what happened in Haiti is over and that he is now safe. Henri then went over to Mom and said that he wanted to make a rainbow with markers. He labeled the black marker as *angry* and the brown one as *bored* (a word sometimes used for a dissociative state) and wanted to throw out those two markers. SW noted that they needed to keep them, along with all the other feelings, because they were very important, and when they were with the other colors/feelings, they would not take over completely, so they and Henri could be safe. When SW noted that it was almost the end of the session, Henri went over to the sand tray, climbed inside on top of the sand and curled up (his feet over the edge because he was too big to fit) and closed his eyes. "Yes, the baby Henri is safe here," SW acknowledged and then mentioned the end of the session again, but there was no response. Mom asked Henri if he would like her to carry him—no response. Mom picked Henri up and carried him out—his eyes never opened.

The trauma processing with Henri was similar to what would have occurred with other trauma-focused therapies—feelings, thoughts, and body sensations were included and then present safety was emphasized at the end. Dissociation-focused therapy allowed Henri—and all of the younger parts of himself—to know that the bad experiences of Haiti were over and that he was now safe. Attention to all feelings, including those that are negative (represented by the black and brown markers), was important. Henri's climbing into the sand tray at the end of the session signified that the younger part of him was present and absorbing a sense of safety. Mom's acceptance of, and response to, Henri's behavior enabled him to experience the present safety and security as both the 6-year-old and as the dissociated, regressed part of himself. Mom reported that Henri was very agitated and hyperactive the afternoon after this session but settled down afterward and did well over the weekend.

The next week Henri came in asking why he had to come to therapy, whereas his brother did not. Mom stated that therapy was to help him get better after all that had happened in Haiti. Henri went over to the doctor's kit and took out the stethoscope. He listened to his heart and then placed it on his forehead. SW asked if he was listening to the robot. Henri asked, "What robot?", and SW reminded him of the robot he had made on the plasticine ball that he had identified as the part of him that didn't do what Mom asked. Henri said that he could not hear any voice in his brain. SW mentioned that they were going to be continuing to talk about his story. At that, Henri again climbed into the sand tray but this time lay on his back rather than curling up. Mom and SW put a pillow under his head. Henri picked up handfuls of sand and let it run through his fingers during the part of the story where the children were hurt at the orphanage. As SW read, Henri started talking about being hurt, not liking being hit, and trying to make good choices but being forced to make bad ones. In the story, SW talked about Henri being so scared and so angry that he had had to not feel those feelings when he was being physically hurt in order to keep himself safe. Henri showed the place on his leg where he had been burned, and SW switched to that part of the story. The story ended with Mom reading to him about being in Canada and his body being healthy now. Henri climbed out of the sand tray and picked up an empty baby bottle from a collection of toy objects. As he pretended to drink from the bottle, SW talked about his letting the "baby him" know that he was now safe and in a new country. Henri talked about having had a bottle when he first came to Canada and how he had shared it with his Canadian brother. When SW noted that it was time to stop, Henri went over to the couch, climbed up, stretched out, and fell asleep—again Mom carried him out. Henri's report of hearing no voices in his head indicated a decrease in his dissociation. Henri's letting the sand run through his fingers was an indication of an increase in his emotional calming skills. Further, Henri engaged in the story, calmed himself with the bottle, and then linked the bottle to his early time in Canada. His falling asleep on this day was like the behavior of a toddler, rather than that of an infant.

Over the following weeks, the review of Henri's life story continued, always ending with an emphasis on the safety of his life in Canada. He continued to find activities that engaged the younger parts of himself. Sometimes SW would approach activities by asking, "How can we tell the 'baby you' about this?" and, at times, Henri directed the activity, as he did when choosing the bottle. Following these sessions, his behavior would be agitated for a day or so, but then he would calm down. For Henri, the third stage of therapy—integration of the trauma and moving on—seemed to occur spontaneously. His hostility toward Mom settled and his intimidating behavior toward others decreased and then disappeared. He would look at SW quizzically when she asked about the robot or the part that sometimes made bad choices. He seemed to find it entirely natural that he had a fully integrated set of feelings, thoughts, and actions, no longer split up into parts.

Conclusion

As the case of Henri illustrates, dissociation-focused therapy for children and adolescents with complex trauma histories begins with assessment and education about dissociation for the child and parent(s), in order to help them gain greater awareness and acceptance of the child's split-off or fragmented emotions and self-states. During trauma memory processing in Stage 2, the monitoring and incorporation of dissociated emotions and self-states enables the therapist to help the child develop an affective and cognitive understanding of past traumatic experiences and an increasingly integrated sense of self. This facilitates Stage 3: resolution of any remaining distressing emotion states and the resumption of healthy, integrated, psychosocial development. Addressing dissociation within any child psychotherapy model thus provides a basis for fostering the reintegration of split-off affects and self-states as well as the resolution of other sequelae of the exposure to, and experiencing of, complex traumatic stressors.

References

American Psychiatric Association. (2013). *Diagnostic and statistical manual of mental disorders* (5th ed.). Arlington, VA: Author.

Armstrong, J., Putnam, F. W., Carlson, E., Libero, D., & Smith, S. (1997). Development and validation of a measure of adolescent dissociation: The Adolescent Dissociative Experience Scale. *Journal of Nervous and Mental Disease, 185,* 491–497.

Bremner, J. D. (2009). Neurobiology of dissociation: A view from the trauma field. In P. F. Dell & J. O'Neill (Eds.), *Dissociation and the dissociative disorders: DSM-V and beyond* (pp. 329–336). New York: Routledge Press.

Brunner, R., Parzer, P., Schuld, V., & Resch, R. (2000). Dissociative symptomatoloty and traumatogenic factors in adolescent psychiatric patients. *Journal of Nervous and Mental Disease, 188,* 71–77.

Buck, J. (1970). *House tree person technique.* Los Angeles: Western Psychological Services.

Carrion, V. G., & Steiner, H. (2000). Trauma and dissociation in delinquent adolescents. *Journal of the American Academy of Child and Adolescent Psychiatry, 39,* 353–359.

Courtois, C., Ford, J., & Cloitre, M. (2011). Best practices in psychotherapy for adults. In C. Courtois & J. Ford (Eds.), *Treating complex stress disorders in adults: Evidence-based guide* (pp. 82–103). New York: Guilford Press.

de Kloet, E. R., & Rinne, T. (2007). Neuroendocrine markers of early trauma: Implications for posttraumatic stress disorders. In E. Vermetten, M. Dorahy, & D. Spiegel (Eds.), *Traumatic dissociation* (pp. 139–156). Washington, DC: American Psychiatric Association.

Diseth, T. (2006). Dissociation following traumatic medical procedures in childhood: A longitudinal follow-up. *Development and Psychopathology, 18,* 233–251.

Farrington, A., Waller, G., Neiderman, M., Sutton, V., Chopping, J., & Lask, B. (2002). Dissociation in adolescent girls with anorexia: Relationship to comorbid psychopathology. *Journal of Nervous and Mental Disease, 190,* 746–751.

Gomez, A. (2013). *EMDR therapy and adjunct approaches with children: Complex trauma, attachment, and dissociation.* New York: Springer.

Grimminck, E. (2011). Emma—from kid actress to healthy child: Treatment of the early sexual abuse led to integration. In S. Wieland (Ed.), *Dissociation in traumatized children and adolescents: Theory and clinical interventions* (pp. 75–96). New York: Routledge.

Herman, J. (1992). *Trauma and recovery.* New York: Basic Books.

Hughes, D. (2009). *Attachment-focused parenting: Effective strategies to care for children.* New York: Norton.

Kluft, R. P. (1984). Multiple personality in childhood. *Psychiatric Clinics of North American, 7,* 121–134.

Lanius, R., Bluhm, R., & Lanius, U. (2007). Posttraumatic stress disorder symptom provocation and neuroimaging: Heterogeneity of response. In E. Vermetten, M.

Dorahy, & D. Spiegel (Eds.), *Traumatic dissociation* (pp. 191–218). Washington, DC: American Psychiatric Association.

Liotti, G. (2009). Attachment and dissociation. In P. F. Dell & J. O'Neill (Eds.), *Dissociation and the dissociative disorders: DSM-V and beyond* (pp. 53–65). New York: Routledge Press.

Lovett, J. (2005, September). *Use of EMDR with traumatized children.* Preconference workshop presented at the 19th meeting of the Eye Movement Desensitization and Reprocessing International Association, Seattle, WA.

Marks, R. P. (2011). Jason—expressing past neglect and abuse: Two-week intensive therapy for an adopted child with dissociation. In S. Wieland (Ed.), *Dissociation in traumatized children and adolescents: Theory and clinical interventions* (pp. 97–140). New York: Routledge.

McKeown, J., & Fine, C. (Trans. & Eds.). (2008). *Despine and the evolution of psychology.* New York: Palgrave Macmillan.

Nijenhuis, E. R. S. (2009). Somatoform dissociation and somatoform dissociative disorders. In P. F. Dell & J. O'Neil (Eds.), *Dissociation and dissociative disorders: DSM-V and beyond* (pp. 259–275). New York: Routledge.

Ogawa, J. R., Sroufe, L. A., Weinfield, N. S., Carlson, E. A., & Egeland, B. (1997). Development and the fragmented self. *Developmental Psychopathology, 9,* 855–877.

Peterson, G., & Putnam, F. W. (1994). Further validation of the Child Dissociation Checklist. *Dissociation, 7,* 204–211.

Putnam, F. W. (1997). *Dissociation in children and adolescents.* New York: Guilford Press.

Ruths, S., Silberg, J. L., Dell, P. F., & Jenkins, C. (2002, November). *Adolescent DID: An elucidation of symptomatology and validation of the MID.* Paper presented at the 19th meeting of the International Society for the Study of Dissociation, Baltimore, MD.

Saunders, B. E., Berliner, L., & Hanson, R. F. (Eds.). (2004). *Child physical and sexual abuse: Guidelines for treatment.* Charleston, SC: National Crime Victims Research and Treatment Center.

Schore, A. (2003). *Affect dysregulation and disorders of the self.* New York: Norton.

Silberg, J. L. (Ed.). (1996). *The dissociative child: Diagnosis, treatment and management.* Lutherville, MD: Sidran Press.

Silberg, J. L. (2011). Angela—finding words for pain: Treatment of a dissociative teen presenting with medical trauma. In S. Wieland (Ed.), *Dissociation in traumatized children and adolescents: Theory and clinical interventions* (pp. 263–284). New York: Routledge Press.

Silberg, J. L. (2013). *The child survivor.* New York: Routledge Press.

Silberg, J. L., & Dallam, S. (2009). Dissociation in children and adolescents. In P. F. Dell & J. O'Neil (Eds.), *Dissociation and the dissociative disorders: DSM-V and beyond* (pp. 67–82). New York: Routledge.

Stolbach, B. (1997). The Children's Dissociative Experiences Scale and Posttraumatic Symptom Inventory. *Dissertation Abstracts International, 58*(03), 1548B.

Trickett, P. K., Noll, J. G., & Putnam, F. W. (2011). The impact of sexual abuse on female development. *Development and Psychopathology, 23,* 453–476.

van der Hart, O., Nijenhuis, E. R. S., & Steele, K. (2006). *The haunted self: Structural dissociation and the treatment of chronic traumatization.* New York: Norton.

van der Kolk, B. A. (2005). Developmental trauma disorder: Toward a rational diagnosis for children with complex trauma histories. *Psychiatric Annals, 35,* 401–409.

Waters, F. S. (2007). *Trauma and dissociation in children: I. Behavioral impacts. II. Issues for interviewing. III. Guidelines for prosecutors.* Nevada City, CA: Cavalcade Productions.

Waters, F. S., & Silberg, J. L. (1996). Promoting integration in dissociative children. In J. L. Silberg (Ed.), *The dissociative child: Diagnosis, treatment and management* (pp. 167–190). Lutherville, MD: Sidran Press.

Wieland, S. (1998). *Issues and techniques in abuse-focused work with children and adolescents: Addressing the internal trauma.* Thousand Oaks, CA: Sage.

Wieland, S. (Ed.). (2011a). *Dissociation in traumatized children and adolescents: Theory and clinical interventions.* New York: Routledge.

Wieland, S. (2011b). Joey—moving out of dissociative protection: Treatment of a boy with dissociative disorder not otherwise specified following early family trauma. In S. Wieland (Ed.), *Dissociation in traumatized children and adolescents: Theory and clinical interventions* (pp. 197–262). New York: Routledge.

Yehuda, N. (2011). Leroy—working with a dissociative child in a school setting. In S. Wieland (Ed.), *Dissociation in traumatized children and andolescents: Theory and clinical interventions* (pp. 285–342). New York: Routledge.

CHAPTER 10

Trauma-Focused Cognitive-Behavioral Therapy

Matthew Kliethermes
Rachel Wamser Nanney
Judith A. Cohen
Anthony P. Mannarino

An alarming number of children are exposed to traumatic events during childhood and adolescence (Finkelhor, Ormrod, & Turner, 2009). Unfortunately, many experience traumatic events that are both chronic and severe—that is, complex trauma. This type of trauma often begins early in life and occurs with such regularity that, for many children and later for adult survivors, coping with trauma becomes a "way of life." Further, the adversity often continues long after the direct traumatization ends, as family environments tend to be chaotic and unsupportive (Cook, Blaustein, Spinazzola, & van der Kolk, 2003). Unsurprisingly, the result of such complex traumatic histories is often severe and can lead to a variety of behavior problems that are best conceptualized as the result of dysregulation, the hallmark impairment associated with a history of complex trauma (van der Kolk, 2005). This chapter focuses on an evidence-based treatment, trauma-focused cognitive-behavioral therapy (TF-CBT; Cohen, Mannarino, & Deblinger, 2006) to address the needs of youth with both trauma-related symptoms and co-occurring behavior problems.

Research indicates that behavior problems are a common symptom after traumatic exposure (Cook et al., 2003; Spinazzola et al., 2005). Although the relationship between behavior problems and trauma is well established, it must be noted that not all behavior problems are trauma related. For many youngsters, behavior problems are the result of the traumatic event; these youngsters may act out as a result of a trauma trigger or an overactive stress response or alarm system (Ford, 2005). For others, the behavior problems precede the traumatic event and thus are unlikely to be a trauma symptom, although traumatic exposure can certainly exacerbate preexisting behavior problems. Some behavior problems are better conceptualized as originating from some other factor (e.g., ineffective parenting strategies, temperament, medical or brain conditions). Indeed, many children who experience or are exposed to traumatic events (especially those that are repeated and chronic) receive diagnoses of oppositional defiant disorder or conduct disorder (Ackerman, Newton, McPherson, Jones, & Dykman, 1998). Such behavior problems often drive treatment referrals and tend to become the focus of assessment, diagnosis, and treatment, with little or no awareness of, or attention to, the child's history of traumatic experiences and symptoms of posttraumatic stress disorder (PTSD). On the other hand, when children displaying problematic behavior are identified as also having PTSD symptoms, treatment for PTSD may not be successful unless the conduct or behavior problems receive significant attention in treatment (Cohen, Berliner, & Mannarino, 2010).

Co-Occurring Behavior Problems and the Implementation of TF-CBT

The presence of behavior problems is likely to disrupt engagement or progress in individual treatment until the traumatized child learns self-management skills and/or the problems that underlie the problematic behaviors are resolved. Additionally, treatment for children with complex trauma histories may be interrupted due to legitimate, yet often unexpected, crises (e.g., change in foster placement, expelled from school). The youth client may be unmotivated and disinterested in treatment, viewing the therapist as yet another authority figure who will judge, punish, or give up on him or her. The youth's caregivers may also be reluctant to engage in treatment especially if they feel "burned out," overwhelmed, or as if they have "tried everything and nothing works."

At the present time, the TF-CBT model is the most researched and best validated evidence-based practice for treating children and adolescents exposed to traumatic events (Cohen, Deblinger, Mannarino, & Steer, 2004). For some youth with behavior problems, the core components of TF-CBT are effective. However, adaptations may be needed for other youth with externalizing behavior problems (Cohen, Berliner, et al., 2010). This chapter first provides an overview of the generic TF-CBT model and then focuses on various adaptations to TF-CBT that have been developed to address the severe child behavior problems that often occur in the aftermath of complex trauma.

An Overview of TF-CBT

TF-CBT is a structured child and parent trauma-focused intervention model. Initial skills-based components (e.g., relaxation skills) are followed by more trauma-specific components; however, gradual exposure to trauma-focused material is incorporated into all components (Cohen et al., 2006). When possible, TF-CBT is conducted with children and primary caregivers in parallel individual sessions wherein both the child and caregiver complete the components, followed by additional conjoint child–caregiver sessions focused on the further consolidation of the knowledge and skills learned in the various components. The TF-CBT components were designed to build upon each other and should typically be completed in the order described by the acronym PRACTICE:

P: **Psychoeducation:** Information about trauma occurrence, impact, and recovery.
P: **Parenting skills:** Working with caregivers to develop effective behavioral management strategies to address trauma-related behavioral difficulties.
R: **Relaxation:** Helping the client and caregiver develop skills (e.g., focused breathing) to manage the physiological manifestations of traumatic stress.
A: **Affective expression and modulation:** Enhancing the child's ability to identify, express, and regulate emotions.
C: **Cognitive coping:** Helping the child and caregiver understand the relationship between thoughts, feelings, and behaviors.
T: **Trauma narrative and processing:** Helping the child and caregiver process memories of the child's trauma to facilitate desensitization to trauma reminders and the modification of trauma-related cognitive distortions.
I: **In vivo mastery of trauma reminders:** Helping the child and caregiver to overcome generalized fear associated with trauma triggers in their current lives.
C: **Conjoint child–parent sessions:** Joint child–caregiver activities to reinforce skills learned in prior components (e.g., practicing focused breathing together).
E: **Enhancing future safety and development:** Safety planning for the future and helping the child and caregiver integrate therapeutic gains into everyday life.

Determining the Appropriateness of TF-CBT

Prior to implementing TF-CBT, the clinician must conduct a comprehensive assessment of the client to determine his or her symptoms and the appropriateness of the TF-CBT model (Cohen, Berliner, et al., 2010). There are times when TF-CBT, even if applied flexibly, may not be feasible or clinically appropriate. This may be the case when behavior problems are extreme (e.g., significant self-injurious behavior or suicidal ideation or gestures, substance abuse, inappropriate sexual behavior, repeated running away from home, severe aggression, or illegal activities) (Child Welfare Information Gateway, 2007). This degree of problematic behavior may call for another strategy, such as parent–child interaction therapy (PCIT; Eyberg & Boggs, 1998), which was developed for younger children with serious externalizing problems and impaired parent–child relationships (see also Urquiza & Timmer, Chapter 17, this volume). With older clients, evidence-based therapies such as dialectical behavior therapy (DBT; Linehan, 1993) may improve youth's behavioral self-regulation (e.g., via mindfulness, distress tolerance), as well as facilitating trauma-focused work during the course of TF-CBT. If TF-CBT is conducted simultaneously with another treatment implemented by another therapist, it is important that both therapists coordinate with each other in order to enhance the synergy and effectiveness of their separate efforts.

The extent to which behavioral difficulties are related to trauma exposure or are due to other causes should also be evaluated. Although the client will likely benefit from the skills taught in TF-CBT, if the behavioral problems are associated with nontrauma-related causes (e.g., attention-deficit/hyperactivity disorder [ADHD]) it is likely that further treatment beyond TF-CBT will be required. During the assessment process, a time line that indicates when behavior problems started in relation to trauma exposure should be developed. Establishing this time line may be challenging in some cases as traumatic exposure may have begun very early in life. However, in these cases, it should be determined if the behavioral difficulties fluctuate in severity in relation to the presence of trauma cues or subsequent trauma exposure. Behavior problems that began or became more severe following a traumatic event are more likely be addressed effectively by TF-CBT than preexisting behavior problems that continue to be maintained by the youth's social environment.

Functional behavioral analysis (FBA; Cohen, Berliner, et al., 2010) therefore is an important strategy to include in the assessment. The basic premise of FBA is that behavior problems are generally triggered and maintained by conditions in the youth's environment. Conducting an FBA then involves studying the context in which the youth's behavioral difficulties occur in order to determine the events immediately preceding problem behaviors and the consequences that occur afterward, as well as the youth's response to these consequences. Completion of an FBA can assist the evaluator in determining if a behavioral difficulty is trauma related or due to some other comorbid condition (e.g., ADHD), or both. If it is trauma related, the information provided by the FBA can inform the implementation of TF-CBT. For example, the FBA may provide information regarding trauma cues present in the environment that are triggering behavior problems.

Using TF-CBT with Co-Occurring Behavior Problems

Structuring TF-CBT Sessions

Typically, the structure of a TF-CBT session involves dividing the time between the youth and his or her caregiver, with the exception of conjoint sessions involving both. Individual time spent with the young client tends to be divided into an initial "check-in" segment, followed by a period of work focused on the appropriate PRACTICE component, and concluded with a period of free time to allow the youth to transition from trauma-focused therapy to everyday life. There are several transitions during the course of a TF-CBT session, and since many youth with behavioral difficulties experience challenges during transitions, the therapist should attempt to minimize them by making the session structure explicit and consistent. It may be helpful to have a visual representation of the different segments of the session, or a kitchen timer that goes off when transitions are about to occur.

The sequencing of the TF-CBT session with the client and caregiver also is important. Often, the therapist meets with the caregiver first to check in on the youth's functioning during the past week in order to address these issues with the client in the subsequent individual work. This order can be switched as needed. For example, some young clients have difficulty transitioning from the waiting room to the office, especially if they have become engrossed in watching a movie or playing a game. In such a case, it might be prudent to meet first before they become absorbed in an outside activity. On the other hand, others may need some time to transition from the "outside world" into the therapist's office, and time spent in the waiting room may serve as a necessary buffer, reducing the likelihood of opposition when the therapist subsequently invites them into the session.

Fostering Engagement

Fostering engagement with a complexly traumatized client who has behavioral difficulties can be challenging (Kliethermes & Wamser, 2012). Beyond establishing rapport, the therapist must establish some degree of trust—the former can usually be accomplished rather quickly, but the latter may take longer. Since these clients are used to being criticized and punished (or worse) by adults in positions of authority, it is common for them to initially perceive the therapist as another hurtful adult authority figure. Prior to addressing problematic behaviors, then, sufficient trust needs to be developed. Therapists may have to pass "tests" of one sort or another to demonstrate that they are trustworthy, safe, and genuinely interested in the client's well-being. Engagement can often be accomplished by developing a therapeutic relationship explicitly based on respect, open sharing of information, empowerment, and the installation of a sense of hope (Pearlman & Courtois, 2005). Because there is "no short-cut to developing trust" (Briere, 2002 pp. 13–14), this stage of treatment may need to be longer than what would typically be allotted in TF-CBT. The therapist may spend up to eight sessions building engagement. During this initial phase, the therapist also should work actively toward stabilization, initiating contact with the other "systems," or other important adults in the youth's life, and address any safety concerns.

Because parents and other caregivers generally bring the youth to treatment, they are often the literal and figurative vehicles for change. Therefore, engaging them in treatment is critical. Behavioral difficulties tend to be more resistant to change in TF-CBT without caregiver involvement (Deblinger, Lippmann, & Steer, 1996). Understandably, due to the demands of parenting a child or adolescent with significant behavioral difficulties, caregivers are often frustrated, overwhelmed, and burned out. Many hope that they can drop off their charge at the therapist's office to be "fixed," much like a car taken to a mechanic. Therefore, they may not be receptive initially to parenting strategies presented by the therapist, or they may exhibit learned helplessness regarding their ability to change the youth's behavior (e.g., "Nothing works," "They just laugh at me when I give them a time out"). It is vital that the therapist normalize and validate the caregiver's experiences and avoid a stance that suggests that therapy "has all the answers." The therapist should also impart hope, stressing that by working together, there is a high likelihood of making significant behavioral changes.

Enhancing Future Safety and Development

Although this component is typically the last PRACTICE component discussed in trainings and papers, we have chosen to prioritize it with youth who exhibit externalizing behavioral difficulties. We have done so because this is also parallel to what commonly happens when implementing TF-CBT with this population. Severe behavioral difficulties often serve to compromise the safety/stability of the client or his or her ability to meet daily functional expectations. These concerns often have to be addressed immediately. For example, a 5-year-old may engage in sexualized behavior with other children in his or her kindergarten class. A 10-year-old may repeatedly run away from home and wander through an unsafe neighborhood when his or her parent/caregiver makes an attempt at discipline. A 16-year-old may drink alcohol or use marijuana daily to alleviate emotional dysregulation and distress. Targeting these behaviors cannot be postponed.

Addressing these safety concerns early in treatment usually involves the development of safety plans (e.g., identifying a safe person/place the 10-year-old can go if he or she decides to run away from home), working to replace potentially dangerous coping strategies with more benign strategies (e.g., teaching the 16-year-old mindfulness skills to replace substance use), and improving the child's problem-solving skills (e.g., teaching the 5-year-old to respond to urges to engage in sexualized behavior by stopping and thinking of other options such a seeking help from a trusted adult). Addressing safety concerns related to behavioral difficulties typically requires the involvement of caregivers and possibly other adults. The adults in the youth's life may need training to address unsafe behavior (e.g., implementing deescalation strategies, safety plans); to process their own reactions, fears, and concerns; and to address any problematic environmental factors such as lack of adequate supervision or support at home or at school.

Sporadic or ongoing safety concerns can emerge throughout the implementation of TF-CBT with these clients. Despite the best efforts of all involved parties, relapses occur. They can be particularly problematic if they occur during the trauma narrative component of treatment, at times making it necessary to temporarily discontinue this component in favor of safety and stabilization efforts. In this situation, the TF-CBT therapist may decide to revisit previously learned skills from other components (e.g., relaxation, safety planning, problem solving).

For example, it may be the case that the substance problems observed in the 16-year-old (mentioned above) decreased during the initial skill-building components of TF-CBT; however, after initiating the trauma narrative, the youth's substance problems reemerge, possibly even more severely than before. Subsequently, the therapist may consider discontinuing the trauma narrative until the substance use can be decreased to a more stable level. However, proceeding in this way is not ideal because it can significantly disrupt the gradual exposure process. The trauma narrative should therefore be suspended only as a last resort, and then in a thoughtful and collaborative manner. The therapist, youth, and caregiver should all agree to temporarily discontinue exposure for a specified number of sessions. During that time, efforts are directed at helping the youth cope more effectively with the situation and working with other resources (e.g., child protective services, schools, mentors) to reduce risk. When sufficient safety and stability have been established, work on the trauma narrative can resume.

Psychoeducation

In addition to information regarding the specific trauma the youth experienced, the youth and caregiver should be educated about the impact of stress and trauma on current functioning, particularly the impact of traumatic stress reactions and coping styles on behavior. Indeed, trauma-related behavioral difficulties need to be explicitly normalized and validated by explaining that they are an understandable outgrowth of chronic trauma exposure. The therapist can also define and discuss stress, common responses to stress and trauma, the adaptive function of stress responses (i.e., to alert an organism to the presence of potential danger), and common coping mechanisms (both healthy and unhealthy). The caregiver should be assisted in conceptualizing emotional and behavioral dysregulation as stress- and trauma-related responses in many instances, rather than as willful misbehavior.

Further, the concept of trauma triggers should be discussed because these youngsters need help in identifying (and wherever possible) avoiding triggers and changing their habitual fight–flight–freeze reactions (Briere & Scott, 2006). The therapist can also note that it is common for individuals who have been interpersonally traumatized to make adaptations in the way they interact with others to promote their own sense of safety and control. Time should be spent helping the client and caregiver identify the adaptive and maladaptive coping strategies the youth is currently implementing. Often, these strategies are intended as self-soothing or distracting, but they take the form of problematic behaviors such as substance abuse and aggressive or sexualized behavior. This discussion can effectively establish the rationale, and increase motivation, for working on the subsequent skill-building components.

Parenting Skills

Throughout treatment, the therapist models appropriate engagement and behavioral management strategies for the caregiver as a way to support his or her parenting and to teach both caregiver and client. As noted, these youth may not have a traditional caregiver, so for this population, the "parenting" component of TF-CBT often needs to be changed to the "systems" component, which includes a caregiver or authority figure who plays a significant role in the youth's life (Kliethermes & Wamser, 2012). The goal is to create a "trauma-informed" system of caregivers and professionals who understand that trauma-related behavioral difficulties are misplaced, excessive, unhealthy survival/coping responses.

Caregivers and other relevant adults should be assisted in developing appropriate engagement, deescalation, and behavior management skills to help reduce the occurrence of these trauma-related behavioral manifestations. These skills may include verbal praise, active ignoring, distraction techniques, contingency plans, consequences, and time-outs. Further, for younger children, the therapist may work toward increasing signals of care from the caregiver to facilitate the development of a stronger attachment between them, which can, in turn, help reduce behavioral difficulties. This component may also enhance the efficacy of later conjoint sessions in TF-CBT.

Some caregivers require extra support in developing positive parenting strategies such as effective engagement or deescalation strategies, the use of praise, and developmentally appropriate discipline strategies. In such instances, the therapist should model these strategies for the caregiver. Parenting or behavior management strategies that can easily be modeled during therapy sessions include the following: establishing "house rules"; giving effective directions; maintaining a calm demeanor when addressing problematic behaviors; and appropriately using time-outs, consequences, praise, and positive reinforcement. Detailed information regarding the development of these skills in caregivers can be found in a variety of sources, including the manuals of evidence-based practice (EBP) strategies explicitly designed to address behavioral difficulties in children. For example, PCIT provides detailed instructions on how to improve the caregiver–child relationship and improve the caregiver's ability to address the child's behavioral difficulties (see Urquiza and Timmer, Chapter 17, this volume).

Relaxation

First the therapist validates the youth's previously developed coping strategies, since they often represent best efforts to deal with traumatic stress, even though they may have been associated with problem behavior and negative consequences (e.g., getting into legal trouble for marijuana possession). The therapist expresses understanding of the use of these strategies, yet observes that some of them may relate directly to behavioral difficulties, leading to the need for treatment in the first place. The relaxation component develops skills that can be used to alleviate distress associated with trauma cues. Physically based activities that accentuate the difference between tension and relaxation (e.g., yoga, stretching, progressive muscle relaxation) may be initially more effective than cognitively based activities (e.g., imagery, positive self-talk). Extended time may be needed to help the youth recognize the difference between "stressed" and "relaxed" states and to defuse his or her neurobiological "alarm" system (Ford, 2005).

Therapists often use movement-based activities as an end-of-session "carrot" for clients who participate during therapeutic activities. A therapist may offer to spend the last 5 minutes of the session playing basketball in exchange for the youth practicing relaxation strategies. Alternatively, incorporating activities based on large muscle movements (e.g., yoga, Hula-Hoop, basketball) into the initial part of sessions can help behaviorally dysregulated youth calm down and improve the focus on therapeutic work.

Self-soothing and distraction techniques are also helpful to emphasize, as these are often familiar and may already be utilized in some fashion, such as listening to music, playing video games, or taking a hot bath. Clients with complex trauma histories may need help using these strategies appropriately and in moderation, including help in developing awareness of the potential overuse of these strategies (e.g., failing to study for a test and not sleeping due to playing video games all night).

Affective Expression and Modulation

Affective regulation is typically focused on increasing awareness of, and ability to express and manage, a range of emotions in day-to-day life, particularly in association with situations that commonly result in behavioral difficulties. These clients may be able to identify only feelings of anger, yet their behavioral difficulties might more often be the product of other feelings such as unacknowledged or unexpressed fear or insecurity. Helping youth identify different emotional states and understand the relationship between emotions and subsequent behavior can greatly increase capacity to regulate those behaviors.

The therapist's use of attunement to help clients identify and express the emotions they experience during session and the therapist's modeling of emotional expression and regulation of his or her own emotions are both very important (Kliethermes & Wamser, 2012). As part of this treatment component, the therapist can introduce some of the following topics:

- The role of emotions in daily life
- The validity and acceptability of all emotions
- The labeling of different emotional states
- The different levels of intensity that can be experienced
- The fact that different and even multiple emotions can be experienced at the same time
- The fact that negative affective states are temporary and that the ability to tolerate them can be learned
- The effective communication of emotions can alleviate their intensity and help secure support from others.

The work of this component may be initially challenging because youth with complex trauma histories often experience emotional numbing or dissociative responses, which were adaptive at one time. The therapist may then have to spend more time highlighting the function of emotions as providing useful information about the environment. Older youth may also benefit from the incorporation of skills from DBT (see also DeRosa & Rathus, Chapter 12, this volume), such as mindfulness to increase awareness of their emotions in the moment.

Active incorporation of an available caregiver in the treatment is critical, particularly for younger children, since the caregiver's improved attunement to the youth's emotional state can result in a decrease in emotional and behavioral outbursts. Close attunement by caregivers allows them to assess the youth's emotional needs and intervene more quickly and effectively, thus decreasing the need to engage in oppositional, disruptive, or aggressive behaviors. Emotional attunement skills such as active listening, acceptance, reflection, and empathy can be taught to caregivers via didactics, role plays, and "live" practice with the client during conjoint sessions. For caregivers in need of more targeted focus in this area, other interventions can also be integrated into TF-CBT (e.g., a family-focused emotion communication training, AFFECT; Shipman & Fitzgerald, 2005).

Cognitive Coping

For traumatized youth with co-occurring behavioral problems, an important aspect of the cognitive coping component is to increase the youth's awareness of his or her thoughts during situations that result in behavioral difficulties. The therapist can teach the cognitive triangle (i.e., the interactive relationship between thoughts, feelings, and behaviors that occurs in response to life situations) and use it to analyze a recently experienced conflict or crisis that resulted in the youth's engagement in a maladaptive behavior. It may be helpful to identify the problematic behavior that occurred (e.g., biting sister) and to "work backward" to determine the situation that initially occurred and the resulting emotions and thoughts that preceded the behavior. In many respects this process is very similar to the "chain analysis" used in DBT (see also DeRosa & Rathus, Chapter 12, this volume) to help clients analyze the events surrounding their behavioral difficulties. Using the cognitive triangle can help clients realize that behavior is directly influenced by thoughts and feelings, and they can then begin to develop cognitive coping strategies (e.g., positive self-talk) that can be used to alter behavioral responses to stressful life events. This process may also help the therapist and adolescent identify various triggers or "signals of danger" that are contributing to distress, which can be processed in detail during the trauma narrative component.

Involving caregivers in this process can enhance their ability to respond proactively to imminent behavioral outbursts. By becoming familiar with the stimuli that are likely to trigger behavioral outbursts, the caregiver can work to prepare the youth for situations that are likely to be challenging, and thereby assist in "breaking the chain" of events that typically culminates in problematic behavior. With this population, it also often beneficial for the caregiver to utilize the cognitive triangle when discussing, with the therapist, situations in which he or she had to engage in disciplinary actions with the youth. The caregiver can then begin to identify and correct any inaccurate or unhelpful beliefs that may be impacting his or her capacity to engage in effective discipline. For example, through the use of the cognitive

triangle, a caregiver may realize that he or she is taking the youth's misbehavior personally, becoming angry, and subsequently yelling at the youth
resulting in the youth's increasing dysregulation.

Trauma Narrative and Processing

Prior to beginning trauma processing, the youth should have made sufficient progress in behavioral stabilization to ensure that interruptions of the
trauma narrative construction activities are unlikely. It is prudent to delay
the initiation of the trauma narrative component if the therapist is aware of
significant upcoming changes or stressors such as a placement change, termination of parental rights, or reunification that may challenge the youth's
capacity to cope effectively. Total life stability, however, is not required, as
"crises of the week" are par for the course. Instead, the client should have
achieved "good enough" stability (Kliethermes & Wamser, 2012). Mild to
moderate behavioral difficulties such as temper tantrums, lying, or minor
physical altercations with siblings can be addressed through parenting
work with the caregiver without disrupting the trauma narrative process.

The caregiver may also need assistance in transitioning to the trauma
narrative component. It can be difficult to change focus from discussing
the youth's behavior problems to processing the youth's trauma exposure.
Further, as some behavior problems may still be present, the caregiver may
continue to regularly bring up behaviorally related incidents and crises in
therapy sessions. The caregiver's concerns regarding the youth's behavior
should be validated and some session time used to address those issues.
The amount of time spent in session addressing these issues should be monitored, however, to ensure that it does not overly reduce the time spent
involving the caregiver in the gradual exposure process.

A primary purpose of completing a trauma narrative is to help the client
break the association between trauma memories and intense negative emotions. Therefore, it is critical that the process of developing a trauma narrative not become emotionally overwhelming for the youth, otherwise it will
only strengthen those associations and, in effect, "retraumatize" him or her.
In turn, this retraumatization may significantly increase the youth's trauma-
related emotional and behavioral difficulties and may also jeopardize his or
her overall safety and stability (e.g., triggering increased suicidal ideation).
This danger is a major reason that TF-CBT implements skill-building components prior to trauma-related components. Specifically, prior to developing a trauma narrative, it is essential for the youth to have developed sufficient self-regulation skills (i.e., relaxation skills, affect modulation skills) to
allow him or her to safely tolerate any possible feelings of distress. Furthermore, trauma-related content is also introduced in a gradually increasing
fashion throughout all of the TF-CBT components to promote safe trauma
processing. Much like easing into a pool of cold water, slowly increasing the
trauma content, session by session, allows the client to gradually become

more capable of tolerating the distress associated with trauma processing. This gradual process also allows the TF-CBT therapist to assess the client's capacity to tolerate trauma processing over time, thereby allowing the therapist to target an appropriate level of processing intensity.

Conducted appropriately, the trauma narrative need not be overwhelming, though it often does cause some increase in distress. For the population under discussion, this distress may result in problematic behaviors characterized by oppositionality, hyperactivity, or even destructiveness or aggressiveness. In many respects, therapists should view these escalations as behaviorally based subjective units of distress score with more extreme behavior indicating more significant distress. Just as hysterical crying or dissociation indicates that a youth has been overwhelmed by the exposure process, so should the throwing of a toy at the therapist or a refusal to follow any directions.

Rather than immediately turning to a discussion of rules and consequences, it is recommended that the therapist use this situation as an opportunity to help the youth identify and express the thoughts and feelings behind the behavior. This is typically accomplished by reflecting the apparent emotion in the behavior (e.g., "It seems like you felt a lot of anger when I asked you that question") and validating/normalizing that emotion (e.g., "This is a really challenging thing to do; a lot of people would feel angry if they were in your shoes"). However, if the misbehavior continues, the client should be reminded of the "house rules" and given the opportunity to "cool down" or take a brief "time-out." The therapist can recommend practicing some relaxation skills but not in a way that becomes a power struggle. If possible, the therapist should try to engage the client in another brief period of exposure work following the completion of the cooldown to continue the development of a sense of mastery related to traumatic memories. As the trauma narrative process continues, behavioral difficulties related to the trauma should consistently decrease. Since behavioral difficulties that occur during session are not all trauma related, some may continue even after the completion of the trauma narrative work.

Traumatized youth with co-occurring behavioral difficulties often present with physical agitation and hyperactivity. Subsequently, much like completing a school writing assignment that involves working on a "pencil-and-paper" project for an extended period of time, these youth may particularly struggle with the trauma narrative if the process involves sitting in one place with little or no physical movement. Consequently, it is helpful to consider working in short bursts that are punctuated by breaks with physical movement. Similarly, it is often possible to incorporate movement directly into the development of the trauma processing. For example, some youth may be interested in utilizing dance, music, acting, or role playing as part of the gradual exposure process. It is also possible to incorporate gradual exposure into games that involve movement. An example might involve playing "Simon says" and integrating gradual exposure "commands" (e.g.,

"Simon says, 'Tell me about what you were thinking when your uncle hit you with the belt'") with more generic commands (e.g., "Simon says, 'Touch your toes'"). This approach also allows the therapist to titrate the level of exposure.

Finally, it is important to assist the client in developing a sense of meaning related to traumatic experience. Adolescents are more likely than younger children to experience extreme forms of guilt. Clearly, taking some responsibility for past actions or a failure to act may be appropriate; however, there are times that this self-blame may be inaccurate or excessive. For example, a youth may say that he deserved being scalded with boiling water because he talked back to his mother, or may state that she is responsible for being gang-raped at a party because she went to the party without her parents' permission. Often, the issue of responsibility is key. It is important to introduce the concept of *accidents* and *random occurrences* and the difference between *regret* and *responsibility*. The therapist can help the youth who accidentally woke up his stepfather, for example, to consider how this is different from intentionally disrupting someone's sleep, as well as whether a person who does something accidentally deserves to be punished. The therapist can also help the youth consider whether an intentional action was severe or blameworthy enough to justify the adverse consequences. For the teenager who was raped when attending a party without permission, the therapist could help her consider the possibility that she could regret going to the party without being responsible for her getting raped. And it would be important to help her consider that the perpetrators are responsible for harming her, regardless of whether she should have been at the party or not. This process can be facilitated by creating dissonance—for example, by asking the teenager if she knew other peers who had skipped school and had not been subsequently raped, leading to a discussion of what made her situation different from that of her peers (i.e., the presence of the assailants).

In Vivo Mastery of Trauma Reminders

The process of facilitating *in vivo* mastery is devoted to exposing the client to innocuous trauma cues to help him or her develop the capacity to tolerate them. As is the case with the trauma narrative, the client may use behavior to express distress in these situations. Unfortunately, parents and other caregivers may focus on internal causes of misbehavior (e.g., the youth is refusing to go to tutoring because he would rather play video games) instead of considering the possibility of external influences on the youth's behavior (e.g., the youth feels uncomfortable around the tutor because he wears the same cologne as his abuser wore). If misbehavior consistently occurs in the same situation, it is important to assess for possible trauma cues and to consider implementing *in vivo* mastery work to address the underlying distress. This work often requires educating other caregivers or resource persons (e.g., teacher, principal, tutor) about the impact of trauma triggers and involving them in this process.

In vivo mastery work can be used to help clients deal with the unfortunately common experience of disciplinary action. Because disciplinary actions are often ripe with trauma cues (e.g., angry tone of voice, criticism, authority figures), they may result in clients' experiencing additional distress and acting out. Role plays of disciplinary action can be conducted in the therapist's office or *in vivo*. For example, a youth who becomes distressed when sent to the principal's office might start by sitting outside the office for a few minutes, work up to sitting in the office alone, and finish by having a discussion with the principal. As mentioned above, involvement of other caregivers or resource persons will typically be required to conduct *in vivo* work of this kind.

Completing Trauma Processing

Determining when traumatic memories have been sufficiently processed can itself be a complex process. Generally speaking, when PTSD symptoms no longer disrupt daily functioning, this component of treatment is viewed as complete (Cohen et al., 2006; Ford, Courtois, Steele, van der Hart, & Nijenhuis, 2005). This is also true of behavioral manifestations of trauma-related distress (e.g., the youth no longer engages in substance use to manage PTSD symptoms). Clients should be able to recognize and experience trauma cues without lapsing into significant behavioral difficulties. They should also have a sense of meaning regarding their traumatic experiences and their subsequent behavioral manifestations. In essence, the goal is the ability to identify trauma exposure as only a part of life rather than its totality. Significantly, trauma-related misbehavior is reinterpreted as an understandable reaction to a horrifying experience and not an indication of clients' identity or their worth.

Conjoint Child–Parent Sessions

Again, youth with co-occurring behavior problems may not present for treatment in the company of a traditional caregiver, and other responsible adults may serve as substitutes and be involved in treatment. A problem can arise if the youth doesn't have a secure, trusting relationship with available caregivers such that he or she is reluctant to disclose details of the trauma history. It is the therapist's responsibility to ensure that the identified caregivers possess adequate self-regulation skills and are capable of giving an appropriate and supportive response to the youth during conjoint sessions. Though the involvement of an appropriate caregiver is optimal, the option of not having a caregiver is considered if the client does not feel comfortable.

Assuming the presence of a caregiver, conjoint work in TF-CBT is also used to facilitate behavioral stabilization. However, due to disrupted attachment, the relationships between traumatized youth (especially those with co-occurring behavioral difficulties) and their caregivers are often strained and dysfunctional (Briere & Spinazzola, 2005). Furthermore, as mentioned earlier, youth with complex trauma histories often enter into interactions with adult caregivers expecting criticism and punishment. For this population, the simple act of engaging with a caregiver may result in dysregulation.

Conjoint sessions then provide valuable *in vivo* opportunities to gradually expose the youth to these cues and to further the development of a supportive, appropriate caregiving relationship that will help to address behavioral dysregulation. These sessions are used to practice decreasing "signals of danger" while increasing "signals of care" (Saxe, Ellis, & Kaplow, 2007), and allow the therapist to model appropriate supportive behavior. Consistent contact with a supportive caregiver facilitates counter-conditioning of the youth's experience of having been victimized by prior caregivers. Conjoint sessions can further facilitate the caregiver's ability to coach the youth in using coping skills; these sessions help to increase communication about stressful situations with the caregiver, including information about the various trauma triggers they have identified. In this way, the sessions help the caregiver to better understand the factors behind the youth's self-regulation difficulties. This understanding may also help caregivers identify ways they can change their approaches to facilitate the youth's ability to regulate behavior. Once these new approaches have been identified, conjoint sessions can involve practicing them, and, if successful, can also decrease the youth's reluctance to discuss future self-regulation difficulties with the caregiver.

Enhancing Future Safety and Development

It is critical to revisit the client's perceived sense of safety and his or her healthy development following the completion of all other components. Youth exposed to traumatic events are at increased risk for further victimization (Finkelhor et al., 2009). It is therefore essential to provide these youngsters with appropriate safety and prevention skills that can be applied to future life situations (e.g., dating, moving away from home). This component focuses on the primary safety/prevention skills of danger awareness, assertiveness, problem solving, and seeking help. If developmentally appropriate, it is also essential to provide these clients with information regarding healthy relationships and sexuality.

It is noteworthy that many of these clients still present with significant behavioral difficulties following completion of TF-CBT. For example, it may be determined that the youth's inattentiveness, hyperactivity, and impulsivity were not all related to trauma exposure and instead might be related to ADHD. Furthermore, behaviors that initially started as a response to trauma exposure may come to be maintained by other factors (e.g., substance abuse, sexualized behavior) and remain present even after completion of TF-CBT. At the end of treatment, clients often return to environments that label them as *problems* or *troublemakers*. This labeling may persist even if they achieve significant behavioral improvement. It is still likely they will continue to be confronted by people who expect them to relapse into their former behavioral patterns. Peers may actually encourage them to do so and will likely express disappointment if they do not. They will also be confronted by adults who may inadvertently create a "self-fulfilling prophecy" by acting as if the youth were still behaving in problematic ways. If enough people predict misbehavior, it is likely to occur, underscoring the importance of devoting a portion of this concluding phase of therapy to "image rehabilitation," coping with peer pressure, and strategies to overcome negative expectations.

To facilitate this process, the therapist can work with relevant caregivers and professionals to identify appropriate expectations and responsibilities for the youth who is moving toward adulthood. Many caregivers have difficulty trusting the youth's capacity to handle situations without engaging in misbehavior and may need encouragement to allow him or her more freedom and responsibility within appropriate limits. On the opposite end of the spectrum, some caregivers may expect too much of the client and take a "sink or swim" approach to future endeavors taken on by the youth. Helping caregivers provide a balance of support and challenge/freedom is often essential. Caregivers may remain hypervigilant to warning signs that misbehavior is on an increase. Helping involved adults focus on successes rather than ruminating on the youth's past or current difficulties can go a long way toward reducing self-fulfilling prophecies. On a related note, it is critical to normalize the occurrence of occasional mistakes and misbehavior in the future. Caregivers and youth should be made aware that occasional misbehavior is developmentally appropriate and is not always indicative of renewed trauma-related or behavioral difficulties. Recognizing that these "bumps in the road" will occur keeps caregivers and youth from overreacting to misbehaviors and inadvertently worsening them.

Ending Treatment

In light of the youth's previous interpersonal experiences, the termination of the treatment relationship is very important and may constitute a first healthy experience of saying "good-bye." A couple of considerations are important when preparing to end the treatment. First, as noted above, it is not unusual for behavioral difficulties to reappear, though usually to a less severe degree and often as an indication of the youth's distress over the end of treatment and the relationship with the therapist. Clients can be helped to understand their emotions as normal responses to a relationship changing significantly or coming to an end. Validation of this sort can open the door for the therapist to address the youth's underlying thoughts and feelings regarding termination. Second, the conclusion of treatment may elicit anxiety about not being able to maintain improved behavior without the therapist. Again, the therapist can validate and normalize this anxiety and help the client consider the fact that he or she has already demonstrated an ability to regulate behavior in a variety of settings without the therapist's being present (e.g., between sessions). The end of treatment is the time to highlight the role of the caregiver who now knows much of what the therapist knows and is capable of assisting the client in maintaining his or her self-regulation abilities.

Conclusion

Working with behaviorally dysregulated youth can certainly be taxing, even given the fact that TF-CBT has been shown to be effective for youth who have experienced multiple traumas and co-occurring behavioral problems (Cohen et al., 2004). This efficacy is not surprising, given that TF-CBT was specifically designed to address trauma-related difficulties, including those that are behavioral. However, some adaptations of the TF-CBT model may be warranted when co-occurring behavioral difficulties are of a more severe and chronic nature. TF-CBT is a highly flexible model, making it possible to incorporate aspects of other EBPs, specifically designed for addressing behavioral difficulties (e.g., PCIT, DBT), into the model's basic components without compromising the trauma-focused nature of the model. With creativity and flexibility, a TF-CBT therapist can successfully address persistent trauma-related behavioral difficulties and reduce the severity of preexisting or comorbid behavioral difficulties.

References

Ackerman, P. T., Newton, J. E. O., McPherson, W. B., Jones, J. G., & Dykman, R. A. (1998). Prevalence of post traumatic stress disorder and other psychiatric diagnoses in three groups of abused children (sexual, physical, and both). *Child Abuse and Neglect*, 22(8), 759–774.

Briere, J. (2002). Treating adult survivors of severe childhood abuse and neglect: Further development of an integrative model. In J. E. B. Myers et al. (Eds.), *The APSAC handbook on child maltreatment* (2nd ed., pp. 175–202). Newbury Park, CA: Sage.

Briere, J., & Scott, C. (2006). *Principles of trauma therapy: A guide to symptoms, evaluation, and treatment*. Thousand Oaks: Sage.

Briere, J., & Spinazzola, J. (2005). Phenomenology and psychological assessment of complex posttraumatic stress. *Journal of Traumatic Stress*, 18(5), 401–412.

Child Welfare Information Gateway. (2007). *Trauma-focused cognitive behavioral therapy: Addressing the mental health of sexually abused children*. Washington, DC: U.S. Department of Health and Human Services.

Cohen, J. A., Berliner, L., & Mannarino, A. P (2010). Trauma-focused CBT for children with co-occurring trauma and behavior problems. *Child Abuse and Neglect*, *34*, 215–224.

Cohen, J. A., Bukstein, O., Walter, H., Benson, R. S., Chrisman, A., Farchione, T. R., et al. (2010). Practice parameters for the assessment and treatment of children and adolescents with posttraumatic stress disorder. *Journal of the American Academy of Child and Adolescent Psychiatry, 49*(4), 414–430.

Cohen, J. A., Deblinger, E., Mannarino, A. P., & Steer, R. (2004). A multisite, randomized controlled trial for children with sexual abuse-related PTSD symptoms. *Journal of the American Academy of Child and Adolescent Psychiatry, 43*, 393–402.

Cohen, J. A., Mannarino, A. P., & Deblinger, E. (2006). *Treating trauma and traumatic grief in children and adolescents*. New York: Guilford Press.

Cook, A., Blaustein, M., Spinazzola, J., & van der Kolk, B. A. (Eds.). (2003). *Complex trauma in children and adolescents*. National Child Traumatic Stress Network. Available online at *www.NCTSNet.org*.

Deblinger, E., Lippmann, J., & Steer, R. (1996). Sexually abused children suffering posttraumatic stress symptoms: Initial treatment outcome findings. *Child Maltreatment, 1*, 310–321.

Eyberg, S. M., & Boggs, S. R. (1998). Parent–child interaction therapy for oppositional preschoolers. In C. E. Schaefer & J. M. Briesmeister (Eds.), *Handbook of parent training: Parents as co-therapists for children's behavior problems* (2nd ed., pp. 61–97). New York: Wiley.

Finkelhor, D., Ormrod, R. K., & Turner, H. A. (2009). Lifetime assessment of poly-victimization in a national sample of children and youth. *Child Abuse and Neglect, 33*, 403–411.

Ford, J. D. (2005). Treatment implications of altered affect regulation and information processing following child maltreatment. *Psychiatric Annals, 35*(5), 410–419.

Ford, J. D., Courtois, C. A., Steele, K., van der Hart, O., & Mijenhuis, E. R. S. (2005). Treatment of complex posttraumatic self-dysregulation. *Journal of Traumatic Stress, 18*(5), 437–447.

Kliethermes, M., & Wamser, R. (2012). Adolescents with complex trauma. In J. A. Cohen, A. P. Mannarino, & E. Deblinger (Eds.), *Trauma-focused CBT for children and adolescents: Treatment applications* (pp. 175–196). New York: Guilford Press.

Linehan, M. M. (1993). *Cognitive-behavioral therapy of borderline personality disorder*. New York: Guilford Press.

Pearlman, L. A., & Courtois, C. A. (2005). Clinical applications of the attachment framework: Relational treatment of complex trauma. *Journal of Traumatic Stress, 18*(5), 449–459.

Saxe, G. N., Ellis, B. H., & Kaplow, J. B. (2007). *Collaborative treatment of traumatized children and teens: The trauma systems therapy approach*. New York: Guilford Press.

Shipman, K., & Fitzgerald, M. M. (2005, April). *A family-focused emotion communication training module (AFFECT)*. Paper presented at the preconference biennial meeting of the Society for Research on Child Development, Atlanta, GA.

Spinazzola, J., Ford, J. D., Zucker, M., van der Kolk, B., Silva, S., Smith, S. F., et al. (2005). Survey evaluates complex trauma exposure, outcome, and intervention among children and adolescents. *Psychiatric Annals, 35*(5), 433–439.

van der Kolk, B. A. (2005). Developmental trauma disorder. *Psychiatric Annals, 35*(5), 401–408.

CHAPTER 11

Eye Movement Desensitization and Reprocessing

Debra Wesselmann
Francine Shapiro

Eye movement desensitization and reprocessing (EMDR) is an integrative psychotherapy approach used to treat a wide range of clinical complaints through the reprocessing of disturbing events that are viewed as etiological to pathology (Shapiro, 2001). Numerous practice guidelines have designated EMDR therapy as an empirically validated psychological treatment of trauma (e.g., Bisson & Andrews, 2007; U.S. Department of Veterans Affairs & Department of Defense, 2004, 2010; Foa, Keane, Friedman, & Cohen, 2009). Although EMDR therapy procedures contain elements that are compatible with other orientations, the treatment emphasizes the brain's information-processing system and the physiologically stored memory networks as the foundation for psychological treatment. Deficits in relational, cognitive, emotional, somatic, and behavioral functioning are identified and initially attended to by ascertaining and then processing the memories that are viewed as both causal and contributory to dysfunction. Unlike other empirically supported treatments of trauma, neither cognitive challenges nor behavioral manipulations are used as the primary agents of change. Rather, the pathological responses are viewed as manifestations of inadequately processed memories, and change is facilitated through procedures that engender internal associations through stimulation of the brain's intrinsic information-processing system.

The application of EMDR therapy to complex traumatic stress disorders involves comprehensive attention to the experiences stored in memory that are the basis of posttraumatic dysfunction. In addition, therapeutic interactions are combined with standardized processing procedures to facilitate learning and encode positive memory experiences in order to address developmental and relational deficits. This approach to psychotherapy is guided by the adaptive information-processing (AIP) model (Shapiro, 2001; described below), which emphasizes the importance of a wide range of experiential contributors to pathology. Therefore, comprehensive EMDR treatment is not limited to the processing of "Criterion A" events needed to diagnose posttraumatic stress disorder (PTSD). Recent research has supported this therapeutic approach. For instance, Mol et al. (2005) report that "life events can generate at least as many PTSD symptoms as traumatic events" (p. 494). Research focusing on adverse life experiences in children has also "established that environmental adversity can have a deleterious effect on children's functioning. . . . Exposure to adverse, stressful events, such as marital conflict, maternal depression, and financial stress, has been linked to socioemotional behavior problems and cognitive deficits" (Obradović, Bush, Stamperdahl, Adler, & Boyce, 2010, p. 270). Consequently, the EMDR treatment of complex PTSD in children addresses the full range of negative experiences that are hampering comprehensive adaptive functioning.

The AIP Model

The AIP theoretical model (Shapiro, 2001) posits that all humans have a natural information-processing system that is designed to take disturbance to resolution and adaptation. Unimpeded information processing allows learning to take place as new experiences are assimilated within already existing memory networks. What is useful is incorporated and what is useless is discarded. Stressful events experienced throughout the course of life are generally processed naturally throughout the day and during the rapid eye movement (REM) stage of sleep. However, this natural information-processing system may become overwhelmed by high levels of stress, trauma, and their associated reactions. When this occurs, unprocessed memories are believed to be stored along with their associated negative emotions, body sensations, and cognitions, and are prevented from being integrated with positive experiences or changing over time (Shapiro, 2001, 2012, 2013). Present-day events, images, smells, sounds, or thoughts can trigger the unprocessed memories, causing the reexperiencing of stored negative images, cognitions, emotions, or sensations. Reexperiencing (i.e., intrusion of unprocessed memory) can happen consciously or subconsciously, driving behavioral reactions that can negatively affect everyday functioning.

The AIP model emphasizes naturalistic processing by fostering a spontaneous internal associational process through the use of standardized procedures with minimal clinical intrusion. The client is prepared to "simply notice" what occurs internally as the traumatic memory is accessed and the information-processing system stimulated. This processing occurs through self-focused attention during consecutive sets of bilateral eye movements or other forms of dual attention stimulation (i.e., taps or tones). Other trauma treatments expose clients to their trauma memories in ways that prevent behavioral avoidance in order to process the emotions associated with them. They do so using such methods as detailed verbal or written narratives of the event to challenge or correct dominant beliefs the client developed in the aftermath of the trauma. However, in EMDR therapy such detailed descriptions are not employed since they would interfere with the spontaneous associations fostered during the sets of bilateral stimulation. More than 20 randomized controlled trials have reported positive effects for the eye movement component, including a rapid reduction of negative emotions and increased recollection and recognition of true information (e.g., Christman, Garvey, Propper, & Phaneuf, 2003; Parker, Buckley, & Dagnall, 2009; Schubert, Lee, & Drummond, 2011; van den Hout et al., 2011).

During the reprocessing phases of treatment the targeted memory connects and integrates with already stored memory networks as learning takes place. This causes positive changes to occur on cognitive, affective and somatic levels. For instance, the traumatic and distressing memories of children who have been abused are stored in an unprocessed form, along with disturbing emotions, related somatic sensations, and negative beliefs regarding self, others, and overall safety. In this form, environmental reminders easily trigger the affect and cognitions. During the reprocessing phase of EMDR, the child's abuse memories may associate and integrate with positive memories related to care from the adults who stopped the abuse and other experiences of protection or nurturing, moving the child's perspective and insight toward adaptive resolution and removing the emotional charge of the abuse memories.

Whereas exposure therapies have been posited to cause the creation of a new memory that competes with the originally targeted event through neurobiological processes of extinction (Craske, Herman, & Vansteenwegen, 2006; Suzuki et al., 2004), EMDR therapeutic effects are posited to be based upon reconsolidation, a neurobiological process through which the original memory is accessed, altered, and restored (Solomon & Shapiro, 2008). Through EMDR reprocessing of earlier disturbing events and current situations, the client's frame of reference regarding troubling memories is transformed to one of learning experiences that become the basis of a new sense of self and resilience.

The Eight Phases of EMDR Therapy

EMDR therapy is composed of eight phases, all of which are considered mandatory for comprehensive treatment (Shapiro, 2001). These phases incorporate a three-pronged approach that targets past memories, current triggers, and positive responses for the future. During the *first phase of EMDR (history taking)*, the therapist identifies the clinical complaints and present-day situations that result in problematic/negative affective, cognitive, somatic, and behavioral responses, and the skills needed for future adaptive responses. A variety of techniques is used in order to identify the etiological situations and events related to the current problems and situations. The therapist determines the client's readiness for EMDR by looking for symptoms of self-harming, suicidality, dissociation, or other signs of severe emotional dysregulation that may require more extensive preparation and stabilization prior to EMDR. However, from an AIP perspective, it is recognized that volatile moods and emotional instability are generally caused by the unprocessed memories, which contain a "volcano" of unresolved distressing affects. Therefore, in many cases stabilization can be facilitated through the judicious processing of the physiologically stored memories (e.g., Brown & Shapiro, 2006).

During the *second phase (preparation)*, the client is educated about the processing procedures. Children especially enjoy being introduced to the various forms of bilateral stimulation, and EMDR is explained to them as "a method for connecting big feelings and upsetting memories with helpful and truthful information." It is easy for children to understand that EMDR "makes upset feelings smaller and positive feelings bigger" and that it "helps the brain get stronger." Children are assisted to develop a vocabulary of "feelings words" and skills (e.g., breathing and mindfulness skills) that help them to maintain a "dual awareness," allowing a sense of safety in the present while "just noticing" what occurs when the past events are accessed and reprocessed. Part of the preparation phase, in AIP terminology, involves ensuring the presence of adequate positive memory networks—a prerequisite to adaptive integration of unprocessed memories. When working with children who have a history of extreme childhood abuse, especially those where no supportive relationships existed, experiences of feeling supported or nurtured in present-day relationships and also recent experiences of resilience, courage, or strength can be reinforced with bilateral eye movements or other forms of bilateral stimulation. By this means the experiences are encoded into positive memory networks. In addition, the use of bilateral stimulation can be used to strengthen and increase access to a "safe" or "calm" place for assisting the child or adult client with self-regulation.

The *third phase (assessment)*, involves identifying a specific target memory of a traumatic event or distressful life experience along with "the worst picture" associated with the memory, related emotions and sensations, negative cognitions, and desired positive cognitions. A baseline measure of the "validity of cognition" (VOC) related to the positive cognition is determined by instructing the client to bring up the disturbing picture and then asking him or her, "How true do the words [insert the positive cognition] feel to you on a scale from 1 to 7, with 7 meaning totally true, and 1 meaning not true at all?" A "subjective unit of distress" (SUD) is taken by instructing the client to bring up the disturbing picture and asking, "How much distress do you feel right now on a scale from 0 to 10, with 10 being the worst distress you could ever imagine and 0 representing no distress at all?" The assessment phase can be simplified with younger children by asking them to show the size of their distress or the strength of the positive thought by moving their hands close together or holding them a distance apart.

During the *fourth phase (desensitization),* the EMDR therapist assists the client in accessing the traumatic memory and associated emotions, sensations, and thoughts, followed by commencement of bilateral stimulation through eye movements (tactile or auditory modalities can also be utilized). Although the client is instructed to bring up the memory prior to bilateral stimulation, he or she is encouraged to "let whatever happens, happen" and "just notice" any thoughts, feelings, images, or sensations that surface during the eye movements. The client is not directed to remain focused on the target memory (as in cognitive-behavioral therapy [CBT] exposure therapies), since the bilateral stimulation facilitates the client's own natural associative processing. A typical set of eye movements involves about 24 "round trips" (side to side), although the therapist watches the client's face to determine if there is an insight or shift of some sort prior to ending the set of eye movements. Children may shift after as few as 11 or 12 "round trips." After asking the client to "Take a breath and let it go," the therapists asks, "What's there now?" and then, depending upon the response, generally instructs the client to "Go with that" before commencing another set of eye movements. When processing occurs, new insights and emotional shifts spontaneously take place as a result of the activation of the client's intrinsic associative processes. If processing stalls, the clinician uses a variety of procedures to activate it again (see Shapiro, 2001). During the processing, the EMDR therapist intervenes as minimally as possible in order to "stay out of the client's way" while the client associates naturally to the thoughts, memories, emotions, and sensations that arise. The desensitization phase is complete when the emotional "charge" or reactivity related to the target event has been eliminated, and new insights have emerged.

The *fifth phase* involves strengthening the positive cognition until it feels "completely true," and *phase six* involves scanning the body and processing any remaining somatic reactivity. During the *seventh phase, closure,* the client is assessed and, if necessary, helped to feel safe and calm prior to leaving the session. Instructions are given for maintaining stability between sessions and to note any disturbance for targeting during future sessions. In the *eighth phase, reevaluation,* the therapist reaccesses the troubling memory to ascertain if any other avenues need to be addressed in subsequent sessions.

In children (e.g., de Roos et al., 2011) and adults (e.g., Wilson, Becker, & Tinker, 1995) a single trauma is typically resolved within three EMDR sessions. Decreases in posttraumatic stress symptoms have been maintained subsequent to treatment through 12- to 15-month follow-ups (e.g., Kemp, Drummond, & mcDermott, 2010; Wilson et al., 1995). Children and adults with a history of multiple traumas and relational traumas require more extensive EMDR treatment (Shapiro, 2001; Wesselmann, 2013). However, rather than having to treat each trauma, one event is chosen to represent a "cluster" of similar events, and positive reprocessing effects often generalize from the targeted event to other associated memories.

EMDR in Practice with a Traumatized Adolescent

The following is a sample transcript illustrating spontaneous reprocessing during sequential sets of eye movements while targeting multiple traumatic losses experienced by 13-year-old "Susan" (name and personal information disguised). Susan was placed into care as a toddler due to neglect related to her biological parents' drug use. She remained with a foster mother until age 4, at which time she was moved to a single-parent adoptive home. Susan and her adoptive mother were referred to treatment due to Susan's escalating behaviors at home and school, including arguing, defiance, fighting with peers, disrupting the classroom, and refusal to complete school assignments. She had attended traditional supportive individual therapy for 2 years prior to the referral.

Susan's starting image for the following reprocessing session was a memory of leaving the foster home at age 4. This experience had been traumatic for Susan, as she had been with her foster mother for 2 years and felt secure with her. Her negative cognition was "I'm bad," and her desired positive cognition was "I didn't do anything wrong." She rated the validity of the desired cognition as 2 on a 7-point scale and her disturbance as 8 on an 11-point SUD scale. She described sadness in her heart.

At the beginning of each set, the therapist helped Susan focus her attention, and after each set instructed her to "Let it go and take a breath." She was then asked to report what had emerged during the set. The sets of eye movements and the therapist's prompt are indicated by < < < < <.

> < < < < < SUSAN: The first people I loved didn't want me either—my birth parents.

> < < < < < SUSAN: I wonder what it would have been like if I had stayed with my birth parents.

< < < < < SUSAN: I wonder what it would have been like to stay with Betty. [her first foster mother].

< < < < < SUSAN: What would it have been like to stay with my biological brother? *(With tears, while adoptive mom puts her arm around her supportively.)*

< < < < < SUSAN: I'm really good with little kids!

< < < < < SUSAN: I have two older brothers in my home now, but I wonder what it would have been like to have a younger brother. *(More tears, with Mom's support.)*

< < < < < SUSAN: I'm really close to my two brothers. If anything happened to them, it would be terrible!

< < < < < SUSAN: Mom says my foster mom was too old to adopt me. But if I had been good, maybe Betty would have kept me. I remember I was naughty. *(With more tears.)*

< < < < < SUSAN: I think I was just upset because of my birth parents.

< < < < < SUSAN: My birth parents wouldn't stop using drugs. It's stupid to use drugs!

< < < < < SUSAN: Someday they are going to get killed! *(With more tears.)*

< < < < < SUSAN: I am so mad at whomever gave them those drugs in the first place!

< < < < < SUSAN: I'm lucky I didn't stay with them.

< < < < < SUSAN: I'm lucky I have a good home now!

At this point, Susan reported her disturbance at a 2, but she continued reprocessing until SUD = 0. At that point, she decided she wanted to strengthen the belief "I didn't do anything wrong, and I'm lucky I have a good home now," which at conclusion she rated as a "7" (completely true) on the validity scale.

Susan and her mother attended both family therapy and EMDR therapy once a week for 3 months, followed by a session with each therapist twice per month for 3 months. In addition to the memory of leaving her foster home, EMDR targets included recent events that had triggered misbehavior, including teasing by peers, redirection from teachers, and Mom saying "no." Finally, Susan was assisted in developing an imagined picture of herself behaving in a positive way during triggering situations, including being told "no" or redirected. The positive image was reinforced with bilateral eye movements. At the end of the 6 months (18 sessions of EMDR), Susan's mother described Susan as "fun to be around for the first time ever." Her scores on the Attachment Disorder Assessment Scale—Revised moved from a 66 ("Significant Attachment Issues") pretreatment to −1 (below "Minimal Attachment Issues") at 24 weeks.

Review of Research

Five randomized controlled studies with children and adolescents, ages 4–18 (Ahmad, Larsson, & Sundelin-Wahlsten, 2007; Chemtob, Nakashima, & Carlson, 2002; de Roos et al., 2011; Jaberghaderi et al., 2004; Kemp et al., 2010), have supported the effectiveness of EMDR therapy in the treatment of PTSD. The two studies directly comparing EMDR therapy and CBT (de Roos et al., 2011; Jaberghaderi et al., 2004) found EMDR to be more efficient, in that it required fewer sessions and little homework. In a randomized comparison of EMDR and CBT treatment of 26 children, EMDR and CBT both showed improvement in self-esteem, and there was evidence of statistically significant improvement in behavioral problems in the EMDR group (Wanders, Serra, & de Jongh, 2008). In addition, 10 open trials evaluating EMDR therapy with traumatized children have reported positive effects (see *www.emdrhap.org*). Three of the studies appraising the EMDR group therapy protocol for children traumatized by natural or human-made disasters (Aduriz, Bluthgen, & Knopfler, 2009; Fernandez, Gallinari, & Lorenzetti, 2004; Jarero, Artigas, & Luber, 2006) reported pronounced and rapid treatment effects after only one session.

A meta-analysis found a significant reduction in PTSD symptoms in traumatized children ages 4–18 years following treatment with EMDR, compared to therapy-as-usual or no-treatment control groups. In studies that compared CBT with EMDR, both therapeutic approaches were effective. However, "when the children treated with EMDR were compared to the children treated with established trauma treatments (CBT), EMDR adds a small but significant incremental value" (Rodenburg, Benjamin, de Roos, Meijer, & Stams, 2009, p. 604). The California Evidence-Based Clearinghouse for Child Welfare *(www.cebc4cw.org)* reported that EMDR and trauma-focused CBT are both considered "Well-Supported by Research Evidence."

In a small, nonrandomized trial (Zaghrout-Hodali, Alissa, & Dodgson, 2008), a representative group of Palestinian children experiencing ongoing traumatic conditions were successfully treated with a group EMDR therapy protocol. Seven children, ages 8–12 years, were referred to treatment 5 days after a shooting had occurred. They were treated with a group protocol developed in Mexico to work with groups of traumatized children after a natural disaster (Jarero et al., 2006). Four sessions were initially planned for treatment. However, after the second session the children were subjected to an additional violent incident in which masked men invaded their homes and separated them from their parents. Despite this unexpected event, the children showed no sign of traumatization, easily processed the new memory, and completed treatment of the original incident. According to reports from the parents, the children's remission of symptoms remained stable at 4- to 5-month follow-up, despite ongoing threats of violence. The overall results indicated increased resilience and resistance to further traumatization.

Conceptualizing Complex Trauma in Children Using EMDR and Attachment Models

Shapiro's AIP model is consistent with attachment theory and the internal working model (IWM) construct, providing an explanation for insecure attachments and the tenacity of a negative IWM by positing that beliefs present at the time of distressing events are stored in memory networks in unprocessed form. From the AIP point of view, multiple distressing caregiver experiences become part of a network of physiologically stored and related memories. Later potentially healthy relationships can become a quagmire of triggers, tapping into the store of negative images, emotions, sensations, and thoughts, and leading to maladaptive behavioral reactions. Consistent with the AIP perspective, children with complex trauma histories often exhibit symptoms that are extremely challenging to their caregivers, including severe emotional and behavioral reactivity, aggression, impulsivity, poor interpersonal skills, and poor sense of self (Ide & Paez, 2000; van der Kolk, 2005; van der Kolk et al., 1996).

Through reprocessing, leading to the integration of unmetabolized memories, EMDR is postulated to reorganize and change the negative IWM, remove the emotional charge from relationship triggers, and improve interpersonal functioning. EMDR treatment appears to have a positive effect on attachment status in adulthood (Potter, Davidson, & Wesselmann, 2013; Wesselmann & Potter, 2009) and on parent–child attachment (Gomez, 2012; Madrid, Skolek, & Shapiro, 2006; Wesselmann, 2013; Wesselmann et al., 2012). In one nonrandomized study, EMDR eliminated PTSD symptoms and improved attachment to mothers of 28 children who had been exposed to domestic violence (Robredo, 2011). Ongoing research indicates that children with a history of abuse and/or foster or orphanage care show significant improvement in scores on behavioral and attachment measures following 36 weeks of integrated EMDR and family therapy treatment (Attachment and Trauma Center of Nebraska, 2011).

Application of EMDR to Children with Complex Trauma Histories

By its nature, EMDR therapy is a gentle and client-centered experiential approach. As opposed to asking children or adults to verbally describe their traumatic memories, clients are encouraged instead to focus on them for short periods of time. The EMDR therapist "stays out of the client's way" as the eye movements help facilitate a natural associative process. Emotional abreaction or reliving of the trauma is not an EMDR goal, and steps to reduce the risk of acute dysregulation are part of the EMDR basic procedures. For example, clients are encouraged to "notice it all pass by" as if they were "watching through a window of a moving train" or "viewing a recording of the memory on a television screen." EMDR therapists instill a sense of control by encouraging children and adults to use a "stop signal" any time they want to take a break during reprocessing (Shapiro, 2001). In addition, training in EMDR instructs therapists in ways to ensure adequate preparation with the client prior to memory reprocessing. If needed, a variety of positive affect states (e.g., courage, strength, calm) are made available through state change techniques, which provide adequate stability and ongoing equilibrium to the client via a process labeled *resource installation* (Korn & Leeds, 2002; Shapiro, 2001, 2012). For example, one child recalled feeling mature when she helped her elderly neighbor with some chores. She was assisted in accessing the memory and noticing the associated positive emotions and sensations while the therapist implemented slow bilateral stimulation to strengthen the affect state as a positive resource.

EMDR also guides therapists in helping clients reduce their anxiety between sessions. For example, children are encouraged to "let the memories go for now" or to "put them in a container" between sessions. Homework is not part of EMDR, as the reprocessing changes are achieved during the therapy sessions. The absence of homework reduces the amount of safety and stabilization precautions that need to be employed, since there is no deliberate exposure to trauma material outside the presence of the therapist. In addition, since homework is not required, EMDR therapy can be conducted on consecutive days, allowing treatment to proceed rapidly, which can be particularly desirable in turbulent family situations or in other acute states. Further, during EMDR reprocessing, associations are often made, both consciously and unconsciously, to other incidents, and targets are often chosen to represent a "cluster" of similar events (e.g., multiple memories of abuse). After completing a reprocessing session on a particular distressing event, clients often find that treatment effects have generalized, and other similar events do not have to be separately targeted. This simultaneous reprocessing increases the efficiency of EMDR therapy with clients suffering from multiple traumas.

Additional adaptations are made, as needed, during the preparation and EMDR reprocessing phases for children affected by complex trauma. For example, Gomez (2010, 2012) suggests using bilateral stimulation to strengthen olfactory cues, using scents from lotions or candles to further reinforce the calming effect during EMDR incorporation of a "safe" place. Eckers (2010) describes the use of bilateral stimulation to reinforce positive feelings associated with play, interspersed by brief glances at a drawing of the traumatic memory in order to strengthen the child's tolerance prior to EMDR reprocessing. Parents can be coached to provide supportive touch and a silent but compassionate presence to help children stay regulated during EMDR reprocessing (Attachment and Trauma Center of Nebraska, 2011; Wesselmann, 2007; Wesselmann, Schweitzer, & Armstrong, 2013). Adler-Tapia and Settle (2008) simplify the language of the questions involved in the EMDR procedure to reduce anxiety and confusion during EMDR with children, and they incorporate sand tray and play dough to help children express their thoughts and feelings.

Often in reprocessing sessions, there is a rapid movement through the associated memory networks to an adaptive resolution. However, if clients become blocked during reprocessing, due to a lack of important relevant information, EMDR therapists utilize the "cognitive interweave"—which, in AIP terms, either accesses the next bit of relevant information already existing within the client's memory networks, or provides information needed due to lack of appropriate education or positive past experiences. Depending upon the client's need, the therapist's instructions can involve a request to focus on a picture, thought, or somatic response (Shapiro, 2001). For children, the most common form of cognitive interweave is the initiating of empowering imagery.

EMDR Therapy in a Case of Complex Trauma

In the following case, a team model integrated family therapy with EMDR to manage family crises and improve caregiver support, which allowed EMDR to be implemented safely on a weekly basis (Attachment and Trauma Center of Nebraska, 2011; Wesselmann et al., 2013).

Phase 1 (History Taking)

Amy (name and identifying details have been changed) was a 9-year-old child referred for EMDR by a colleague who was conducting family therapy. Amy was living with a foster mother who was willing to adopt her if Amy's behaviors could be stabilized. During history taking, the mother reported that Amy had been removed by the state from the home of her biological parents at age 3. Her biological mother had given birth at age 14 and had been a drug and alcohol abuser. Amy had been physically abused and neglected by both her mother and her mother's boyfriend, who had also sexually abused her. Amy had experienced six placements, including three adoptive attempts that failed. A younger sister had been adopted in the first placement.

The early abuse and multiple disrupted placements had taken a serious toll on Amy, whose symptoms included rages that lasted for hours; physical abuse of pets and younger children; sexual acting out toward younger children; self-harm with sharp objects; eating and drinking soaps, shampoos, and toothpaste; and urinating and defecating in her room and in her shoes. She suffered from flashbacks, complained of pain in her genital area, and compulsively inserted sharp objects in her vagina. In addition, Amy expressed negative feelings toward infants. The mother reported, for example, that when a premature infant had been placed briefly in the home, Amy had remarked, "I wish I could squeeze her head and pop it like a pimple."

From an AIP perspective, it was hypothesized that Amy's traumatic memories of abuse were triggered by present-day attachment figures and that the aggression toward herself and others was driven by the attendant feelings of anxiety, fear, and anger, disturbing body sensations, and associated negative beliefs regarding caregivers, herself, and the world. A plan was made for Amy and her foster mother to meet with the EMDR therapist and the family therapist once per week.

The therapist asked the foster mother to help hypothesize possible negative beliefs held by Amy by thinking about the child's early history and current behaviors. The following list was created:

- "Moms can't be trusted."
- "I will always be hurt."
- "I will always be abandoned."
- "Something is wrong with me."
- "The world is not safe."
- "Others deserve to hurt."
- "It's not safe to be close to people."
- "If you don't see me and hear me, I will disappear."
- "Others are out to get me."
- "I have to be in control."
- "Others deserve to feel what I feel."
- "I'm bad. I'm wrong. I'm defective."

The list assisted the EMDR therapist in looking for the earliest "touchstone" events or situations during which Amy's thoughts may have developed (Shapiro, 2001, 2012). In EMDR therapy, beliefs such as these are not directly challenged, but are used as a way to identify appropriate targets for processing. An additional benefit of developing Amy's list was that it assisted the foster mother in becoming more attuned to Amy's thoughts and feelings and to respond with greater sensitivity to her behaviors.

Phase 2 (Preparation)

Bilateral eye movements were used with Amy throughout the EMDR. Most commonly, EMDR therapists implement eye movements by holding up two fingers and instructing children to watch their fingers and follow the movement, side to side, with their eyes. This therapist utilized a light bar attached to a tripod, which allowed Amy to follow a light that moved bilaterally. In the preparation phase protocol, the bilateral eye movements were used to develop and reinforce a positive felt sense related to nurturing imagery, as part of the Attachment Resource Development protocol for children with attachment disorder (Attachment and Trauma Center of Nebraska, 2011; Wesselmann et al., 2013). The therapist utilized slow bilateral eye movements during resource development, because rapid saccadic eye movement can sometimes cause associations to other unprocessed memories that may contain negative content. Amy was asked to visualize herself as a young child in a safe and comfortable place with her present-day foster mother tending to her:

THERAPIST: Amy, how old is that part of you that is so sad and mad?

AMY: Two years old.

THERAPIST: Amy, I would like you to see if you can picture a place inside of you, inside your heart, where the 2-year-old you can feel safe.

[In a short discussion with the therapist, Amy remembers a past group home as a place where she had felt safe. The therapist asks Amy to follow the slow, bilateral moving light on the light bar with her eyes for approximately five round trips.]

AMY: I can see the 2-year-old me in the courtyard at the group treatment home. I remember I liked that courtyard. It was pretty, with lots of flowers.

THERAPIST: That sounds like a wonderful place for the little 2-year-old you. Who could take care of the little you there? Someone who is protective and loving . . .

AMY: Danielle and John from the treatment home.

THERAPIST: Picture the 2-year-old you there, in the courtyard, with the pretty flowers, and with Danielle and John there watching over her. (Amy follows the slow, bilateral lights for another five round trips.) How did that go?

AMY: It gave me a happy feeling.

THERAPIST: Is it OK if Mom helps John and Danielle care for the little you?

AMY: Yes.

THERAPIST: Mom, describe how you see yourself caring for little Amy, right now, in the safe place. (Instructs Amy to follow the slow, bilateral moving lights while she listens to her mother speak.)

MOM: I see myself holding her on my lap and giving her a sippy cup of milk. We're singing songs and doing silly finger plays together. I see myself rocking her in a rocking chair as she gets sleepy, falling asleep in my arms.

[At this point, Amy describes feelings of warmth and safety, which are further increased when the therapist again suggests that she watch the light as it moves slowly, side to side.]

Four weeks were devoted to the preparation phase, involving the use of EMDR to develop feelings of closeness and safety, as well as family sessions geared to increase the emotional support provided by the foster mother. Next, the EMDR therapist hypothesized with Amy and her mother about the relationship between Amy's behavioral reactivity and the past traumatic events. Current triggers for Amy's "big feelings" were identified, and as therapy progressed, Amy gradually shared memories.

Phase 3 (Assessment)

As memories were addressed one by one, each was assessed prior to reprocessing. Following is an example of the assessment phase related to a memory of sexual abuse by her biological mother's boyfriend. Amy was asked to identify the most disturbing picture associated with the memory and then was asked to identify an "upsetting thought." Amy said that the memory made her think, "Men are not safe," and she described her "wished-for" thought as "Most men are safe." She said that the memory made her feel "weird" and that she had an "uncomfortable" sensation in her stomach. On the SUD scale, where 0 = neutral and 10 = the highest disturbance imaginable, she reported a "5," and on the VOC scale, regarding the desired positive cognition, where 1 = false and 7 = completely true, she reported a "2."

Reprocessing: Phase 4 (Desensitization)

During the desensitization phase, the foster mother was encouraged to stay physically close and quietly supportive in order to help Amy stay grounded and regulated. Amy was instructed to follow the moving light on the light bar with her eyes at a speed that was rapid, but not uncomfortable. (More rapid eye movements appear to result in faster, spontaneous associations to memories and other stored information.) Following is a portion of the transcript during the desensitization phase of the sexual abuse memory that demonstrates the use of the "cognitive interweave" when processing becomes stalled. Note the changes that Amy reports after each set of eye movements. Reprocessing shifts may include new thoughts, images, emotions, or feelings.

At the beginning of each set the therapist helped Amy focus her attention, and after each set instructed her to "Let it go, and take a breath." She was then asked to report what emerged during the set. Amy's starting image was a picture of herself sitting on the lap of the perpetrator. The therapist's prompts and sets of eye movements are indicated by < < < < <.

THERAPIST: Take a breath. That's right. Let it go. OK, what's there now?

AMY: Pushing away. Telling him to stop.

< < < < < AMY: He throws me. I scream. I can't breathe.

< < < < < AMY: I thought I was going to die.

< < < < < AMY: Heartburn feeling.

< < < < < AMY: Can see him hurting me. It hurts. I can feel it inside.

< < < < < AMY: It's still the same. I can feel it inside.

[Amy's reprocessing is stalled, so the therapist decides to utilize a cognitive interweave involving imagery.]

THERAPIST: You have permission, Amy, if you want, to go there as your big 9-year-old self—to do anything you want to do—to bring anyone or anything you want along with you.

AMY: I'd bring Mom, the police, Uncle Bill, a tiger, a first-aid kit, blankets, clothes, and diapers.

< < < < < AMY: *(addressing the perpetrator)* Put her down!

< < < < < AMY: *(addressing the younger self)* He did a lot of bad things to you and we're going to take you home. [Note that spontaneous processing is resuming.]

< < < < < AMY: The police are arresting him. I'm using the first-aid kit. The tiger is protecting me. I will call little Amy by my middle name—it means "beautiful song." I will take her to the safe place.

< < < < < AMY: The pain is gone.

Amy was asked to think again of the original picture. She now reported a small sensation in her chest. Reprocessing was continued until Amy reported that her body was clear and her disturbance on the SUD scale was a 0.

Reprocessing: Phase 5 (Installation)

After the disturbance reached a 0, the desired positive cognition was strengthened.

THERAPIST: Does the positive statement, "Most men are safe" still feel like the belief you want to have, even when you think back to what happened when you were younger?

AMY: Yes. I want to be able to visit my new grandpa without getting so nervous.

THERAPIST: Yes, I remember, you and I have talked about your nervous feelings with Grandpa. OK, I would like you to think of the memory we worked on today and hold the following thought in your mind: "Most men are safe." Look at the scale on this card. Show me how true it feels to you right now. *(Amy points to a 6 on the 7-point VOC scale.)* OK, hold the memory in mind and the words "Most men are safe." Then follow the light on the light bar with your eyes. [The paired image, thought, and sets of eye movements are repeated several times until the cognition is fully installed.] What are you getting now?

AMY: Yes, it feels good. It feels really true.

Phases 6, 7, and 8 (Body Scan, Closure, and Reevaluation)

Amy was guided to scan her body one more time, looking for any remaining disturbance (Phase 6). If any existed, it would have been the focus of reprocessing. Since Amy reported no disturbance, the therapist closed the session by encouraging Amy to "let it go now," but to tell her mom if anything bothered her during the week (Phase 7). Amy was also encouraged to use her "safe place" if any disturbance emerged. At the following session, the therapist asked Amy to bring up the incident again and look for any disturbance in her body, emotion, or thoughts (Phase 8). Amy reported that it was "all clear," so the next disturbing memory was targeted. The full, three-pronged (past–present–future) approach was utilized in treatment.

Memories subsequently targeted with EMDR for Amy included:

- Birth mother's failure to attend scheduled visits.
- Physical abuse by birth mother's boyfriend.
- Memory of sexual abuse by birth mother's boyfriend.
- Memory of domestic violence between birth mother and boyfriend.
- Removal from each of the previous adoptive homes.
- Memory of being left alone.
- Memory of her own sexualized behavior toward younger children— Amy felt shame about these memories and viewed herself as "bad" and "evil."

Recent and current triggers were also identified and reprocessed along with the associated negative beliefs, including:

- Anxiety triggered when Amy was cuddling with foster mom at home. NC: "I will be hurt!"
- Anger related to foster mom going out for the evening. Negative cognition (NC): "I will be abandoned."

- Sadness related to seeing an infant being cared for. NC: "Something was wrong with me!"
- Film at school about domestic violence, associated to memory of the boyfriend hitting birth mom. NC: "I'm not in control."
- Mom saying *no* to sweets before meals. NC: "She's out to get me—I have to be in control."

In order to reinforce positive responses to challenging situations in the future, the therapist and Amy made a list of positive behaviors. Guidance/education regarding the behaviors was given, as necessary, and the behaviors were reinforced through imagery (using positive "future template" procedures; Shapiro, 2001) enhanced with sets of eye movements. Behaviors included:

- Doing chores responsibly.
- Saying "OK" when Mom says "no."
- Doing schoolwork at the appropriate time.
- Using appropriate, assertive behavior with friends.
- Presenting calm, cooperative behavior on each holiday.
- Presenting calm, cooperative behavior with a babysitter.

Conclusion of Therapy

EMDR and family therapy were continued on a nearly weekly basis for 1 year, targeting and reprocessing past events, current and recent difficulties, and reinforcing positive future cognitive and emotional templates. The adoption was finalized 9 months after the beginning of therapy. At that time, the flashbacks and body sensations had stopped; fear and anxiety were no longer evident; the urination and defecation behaviors, self-harming, and inappropriate sexual talk as school had all ceased. Amy reportedly still whined and had occasional tantrums consistent with her chronological age. In sum, all of the presenting symptoms were eliminated, and Amy functioned much better at home and school.

As a follow-up, Amy was interviewed at 13 years of age, 3 years after completing her EMDR therapy. In the interim, Amy had attended 12 supportive counseling sessions for adjustment issues related to a move, a school change, and challenges with foster children who had joined the family. A portion of the interview of this representative case is included in order to emphasize the broad range of goals that can be achieved through comprehensive treatment of even the most severely abused children. The transcript of the interview shows evidence that Amy now holds a secure attachment style, with coherence of speech and evidence of a sense of forgiveness, an ability to talk on an emotional level without becoming overwhelmed, and a lack of blaming toward either self or others.

THERAPIST: When you first came to your mom's, you were all of—how old?

AMY: Eight—when I first came to my mom's.

THERAPIST: Eight, OK. You threw some pretty hefty tantrums, do you remember?

AMY: Yes.

THERAPIST: Do you remember what kinds of things you would do when you threw those tantrums?

AMY: Try to break the window.

THERAPIST: Wow. And you kind of went on for hours, didn't you?

AMY: Yeah, I definitely went on for hours.

THERAPIST: Thinking back on it now, do you think you didn't have any control over it at the time?

AMY: Well, I think it's probably because I'd been through so much, and going to a different home, it was kind of frustrating for me, so, throwing the temper tantrums, I guess, was just to get the anger out.

THERAPIST: You were just really, really mad. Do you remember that feeling?

AMY: Yeah. I remember just a couple days before I had come [to this home] I had put soap all over the people's toothbrushes, and they didn't know, and . . . it didn't turn out so good.

THERAPIST: So when we did our EMDR, we did our EMDR on all the bad stuff that had happened to you. It was really painful for you at the time to think about it, to work on it. Is it easier now for you to talk about your life?

AMY: Yeah, it is easier, it's just a whole lot easier. It's kind of like—it's just a lot easier because when I was doing that (points to the light bar which she and her therapist had used to guide her eye movements)—it helped.

THERAPIST: That's so cool. You remember, when I worked with you, you remembered what happened in your birth home. You had some pretty bad experiences there.

AMY: Yeah. It's like, if someone asked me, do you want to go see your parents? It would probably be like, yes, but at the very same time, no, because of the stuff that they did, and yet, I still love them.

THERAPIST: Sure. That makes perfect sense. And then you were in three other homes that were supposed to adopt you, but didn't. And you had a lot of pain about that.

AMY: Yeah.

THERAPIST: Yeah, a lot of sadness, pain, and hurt.

AMY: Thinking I'm going to stay in that home, and of course, no. It's not going to happen.

THERAPIST: What is your understanding of that now?

AMY: My understanding of that now would probably be that the parents didn't know what they were doing. Probably thinking that they knew what they were doing, but probably not knowing that when you adopt a child from a different place . . .

THERAPIST: Like from abuse?

AMY: Yes, from abuse and stuff. They probably didn't know what's going to happen—what the problems are going to be at home.

THERAPIST: Yes.

AMY: Yes, they probably weren't ready for that. They probably thought, "Oh, this is a fine kid." But it's probably not. It's really not.

THERAPIST: Yes, they weren't prepared for the problems, yeah. And of course you had problems.

AMY: Yeah.

[Toward the end, the conversation shifts to Amy's excitement over her mother's pregnancy. It reveals a distinct difference from her pretreatment desire to squeeze and pop a visiting infant's head.]

AMY: Sometimes when you look really closely at my mom's stomach, you can see the kick. It's really fun.

THERAPIST: Are you excited to be a big sister?

AMY: Yeah.

THERAPIST: I'll bet you'll be a big help to your mom, too.

AMY: Yeah. And my mom wanted a boy and I wanted a girl, and since we're going to adopt a boy, I kind of say, well, you can adopt the dude . . . you get the man, and I get the lady.

Conclusion

EMDR is adapted for children and adolescents suffering from complex trauma through more emphasis on client preparation (Phase 2); assistance with expression of thoughts, feelings, and sensations (Phase 3); and cognitive interweaves, as needed, during reprocessing (Phase 4). For children removed from biological homes due to mistreatment, collaboration with a family therapist can help ensure that present-day caregivers provide appropriate support during EMDR. In addition, it can be useful to evaluate the parental response to determine if it is appropriate, and whether EMDR therapy is needed to ensure that the caregiver can be both present and an adequate attachment figure for the child. The delineation of EMDR and family therapy roles ensures that EMDR can be implemented every week (Attachment and Trauma Center of Nebraska, 2011; Wesselmann et al., 2013).

The EMDR practitioner can help traumatized children and adolescents by targeting and reprocessing memories to allow comprehensive changes in cognitive, affective, and somatic domains, leading to earned secure attachments and an integrated sense of self. By reprocessing targets involving past, present, and future, EMDR can help hurt children discover a new perspective regarding themselves, others, and their world. Timely treatment can prevent a lifelong trajectory of dysfunction and help end the transgenerational transmission of abuse and victimization fed by the unprocessed memories.

References

Adler-Tapia, R., & Settle, C. (2008). *EMDR and the art of psychotherapy with children*. New York: Springer.

Aduriz, M. E., Bluthgen, C., & Knopfler, C. (2009). Helping child flood victims using group EMDR intervention in Argentina: Treatment outcome and gender differences. *International Journal of Stress Management, 16*, 138–153.

Ahmad, A., Larsson, B., & Sundelin-Wahlsten, V. (2007). EMDR treatment for children with PTSD: Results of a randomized controlled trial. *Nordic Journal of Psychiatry, 61*, 349–354.

Attachment and Trauma Center of Nebraska. (2011). *EMDR integrative team treatment for attachment trauma in children: Treatment manual*. Omaha, NE: Author.

Bisson, J., & Andrew, M. (2007). Psychological treatment of posttraumatic stress disorder (PTSD). *Cochrane Database of Systematic Reviews 2007*.

Brown, S., & Shapiro, F. (2006). EMDR in the treatment of borderline personality disorder. *Clinical Case Studies, 5*, 403–420.

Chemtob, C. M., Nakashima, J., & Carlson, J. G. (2002). Brief treatment for elementary school children with disaster-related PTSD: A field study. *Journal of Clinical Psychology, 58*, 99–112.

Christman, S. D., Garvey, K. J., Propper, R. E., & Phaneuf, K. A. (2003). Bilateral eye movements enhance the retrieval of episodic memories. *Neuropsychology, 17*, 221–229.

Craske, M., Herman, D., & Vansteenwegen, D. (Eds.). (2006). *Fear and learning: From basic processes to clinical implications*. Washington, DC: American Psychological Association.

de Roos, C., Greenwald, R., den Hollander-Gijsm, M., Noorthoorn, E., van Buuren, S., & de Jongh, A. (2011). A randomized comparison of cognitive behavioural therapy. *European Journal of Psychotraumatology, 2*, 5694–5704.

Eckers, D. (2010). The method of constant installation of present orientation and safety (CIPOS) for children. In M. Luber (Ed.), *EMDR scripted protocols: Special populations* (pp. 51–58). New York: Springer.

Fernandez, I., Gallinari, E., & Lorenzetti, A. (2004). A school-based EMDR intervention for chidren who witnessed the Pirelli building airplane crash in Milan, Italy. *Journal of Brief Therapy, 2,* 129–136.

Foa, E. B., Keane, T. M., Friedman, M. J., & Cohen, J. A. (2009). *Effective treatments for PTSD: Practice guidelines of the International Society for Traumatic Stress Studies.* New York: Guilford Press.

Gomez, A. M. (2010). Using olfactory stimulation with children to cue resource development and installation (RDI). In M. Luber (Ed.), *EMDR scripted protocols: Special population* (pp. 19–30). New York: Springer.

Gomez, A. M. (2012). *EMDR therapy and adjunct approaches with children: Complex trauma, attachment and dissociation.* New York: Springer.

Ide, N., & Paez, A. (2000). Complex PTSD: A review of current issues. *International Journal of Emergency Mental Health, 2,* 43–49.

Jaberghaderi, N., Greenwald, R., Rubin, A., Dolatabadim, S., & Zand, S. O. (2004). A comparison of CBT and EMDR for sexually abused Iranian girls. *Clinical Psychology and Psychotherapy, 11,* 358–368.

Jarero, I., Artigas, L., & Luber, M. (2011). The EMDR protocol for recent critical incidents: Application in a disaster mental health continuum of care context. *Journal of EMDR Practice and Research, 5,* 92–94.

Kemp, M., Drummond, P., & McDermott, B. (2010). A wait-list controlled pilot study of eye movement desensitization and reprocessing (EMDR) for children with posttraumatic stress disorder (PTSD) symptoms from motor vehicle accidents. *Clinical Child Psychology and Psychiatry, 15,* 5025.

Korn, D., & Leeds, A. (2002). Preliminary evidence of efficacy for EMDR resource development and installation in the stabilization phase of treatment of complex posttraumatic stress disorder. *Journal of Clinical Psychology, 58,* 1465–1487.

Madrid, A., Skolek, S., & Shapiro, F. (2006). Repairing failures in bonding through EMDR. *Clinical Case Studies, 5,* 271–286.

Mol, S. S. L., Arntz, A., Metsemakers, J. F. M., Dinant, G., Vilters-Van Montfort, P. A. P., & Knottnerus, A. (2005). Symptoms of post-traumatic stress disorder after non-traumatic events: Evidence from an open population study. *British Journal of Psychiatry, 186,* 494–499.

Obradović, J., Bush, N. R., Stamperdahl, J., Adler, N. E., & Boyce, W. T. (2010). Biological sensitivity to context: The interactive effects of stress reactivity and family adversity on socioemotional behavior and school readiness. *Child Development, 1,* 270–289.

Parker, A., Buckley, S., & Dagnall, N. (2009). Reduced misinformation effects following saccadic bilateral eye movements. *Brain and Cognition, 69,* 89–97.

Potter, A. E., Davidson, M., & Wesselmann, D. (2013). *Utilizing dialectical behavior therapy and eye movement desensitization and reprocessing as phase-based trauma treatment: A case study series.* Manuscript submitted for publication.

Robredo, J. (2011, June). *EMDR and gender violence: Brief and intensive treatment for children exposed to gender violence.* Paper presented at the annual meeting of the EMDR Europe Association, Vienna, Austria.

Rodenburg, R., Benjamin, A., de Roos, C., Meijer, A. M., & Stams, G. J. (2009). Efficacy of EMDR in children: A meta-analysis. *Clinical Psychology Review, 29,* 599–606.

Schubert, S. J., Lee, C. W., & Drummond, P. D. (2011). The efficacy and psychophysiological correlates of dual-attention tasks in eye movement desensitization and reprocessing (EMDR). *Journal of Anxiety Disorders, 25,* 1–11

Shapiro, F. (2001). *Eye movement desensitization and reprocessing: Basic principles, protocols and procedures* (2nd ed.). New York: Guilford Press.

Shapiro, F. (2012). *Getting past your past: Take control of your life with self-help techniques from EMDR therapy.* New York: Rodale.

Shapiro, F. (2013). Redefining trauma and its hidden connections: Identifying and reprocessing the experiential contributors to a wide variety of disorders. In M. Solomon & D.S. Siegel (Eds.), *Healing moments in psychotherapy.* New York: Norton.

Solomon, R. M., & Shapiro, F. (2008). EMDR and the adaptive information processing model: Potential mechanisms of change. *Journal of EMDR Practice and Research, 2,* 315–325.

Suzuki, A., Josselyn, S. A., Frankland, P. W., Masushige, S., Silva, A. J., & Satoshi, K. (2004). Memory reconsolidation and extinction have distinct temporal and biochemical signatures. *Journal of Neuroscience, 24,* 4787–4795.

U.S. Department of Veterans Affairs & Department of Defense. (2004, 2010). *VA/DoD clinical practice guideline for the management of post-traumatic stress.* Washington, DC: Author.

van den Hout, M. A., Engelhard, I. M., Rijkeboer, M. M., Koekebakker, J., Hornsveld, H., Leer, A., et al. (2011). EMDR: Eye movements superior to beeps in taxing working memory and reducing vividness of recollections. *Behaviour Research and Therapy, 49*(2), 92–98.

van der Kolk, B. (2005). Developmental trauma disorder: Toward a rational diagnosis for children with complex trauma histories. *Psychiatric Annals, 35*(5), 401–408.

van der Kolk, B. A., Pelcovitz, D., Roth, S., Mandel, F. S., McFarlane, A. C., & Herman, J. L. (1996). Dissociation, somatization, and affect regulation: The complexity of adaptation to trauma. *American Journal of Psychiatry, 153*(7), 83–93.

Wanders, F., Serra, M., & de Jongh, A. (2008). EMDR versus CBT for children with self-esteem and behavioral problems: A randomized controlled trial. *Journal of EMDR Practice and Research, 2,* 180–189.

Wesselmann, D. (2007). Treating attachment issues through EMDR and a family systems approach. In F. Shapiro, F. W. Kaslow, & L. Maxfield (Eds.), *Handbook of EMDR and family therapy processes* (pp. 113–130). Hoboken, NJ: Wiley.

Wesselmann, D. (2013). Healing trauma and creating secure attachments with EMDR. In M. Solomon & D. S. Siegel (Eds.), *Healing moments in psychotherapy: Mindful awareness, neural integration, and therapeutic presence.* New York: Norton.

Wesselmann, D., Davidson, M., Armstrong, S., Schweitzer, C., Bruckner, O., & Potter, A. (2012). EMDR as a treatment for improving attachment status in adults and children. *European Review of Applied Psychology, 62,* 223–230.

Wesselmann, D., & Potter, A. E. (2009). Change in adult attachment status following treatment with EMDR: Three case studies. *Journal of EMDR Practice and Research, 3,* 178–191.

Wesselmann, D., Schweitzer, C., & Armstrong, S. (2013). *Integrative team treatment for attachment trauma in children: Family therapy and EMDR.* New York: Norton.

Wilson, S., Becker, L., & Tinker, R. (1995). Eye movement desensitization and reprocessing (EMDR) treatment for psychologically traumatized individuals. *Journal of Consulting and Clinical Psychology, 63,* 928–937.

Zaghrout-Hodali, M., Alissa, F., & Dodgson, P. (2008). Building resilience and dismantling fear: EMDR group protocol with children in an area of ongoing trauma. *Journal of EMDR Practice and Research, 2,* 106–113.

CHAPTER 12

Dialectical Behavior Therapy with Adolescents

Ruth R. DeRosa
Jill H. Rathus

Dialectical behavior therapy (DBT), originally developed for borderline personality disorder (BPD) in adult women, has been extensively researched, resulting in a great deal of empirical support, including randomized controlled trials (see Lynch, Trost, Salsman, & Linehan, 2007; Linehan, Armstrong, Suarez, Allmon, & Heard, 1991; Linehan et al., 2006). DBT is a flexible, principle-driven, manualized treatment that incorporates behavioral and cognitive-behavioral therapy principles with mindfulness-based practices (Linehan, 1993). It has demonstrated success with adults in increasing emotion regulation capacities as well as decreasing inpatient hospitalizations, suicidal behaviors, and nonsuicidal self injury, anger, and symptoms of depression (Axelrod, Perepletchikova, Holtzman, & Sinha, 2011; Lynch, Morse, Mendelson, & Robins, 2003; Linehan, McDavid, Brown, Sayrs, & Gallop, 2008; Neacsiu, Rizvi, & Linehan, 2010). Over time, DBT has been successfully implemented and/or adapted with a variety of other populations, including adults diagnosed with substance abuse, eating disorders, depression, and comorbid BPD and posttraumatic stress disorder (PTSD) (Axelrod et al., 2011; Courbasson, Nishikawa, & Dixon, 2011; Harned, Jackson, Comtois, & Linehan, 2010; Lynch et al., 2003).

There is evidence that the dimensional features of BPD (negative affectivity, impulsivity, and interpersonal aggression) may emerge in childhood and remain over time (Stepp, Pilkonis, Hipwell, Loeber, & Stouthamer-Loeber, 2010). Interestingly, the most stable BPD criterion, according to longitudinal research, appears to be emotional dysregulation (Gunderson et al., 2011). Moreover, some research suggests that difficulties with emotion regulation and relationships might precede problems with impulse control in adolescent BPD (Stepp, Burke, Hipwell, & Loeber, 2012). In a nontreatment-seeking sample of children, emotional abuse was associated with BP features only among participants who also had significant problems with emotion regulation (Gratz, Latzman, Tull, Reynolds, & Lejuez, 2011). Emotion regulation seems to be a foundational capacity and potentially a protective factor. DBT's approach to enhancing emotion regulation, distress tolerance, and mindfulness may serve a preventive function if provided to adolescents.

DBT treatment for adolescents (Miller, Rathus, & Linehan, 2007) therefore was developed, with a number of modifications designed to suit this developmental period, including a shorter length (16–32 sessions), simplified handouts, a multifamily group skills format to include caregivers, and an additional skills module to address parenting strategies, titled "Walking the Middle Path." A growing body of literature indicates that DBT for adolescents is a promising treatment for youth who exhibit significant emotional dysregulation (Groves, Backer, van der Bosch, & Miller, 2012). Clinical research implementing DBT with adolescents has been conducted in a number of settings, including inpatient, outpatient, residential, and detention centers, with adolescents with BPD, as well as a number of other adolescent populations without current suicidality—including teens with bipolar disorder, substance abuse, eating disorders, oppositional defiant disorder, and attention-deficit/hyperactivity disorder (ADHD) (Goldstein, Axelson, Birmaher, & Brent, 2007; see Klein & Miller, 2011, for a comprehensive review). Although to date no randomized controlled trials with adolescents have been published, two studies are currently underway in Norway and New Zealand (Klein & Miller, 2011). Studies of adolescents with quasi-experimental designs have demonstrated significant reductions in suicidal ideation, nonsuicidal self-injury, BP and depressive symptoms, and fewer inpatient hospitalizations compared to controls (Rathus & Miller, 2002; Katz, Cox, Gunasekara, & Miller, 2004).

DBT may be particularly relevant for the prevention of BPD with traumatized adolescents. As many as 75% of adults with BPD have reported histories of childhood trauma (Zanarini, 2000). Affect regulation and information processing are often altered in the face of chronic child maltreatment, with neurobiological consequences (Ford, 2005). Among survivors of multiple, repeated experiences of child maltreatment, typical clinical adolescent presentations include problems involving self-concept, emotional and behavioral self-regulation, and academic and interpersonal functioning. These adaptations to complex trauma are not fully captured by the diagnosis of PTSD and include difficulty with regulation of the following: (1) affects and impulses (upset or angered easily, trouble calming down, impulsivity, self-destructive behaviors), (2) somatization and physical health (e.g., multiple, chronic physical complaints; autoimmune disorders), (3) attention and information processing (dissociation), (4) self-perception (e.g., self as damaged, shameful, guilty), (5) sense of meaning and purpose in life (hopeless and pessimistic about the future), and (6) interpersonal relationships (e.g., problems with trust, assertiveness, and maintaining stable relationships). This constellation of problems has been described in many ways over time (e.g., as complex PTSD, complex traumatic stress disorders, sequelae of Type II traumas, disorder of extreme stress not otherwise specified (DESNOS), developmental trauma disorder, and complex posttraumatic self-dysregulation; see Courtois & Ford, 2009).

Although there are treatment recommendations for complex trauma cases (Courtois & Ford, 2009) and an emerging consensus across trauma experts in the treatment literature for Complex PTSD (Cloitre et al., 2011), specific treatment protocols are less clear when adolescents present with significant behavioral and emotional dysregulation accompanied by risky, self-injurious, or suicidal behaviors. Lang, Ford, and Fitzgerald (2010) provide a useful algorithm to help clinicians determine whether trauma-focused cognitive-behavioral therapy (TF-CBT) is appropriate for a particular child. These authors point out that evidence for exposure-based treatment is less clear when the child or adolescent is in need of stabilization due to high-risk behaviors. This assessment also coincides with a history of best-practice recommendations in the clinical literature (see Ford & Cloitre, 2009) that outlines a phase-based treatment approach that begins with increasing safety, stabilization, and emotion regulation capacities. DBT, with its focus on establishing safety and behavioral control, may be particularly useful when traumatized adolescents and their parents present with impulsive, dysregulated behavior and emotions, initially precluding narrative work. In a study with adult clients, as many as 68% of participants who would not have been eligible for PTSD treatment due to high-risk behaviors became eligible after 1 year of DBT (Harned, Jackson, et al., 2010).

In the remainder of this chapter, we describe and illustrate central components of DBT that may be especially helpful for treating high-risk adolescents with complex PTSD. DBT for adolescents is a comprehensive program that includes individual therapy, a weekly multifamily 2-hour skills group, phone coaching to support use of the skills between sessions, and weekly DBT consultation team meetings for the clinicians. Adolescents also complete a weekly self-monitoring checklist, referred to as the *diary card,* to track specific behaviors, emotions, and skills used during the week. The DBT model provides therapists with a variety of acceptance and change strategies to teach and assist teens with very painful, overwhelming lives. The focus of treatment with chronically traumatized teens is to address severe emotional dysregulation. When adolescents come to session with multiple pressing problems, DBT helps clinicians prioritize interventions according to its hierarchy of treatment targets. This prioritized order consists of decreasing life-threatening behavior, decreasing therapy-interfering behavior, decreasing quality-of-life-interfering behavior, and increasing behavioral capacities. The DBT model thus provides a "road map" of what to address by focusing both the therapist and the client on priorities for the session. *Life-threatening behavior* refers to suicidal behavior (i.e., ideation, communication, planning, attempts) and nonsuicidal self-injury. If nonsuicidal self-injury is present, it is critical to address this behavior in each session; research suggests that self-injury, even without suicidal intent, is just as likely as a previous suicide attempt to predict future suicidal attempts (Brent, 2011).

The second treatment priority after life-threatening behavior is therapy-interfering behavior. This focus includes actions on the part of the client (e.g., not completing homework, skipping sessions) or on the part of the therapist (e.g., not returning phone calls in timely manner, making an invalidating comment) that interfere with the progress or continuation of therapy. So, if a client comes in after just having had an upsetting fight with a family member or friend, or skipped class because he or she got high last night and overslept, and didn't fill out the diary card, the therapist addresses not doing the diary card first. This sequence is important because assessing and problem-solving the factors that will impede the client's progress can enhance both compliance and the therapy relationship. Of course, one does not assume why the client may not have done the homework; for example, it could be connected to a desire to avoid rating intense emotions, to not remembering or understanding the specific instructions, fear of doing it wrong, feeling overwhelmed, etc.

If life-threatening or therapy-interfering behaviors are not present, clinicians address problems that interfere with clients' quality of life, such as difficulties in school, problems with sleep, dissociation, depression, substance abuse, disordered eating, risky sexual behavior, repeatedly going to places that aren't safe, driving too fast, and tumultuous relationships. The final target is increasing of the client's behavioral skills.

The therapist addresses symptoms of PTSD and complex PTSD in several different places throughout the treatment. In-depth discussions of thoughts, behaviors, and physiological reactivity before, during, and after life-threatening behaviors and urges could reveal reactions to trauma triggers, for example, or efforts to combat numbing, dissociation, or regulate emotions. Discussions of therapy-interfering behaviors might also point to trauma symptomatology—for example, shutting down in session and/or avoidance of trauma reminders. Trauma symptoms can also be included on the diary card, so that clients track the frequency and intensity of specific responses, which increases their ability to label and step back from the experience and facilitates in-session assessment and problem solving.

Examples of skills in DBT that may be especially relevant for adolescents who have experienced chronic interpersonal trauma include mindfulness skills to focus a nonjudgmental attention on the present moment; skills to increase their tolerance of distressing emotions, including specific ways to distract, self-soothe, and use visual imagery and breathing techniques; skills to enhance communication even in the face of distrust or alienation; and skills that would enable them to act the opposite of the urges associated with shame and fear that can compound maladaptive avoidance.

Next, we highlight selected components of DBT that may be especially relevant for adolescents with complex PTSD: engagement strategies (validation, commitment strategies, and addressing therapy-interfering behavior), functional assessment, mindfulness practice, family/caregiver involvement (multifamily skills training group and as-needed family therapy sessions), phone coaching, and the therapist consultation team.

Engagement

The task of gaining the attention and commitment of a despondent, perhaps angry, adolescent can be challenging. Those who work regularly with adolescents know that providing a mixture of genuineness, playfulness, sincerity, validation, frankness, and irreverence balanced with attention to timing, tone of voice, and nonverbal communication is key. One of the benefits of working with teenagers is that they will let you know right away if they think your intervention stinks! In this case, a validating response may be in order while being radically genuine.

> CLIENT: I'm fine. It is none of my parents' business what I do. It's not a big deal an I'm not participating in this &*$#.
>
> THERAPIST: OK. Bad idea. You've had enough of this psychotherapy crap, and you want your parents to leave you alone.
>
> CLIENT: Yes.
>
> THERAPIST: What do you think is most likely to get your parents off your back? Could we work on that?

Validation

Validation is certainly a cornerstone of the therapeutic alliance, engagement, and psychotherapy treatment. Linehan (1993) emphasizes, however, that validation is more than empathy:

> Validation strategies require the therapist to search for, recognize, and reflect to the client the validity inherent in her [sic] response to events. With unruly children, parents have to catch them while they're good in order to reinforce

their behavior; similarly, the therapist has to uncover the validity within the client's response, sometimes amplify it, and then reinforce it. (pp. 222–223)

Validation requires therapists to identify responses that make sense given the client's *current* life circumstances and experiences, not merely in the context of their past experiences. To focus solely or primarily on the past— for example, "It makes sense that you are hurt by your friend's behavior because it feels similar to ways your family treated you"—could actually be experienced as invalidating. Likewise, focusing on change strategies and problem solving without sufficiently communicating the ways in which clients' initial reactions make sense (even if you disagree!) will also likely be ineffective and invalidating. Instead of starting with cognitive restructuring, or problem solving, or a discussion of reasons to live, in the following example the therapist initially focuses on validating the client's wish to die:

> CLIENT: I can't stand the thought of going back to that school and all its &*$%. Everyone is fake and the teachers suck. My parents don't care, and I've been doing this all alone. I feel like something is wrong with me. Sometimes I even think I'd be better off dead.
>
> THERAPIST: You have been alone with this for a long time.
>
> CLIENT: Mmm-hmm.
>
> THERAPIST: No wonder you would want out.
>
> CLIENT: Yeah, I'm tired and I'm done. *(Starts avoiding eye contact, head down.)*
>
> THERAPIST: You are done—you don't want to feel this way anymore.
>
> CLIENT: *(Starts to cry.)* No, I really don't.
>
> THERAPIST: The thing about being dead is that it is a very permanent solution to what I would suggest is a temporary problem. If you are not around, we can't work on making things better.
>
> CLIENT: *(Makes eye contact.)* I don't know what to do.
>
> THERAPIST: OK. Would you be willing for us to think together about how to deal with the school &*$%?
>
> CLIENT: OK.

Needless to say, risk assessment is also an essential part of this session. Now that the therapist has gotten agreement to embark on a problem-solving discussion together, the likelihood of obtaining a commitment to follow through on a plan, and/or a willingness to call the therapist for coaching, may be greatly enhanced. The use of validation in DBT is also very precise and purposeful with attention on both how and when to apply this strategy in session. A recent study that compared the use of validation in DBT to the use of validation in expert nonbehavioral therapy (Bedics,

Atkins, Comtois, & Linehan, 2011) found that participants in DBT who perceived greater warmth, affirmation, and protection from their therapists exhibited significantly fewer nonsuicidal self-injurious behaviors (NSIB), whereas participants in the expert nonbehavioral community therapist condition who perceived greater warmth, affirmation, and protection exhibited *more* self-injurious behavior. The authors proposed that the non-DBT community therapists may have inadvertently reinforced NSIB by being more validating and affirming after self-injurious acts. DBT specifically outlines implementing validation strategies in a strategic manner in order to validate the intention or behavior of the client that the therapist wants to reinforce. The practice of balancing acceptance and change strategies is an integral and explicitly defined component of DBT. This balance of strategies may be of great utility for treating clients with complex trauma histories. On the one hand, their pain and problems with impulses demand change. On the other, the dysregulation of emotions, cognition, biology, relationships, and self-image requires validation to reduce in-session affective arousal, improve information processing, build the alliance, and cultivate sense of self.

Commitment Strategies

The goal of obtaining a pledge to participate in treatment is a part of the engagement definition described above but is also a separate step. Even having successfully engaged a client in some ways doesn't mean that he or she has agreed to actively participate. A perfectly acceptable client goal may be to simply work to get out of treatment or to get caregivers off their backs. A commitment goal can also mean leaving the door open for the future . . . if the clinician cannot obtain full commitment right away. The therapist's tone, facial expression, and timing are critical because with adolescents, it is especially important to be sincere, light, genuine, and at times irreverent.

DBT provides specific strategies to obtain and strengthen adolescents' commitment. These are not strategies used only at the beginning of treatment, but throughout therapy when looking for commitment to try something new or change a behavior, or when engagement in treatment wanes. The decision to exercise, followed by several weeks of working out, for example, does not necessarily sustain a commitment to lifelong physical activity (as many of us know!). It typically requires recommitment. The commitment to continue treatment in the face of life stressors and family conflict can be very difficult and can be strengthened with specific commitment strategies, some of which are outlined below.

FOOT IN THE DOOR/DOOR IN THE FACE

Clinicians might remember learning about the "foot in the door" approach from social psychology class. The therapist asks for just a tiny agreement, with which the client will almost surely comply, which then makes it more likely that the client will agree to do a little more. For example, when clients feel overwhelmed by the idea of a diary card, the therapist might say: "How about filling out one column of the diary card, right here and right now, with me?" The therapist might follow up this exercise with a request to try the next column at home.

The "door in the face" strategy involves asking for an unrealistic amount at once, and then lowering the request to a level to which the client is likely to agree. Example: Just before skills group, the therapist quietly approaches a client who has been withdrawn and sitting away from the group lately, and asks, "Hector, are you willing to come sit at the head of the table and lead us in a mindfulness exercise today?" Hector looks startled and quietly replies, "I don't think so." The therapist asks, "OK, then how about sitting around the table with everyone today instead of off to the side?" Hector looks relieved and replies, "Well, all right, I guess I can do that."

DEVIL'S ADVOCATE

In the devil's advocate strategy, the therapist points out the down side of making a requested change. So, if the client seems agreeable in a manner that appears to happen too quickly or easily, perhaps without thinking it through, the therapist can then ask the client to justify his or her choice. For example:

> THERAPIST: You know there's homework in DBT. Are you up for that?
>
> LUKE: Yeah, sure (answering very quickly, without eye contact).
>
> THERAPIST: Really? Most people are not too thrilled with homework. Why are you are cool with more homework?"

Then the clients make the argument for why it is needed—perhaps nothing else has worked, they feel miserable, they know that turning things around is going to take hard work, and so on.

FREEDOM TO CHOOSE/ABSENCE OF ALTERNATIVES

In this commitment strategy, the therapist highlights the client's freedom to make his or her own choices while pointing out that there are no other options (other than the effective one) for reaching his or her goals. For example, the therapist might say to a client on the verge of a substance relapse: "Look, it is obviously up to you, and only you, if you want to go back to using drugs. It is your choice. But the down side is that continuing to use is never going to be the ticket to building the life I know you said you wanted: school, a job, and a relationship."

PROS/CONS

In this strategy, the therapist asks the client to consider the pros and cons of continuing as is, and the pros and cons of entering therapy (or making another effective decision). This focus helps the client generate the reasons for entering therapy as well as the problems with continuing down the same path. It also provides the therapist with information about what is discouraging the client, so the therapist might be better able to help problem solve. It is useful to write the list together, so both client and therapist can see and read it as they go along, and for the therapist to write down exactly, word for word, the language the client uses (including possible curse words!). This demonstrates that the therapist is truly listening, is nonjudgmental, and is taking the client's point of view seriously. Beginning this process might look like this:

> THERAPIST: *(after orienting to treatment)* So, Alex, what do you think? Does DBT sound like something you are ready to sign up for?
>
> ALEX: I dunno.
>
> THERAPIST: *(taking out a pad of paper and getting ready to write so both of them can see the pros and cons list generated)* Why don't we consider the pros and cons of your continuing as you have been going, versus the pros and cons of starting therapy. Are you willing to do that? It might help us get a better handle on whether this is a good idea right now, and what might be interfering with your getting some help.
>
> ALEX: OK, I guess.
>
> THERAPIST: Good. Why don't we start with the down side of starting therapy now?

SHAPING COMMITMENT

With this strategy, the therapist reinforces small steps in the direction of commitment, rather than demanding commitment to the whole treatment or request at once. The following example takes place during orientation to treatment:

> THERAPIST: So, what are you thinking at this point?
>
> NATASHA: I'm thinking that it sounds OK. I'm willing to try group maybe. I'm just not sure about filling out diary cards every single week . . . that's really too much.
>
> THERAPIST: That's great that you are willing to come to group! That's a big step, and I'm really excited for you to start learning the skills! I understand about the diary card—and it sounds as though

you might be willing to consider it if we can find a way to make it manageable?

LINKING PRESENT COMMITMENT TO PAST COMMITMENT

In this strategy, the therapist links asking for commitment to engage in a particular behavior (e.g., sticking to plan of attending school every day of the week) to the client's prior commitment to treatment goals and long-term goals. Prompting clients' memories of their own goals in their own words helps reenergize their willingness to follow through. For example:

THERAPIST: So, Nikki, I know you don't want to go to school, and I know it's really hard to go. And do you remember what you said to me last month when you almost dropped out?

NIKKI: I know, I know. I said I really wanted to graduate from high school.

THERAPIST: Do you remember why you said that was important to you?

NIKKI: To stay on track with my goal of going to college and then becoming a teacher.

THERAPIST: Is that something that's still important to you?

NIKKI: Yeah, I guess so, I mean, yeah, it is.

THERAPIST: So how about we work together to find a way to get through school? You've got 4 months to go.

NIKKI: What do you think I could do?

THERAPIST: Well, let's look together at all the things that are getting in the way, and see if we can come up with an "experiment" to try this week.

Targeting Therapy-Interfering Behavior

In addition to implementing commitment strategies, DBT therapists directly address behaviors that interfere with the therapy to enhance and maintain engagement in treatment. Perhaps a unique feature of the DBT approach is that actions on the part of both the client *and* the therapist are routinely included in discussions during therapy sessions when either party behaves in a way that could interfere with the treatment and the therapy relationship. Therapy-interfering behaviors include behaviors such as not completing the diary card, missing sessions, not calling for coaching, not completing the homework, and in-session behaviors that interfere with the therapy (e.g., shutting down or dissociating due to anger, shame, or other intense emotions; invalidating comments by the therapist or not starting sessions on time). Working collaboratively to discuss and to solve problems that arise with engaging in treatment also helps to sustain a strong therapeutic relationship and reduce dropout. In the following pretreatment-stage session, a therapist explains therapy-interfering behavior and the importance of discussing difficulties in the therapy relationship:

> CLIENT: I've just been feeling angry at the world . . . everyone is letting me down. I feel like, no one understands what I am going through, and they just don't get it. I don't feel like talking to anyone.
>
> THERAPIST: That sounds really disappointing, and we can definitely work on what is happening with these relationships and see how we can increase your support. And, I've got to say, there is a possibility that I could let you down in some way. I wouldn't mean to, but I might accidentally say or do something that gets you thinking, "Boy, Dr. X is a kind of a jerk!" Could you imagine that happening?
>
> CLIENT: Well, it's not that likely; you seem pretty nice . . . but, I don't know, maybe.
>
> THERAPIST: So, if it does happen, you could have the temptation to withdraw from me as well. What I'd like for us to do is "cope ahead" together and plan what we can do if you start to feel that way, and maybe we can even try to prevent it. In order for me to be helpful to you, it is important that we keep our relationship strong. And so, if you do something that might interfere with our work in therapy together, I will let you know—like, for example, always coming late to appointments. And, just as important, if I am doing something that lets you down, seems insensitive, or otherwise upsets you, I am inviting you to let me know too, to be frank with me about it, so we can work on fixing it. How does that sound?
>
> CLIENT: I guess it sounds OK.
>
> THERAPIST: You'd be willing to let me know?
>
> CLIENT: Sure, I guess.
>
> THERAPIST: Great. Because you and I have to work together well for this therapy to work.

Functional Assessment

In DBT individual therapy, monitoring clients' problems occurs on an ongoing basis as clients fill out a weekly diary card. The diary card is a detailed checklist that requires the client to track targets for change; targets range from high-risk items such as suicidal thoughts and substance use, to dissociation, trauma triggers, fights with friends/family, somatic complaints, and rating emotions such as sadness, shame/alienation, and numbing. Problematic areas identified on the diary card, plus consideration of any therapy-interfering behavior, become the focus of the session. In addition to monitoring problem areas, the diary card also provides an opportunity to identify strengths and positive coping strategies used throughout the week, such as texting friends for support, exercising, listening to music, and communicating assertively. The therapist helps the client conduct a behavioral chain analysis to identify vulnerability factors for, and precipitants of, the highest-priority maladaptive behavior, as well as consequences of the behavior (e.g., relief, numbing, instrumental gains). Thus, DBT therapists assess, rather than assume, the idiographic functions of behaviors for particular clients at particular times. It is not uncommon for family members or others in an adolescent's life to assume that a behavior is "for attention" or that the adolescent is "not motivated" to act differently and needs to "take responsibility" for his or her actions. DBT takes a different stance, not presuming what factors contributed to, or are maintaining, the behavior. Instead, therapist and client engage in a detailed and collaborative process of discovering the moment-to-moment links on the chain (i.e., thoughts, behaviors, body sensations, urges, environmental/situational factors, interpersonal factors) that lead to and follow problematic behaviors. In this way, there is an opportunity to discover that the hours online in the middle of the night are an attempt to cope with intrusions rather than simply being defiant behavior. Therapists and clients also conduct functional analyses after therapy-interfering behavior such as not completing homework. Without this discussion, therapists could assume that lack of motivation was to blame rather than fear of rating emotions and becoming overwhelmed.

An example of a chain analysis might reveal that intense irritability and a subsequent heated argument with family was in response to trauma reminders that elicited painful emotions, was negatively reinforced by providing relief from painful emotions, was positively reinforced by a desired response of a parent, or all of the above. By discovering these connections, the therapist and client now have a number of options for intervening that could include enhancing coping strategies, decreasing invalidating family communications that are triggering, and support caregivers to respond to escalating conflict in a way that is not reinforcing for that particular adolescent. A behavioral analysis may also be able to answer the questions: Are the client's adaptive efforts to respond ignored or inadvertently punished by the caregivers? Or is maladaptive behavior getting reinforced?

Interestingly, the primary functions of NSIB among clients with BPD and PTSD appear to differ from clients with BPD alone (Harned, Rizvi, & Linehan, 2010). Harned, Risvi, et al. (2010) report that individuals with both BPD and PTSD were more likely to engage in self-injury as a means to influence others or communicate and as a means to manage trauma triggers compared to individuals with BPD alone. In a study with adolescents,

Prinstein (2008) found that NSIB often functioned to regulate negative affect or alternatively to induce emotion in the face of emotional numbing. Wagner, Rizvi, and Harned (2007) also highlight the importance of analyzing the function of behaviors among complex trauma survivors, understanding what initiates and maintains maladaptive responses and coping strategies, in order to provide more precise and effective treatment interventions.

With complex trauma cases, the range of symptoms and comorbid diagnoses makes it essential to identify the functions of all problematic behaviors. The therapist can then guide the client through a solution analysis, coming up with links on the chain where other, more skillful behaviors might have been employed toward a more effective outcome. Once the antecedents and consequences are clear, the therapist uses one or more of the behavioral change strategies in DBT—contingency management, problem solving, cognitive restructuring, increasing behavioral skills—to work with the client change key links to prevent recurrences. In the following example, the therapist draws a flow chart, together with the client, which includes a series of events linking thoughts, feelings, and physical sensations:

THERAPIST: Looks like from your diary card that yesterday was a really tough day.

CLIENT: Yeah, I cut when I got home from school.

THERAPIST: So when did things start? Did you decide to cut before you got home?

CLIENT: Yeah, after science.

THERAPIST: What happened in science?

CLIENT: I flipped out and ran to the bathroom.

THERAPIST: Flipped out?

CLIENT: I couldn't breathe, my heart was racing, and I wanted to punch someone. I felt so stupid.

THERAPIST: Why *stupid?*

CLIENT: For getting so upset.

THERAPIST: I'm sure there is a reason—what happened just before you got upset?

CLIENT: We were just starting to go over the homework and then Tracy opened the window...

THERAPIST: Something about the window?

CLIENT: Actually, I smelled cigarette smoke. Coming in from outside. I hate that smell. It reminds me of my uncle. The SOB always reeked of smoke.

THERAPIST: Do you remember what you were thinking?

CLIENT: I gotta get out of here and that stupid teacher better not get in my way.

THERAPIST: You felt trapped.

CLIENT: Totally.

THERAPIST: So how did you get from feeling trapped in science to cutting at home?

CLIENT: I decided in the bathroom that I would do it when I got home.

THERAPIST: What were you thinking?

CLIENT: I'm an idiot. Running out like a little kid. What is wrong with me? Something is wrong with my brain!

THERAPIST: So the smoke was a trigger. And the feeling?

CLIENT: Embarrassed.

THERAPIST: What thoughts were going through your mind when you got home right before you cut?

CLIENT: Kinda like I should be taught a lesson.

THERAPIST: What were you feeling physically?

CLIENT: Heaviness in my chest. Hard to breathe. I knew I'd feel better after.

THERAPIST: Did you?

CLIENT: Yeah, till my mom started banging on the bathroom door. She freaked out and then called my dad to come home early so that we could talk.

The remainder of the session would also include a review of trauma reactions along with problem-solving strategies for different points along the flow chart. Together client and therapist identify coping skills that he or she might be willing to try and topics for discussions with family members regarding nonreinforcing responses to NSIB.

Mindfulness

Mindfulness is a core DBT skill included to help clients practice paying attention in a particular way: "Mindfulness means moment-to-moment, non-judgmental awareness" (Kabat-Zinn & Kabat-Zinn, 1997, p. 24). *Awareness* can refer to noticing internal experiences such as thoughts, feelings, physical sensations, and urges as well as external experiences in the environment and with other people. Clinical research involving treatment outcome studies has demonstrated that mindfulness is a powerful intervention (see Hofmann, Sawyer, Witt & Oh, 2010) and plays a role in engaging in risky behavior. For example, college students who scored lower on mindfulness scales were significantly more likely to text while driving (Feldman, Greeson, Renna, & Robbins-Monteith, 2011).

In DBT, adolescents have the opportunity to practice mindfulness in a number of engaging ways, including, for example, blowing bubbles, mindful eating, listening to music without judging it, and noticing urges to move without acting on those urges (e.g., the urge to shift in their seat, scratch their nose). Teaching adolescents mindfulness skills can address several complex PTSD symptoms. For example, mindfulness can have a powerful influence on affect regulation and impulsivity because being observant and describing one's experiences require that one slow down and therefore be less impulsive. Mindfulness can help adolescents identify the link between emotions and the body that often becomes disconnected as adolescents simply report frequent somatic complaints such as headaches, stomachaches, etc. Exercises to practice mindfulness include several activities that require focused attention. Group members are asked to observe and describe their thoughts or feelings while repeatedly refocusing their attention on the present moment as their minds drift to the past or their plans for the weekend. Mindfulness practice is the key to accessing one's "wise mind" (Miller et al., 2007), otherwise known as intuition. Adolescents learn that this wisdom is something to which everyone has access; they just need practice getting there. This concept can be empowering and runs counter to trauma survivors' negative self-perceptions as permanently damaged and ineffective. Interestingly, adolescents have rated these skills, which are linked to developing acceptance, as among the most helpful skills they learned (Miller, Wyman, Glassman, Huppert, & Rathus, 2000).

Best practices for presenting mindfulness (and teaching skills in general) include starting with a story or engaging introduction and explaining the rationale for the practice in a way that is meaningful to the clients' lives (Rathus & Miller, 2013). The story should illustrate both struggle and success with the skills. For example, when teaching communication skills, the group leader could tell a story about a somewhat upsetting experience of being cut off while standing in line and include the thoughts, urges, and strong emotions he or she had noticed along with the skills—highlighting both the struggles and the benefits of being effective. When leaders self-disclose while being genuine, using a carefully selected personal example in an engaging, perhaps humorous story, adolescents sit up and listen, unlike their posture and unfocused gaze in a dry didactic lecture. More importantly, they seem more likely to remember the material. Another example of a mindfulness practice is called "observe the urge," and the instructions are as follows:

> "Try to get into a comfortable position because once we begin, for the next 2 mintues I am going to ask you to do your best not to move. The task is to notice any urges that you have to move, to scratch, to giggle, etc. Try your best not to act on these urges while noticing what other

urges come up. When your mind wanders and you are distracted by noises in the room or thoughts like 'Why the heck am I doing this?' or 'Man, my nose itches' notice the thought and gently bring yourself back to what is happening now. Being able to observe urges before acting on them can be an incredibly helpful! Saying or doing things impulsively can make the situation worse. For example, you can be really pissed off with your friend without actually screaming at him or her or texting them 20 times. Let's begin now."

After the practice, each group member is asked to describe his or her observations—what he or she noticed during the practice, including emotions.

Family/Caregiver Involvement

Multifamily Skills Training Group

DBT is based on a biosocial theory that holds that chronic emotional dysregulation arises from a transaction between (1) a biological tendency toward emotional vulnerability with an inability to modulate affect and (2) a pervasively invalidating environment. In cases of complex trauma, both of these transactional factors are heightened. For teens still residing in invalidating environments, when appropriate, including caregivers in skills training can enable the caregivers to gain awareness of, and change, their invalidating behaviors, as well as helping them to serve as a role model to encourage the teenager to use the skills. Moreover, caregivers of emotionally dysregulated, high-risk adolescents are often themselves emotionally dysregulated and often parent in a reactive, erratic manner (see Rathus & Miller, 2002). Dysregulated parents may contribute to poor family functioning, which has been found to be associated with suicidal behavior in teens (Wilkinson, Kelvin, Robert, Dubicka, & Goodyer, 2011).

Thus, in DBT for adolescents, we routinely include caregivers in skills training in multifamily groups. Family members learn skills in modules that teach mindfulness, emotion regulation, interpersonal effectiveness (communication strategies), distress tolerance (short-term coping strategies), and walking the middle path (strategies to reduce family conflict). In this last module, caregivers learn validation techniques, behavior change strategies, and dialectics (see Miller et al., 2007). *Dialectics* refers to the notion of finding a synthesis of polarized or extreme positions, whether to reduce family conflict or patterns of extreme thinking and behaving. In this setting, not only would teens with complex PTSD and risk behaviors learn skills to address impulsivity, emotions, attention, self, and relationships, but their caregivers would learn skills alongside of them. This emphasis on improving caregivers' capacities can enhance parenting skills, improve family interactions, and be inherently validating for teens. It also provides a supportive network and normalizes problems of emotional dysregulation for a client population that often experiences increasing social isolation.

As-Needed Family Sessions

Skills training enhances clients' capabilities, and individual therapy helps clients apply skills and increase their motivation. Including caregivers in skills training and in as-needed family sessions helps families become more supportive and rewarding of adaptive behaviors and to remove reinforcement for (or help extinguish) maladaptive behaviors. When problematic family interactions appear on the chain analysis of targeted behaviors, therapists can schedule a family session (see Miller et al., 2007). In family sessions therapists work with parents to increase validation and reduce invalidation, reduce conflict, enhance interpersonally communication, reduce emotional vulnerability, increase effective parenting, and facilitate problem solving. For adolescents with chronic trauma histories, psychoeducation about complex PTSD and the normalization of posttraumatic reactions can be valuable. Sessions are generally scheduled as supplemental every few weeks, as indicated; if the session must replace an individual session, we recommend review of the diary card and safety–risk assessment for the first 15 minutes with the adolescent. We also prioritize validation (and teach it, if necessary) so that sessions remain relatively calm, productive, and *not* retraumatizing.

Phone Coaching

In DBT, therapists are available for telephone coaching outside of sessions, which helps to generalize the DBT skills learned in group. This modality offers clients contact during the moment of crisis and prior to engaging in risk behaviors (and thus ideally preventing a risky behavior), rather than having to wait until the next session when the behavior has already occurred. Therapists then can help clients apply effective skills and other strategies *in vivo*, particularly in situations where emotions are too high for the client to remember what to do or to access previously learned knowledge. Between-session coaching and having the opportunity to connect with the therapist can be especially helpful for clients with complex trauma who may experience frequent and intense emotional dysregulation, struggles with impulses, dissociative states or memory problems, and trust/relationship difficulties. Importantly, phone calls are not only for crisis management or for implementing skills. Phone calls (and sometimes texting) are also encouraged to communicate good news and to discuss any questions or concerns about the therapy relationship or about anything that happened during the session. It is critical that permission to talk with the therapist by phone not be linked only with crises!

Therapist Consultation Team

Because clients with complex trauma who exhibit risky behaviors may present many challenges in treatment, the consultation team model can be a strong source of support for therapists working with this population. The consultation group meets weekly and aims to "treat the therapist." In other words, the team (1) helps therapists stay adherent to the model and assess difficulties conducting the therapy; (2) increases therapists' motivation and skills; (3) reduces burnout; and (4) enhances therapists' ability to formulate empathic, nonjudgmental conceptualizations of client behaviors. Not only can adolescents with complex trauma present with dysregulated affect, emotional pain, and risky behavior, but they may also exhibit features that impede the development of the therapeutic relationship and compliance with treatment, including significant struggles with mistrust, attention, dissociation, and impulsivity. The team approach reduces isolation while helping therapists' to stay balanced and compassionate.

Case consultation begins with a mindfulness exercise led by one of the team members, followed by "good news" about at least one of the clients being treated by the team. Next, therapists write the initials of clients that they would like to discuss on the board and place a number next to each for severity/priority: 3 for the highest, 2 for medium, and 1 for lowest priority. Team members receive consultation based on highest-priority cases. In order to focus the discussion and explicitly describe the help being requested, therapists begin by posing a specific question to the team, instead of starting to talk about the case. For example, a therapist might say:

> "I really need help with decreasing my own stress. I've started having bad dreams after listening to Jayda's experiences over the past several months. I think it really bothers me that the family has become so immobilized, despite all my attempts to reach out to them, leaving her vulnerable and without the support she still really needs. I understand intellectually why her grandmother is not available; however, at the same time it *so* upsetting! So, maybe it's not the nightmares I need help with, but feeling helpless at the end of some of the sessions!"

The team then has the opportunity to provide support and validation; conduct a collaborative, nonjudgmental assessment to identify the factors that are contributing to the therapist's reactions; and subsequently generate strategies to help the therapist reduce feelings of stress and helplessness.

Conclusion

In this chapter we have described how DBT has been adapted as a treatment for adolescent clients who have both complex PTSD and high-risk behaviors. DBT establishes safety and enhances behavioral control, attends to the therapeutic relationship to enhance engagement and reduce dropout, and treats features of complex PTSD such as problems with regulation of affect, attention, and impulses, disturbed sense of self, and problematic relationships. It also relies on a team approach to support and validate the therapist, treat vicarious traumatization, and help therapists adhere to the treatment model with fidelity and compassion. Thus, it may prove to be a useful intervention for traumatized adolescents who may be at risk for the development of BPD.

References

Axelrod, S. R., Perepletchikova, F., Holtzman, K., & Sinha, R. (2011). Emotion regulation and substance use frequency in women with substance dependence and borderline personality disorder receiving dialectical behavior therapy. *American Journal of Drug and Alcohol Abuse, 37*(1), 37–42.

Bedics, J. D., Atkins, D., Comtois, K. A., & Linehan, M. M. (2012). Treatment differences in the therapeutic relationship and introject during a 2-year randomized controlled trial of dialectical behavior therapy versus nonbehavioral psychotherapy experts for borderline personality disorder. *Journal of Consulting and Clinical Psychology, 80*(1), 66–77.

Brent, D. (2011). Nonsuicidal self-injury as predictor of suicidal behavior in depressed adolescents. *American Journal of Psychiatry, 168*(5), 452–454.

Cloitre, M., Courtois, C. A., Charuvstra, A., Carapezza, R., Stolback, B. C., & Green, B. L. (2011). Treatment of complex PTSD: Results of the ISTSS expert clinican survey on best practices. *Journal of Traumatic Stress, 24*(6), 615–627.

Courbasson, C., Nishikawa, Y., & Dixon, L. (2011). Outcome of dialectical behavior therapy for concurrent eating and substance use disorders. *Clinical Psychology and Psychotherapy, 19*(5), 434–439.

Courtois, C. A., & Ford, J. D. (Eds.). (2009). *Treating complex traumatic stress disorders: An evidence-based guide.* New York: Guilford Press.

Feldman, G., Greeson, J., Renna, M., & Robbins-Monteith, K. (2011). Mindfulness predicts less texting while driving among young adults: Examining attention and emotion-regulation motives as potential mediators. *Personality and Individual Differences, 51*(7), 856–861.

Ford, J. D. (2005). Treatment implications of altered affect regulation and information processing following child maltreatment. *Psychiatric Annals, 35*(5), 410–419.

Ford, J. D., & Cloitre, M. (2009). Best practices in psychotherapy for children and adolescents. In C. A. Courtois & J. D. Ford (Eds.), *Treating complex traumatic stress disorders: An evidence-based guide* (pp. 59–81). New York: Guilford Press.

Goldstein, T. R., Axelson, D. A., Birmaher, B., & Brent, D. A. (2007). Dialectical behavior therapy for adolescents with bipolar disorder: A 1 year open trial. *Journal of the American Academy of Child and Adolescent Psychiatry, 46*(7), 820–830.

Gratz, K. L., Latzman, R. D., Tull, M. T., Reynolds, E. K., & Lejuez, C. W. (2011). Exploring the association between emotional abuse and childhood borderline personality features: The moderating role of personality traits. *Behavior Therapy, 42*, 493–508.

Groves, S., Backer, H. S., van den Bosch, W., & Miller, A. (2012). Dialectical behavior therapy with adolescents: A review. *Child and Adolescent Mental Health, 17*(2), 65–75.

Gunderson, J. G., Stout, R. L., McGlashan, T. H., Shea, M. T., Morey, L. C, Grilo, C. M., et al. (2011). Ten-year course of borderline personality disorder: Psychopathology and function from the collaborative longitudinal personality disorders study. *Archives of General Psychiatry, 68*, 827–837.

Harned, M. S., Jackson, S. C., Comtois, K. A., & Linehan, M. M. (2010). Dialectical behavior therapy as a precursor to PTSD treatment for suicidal and/or self-injuring women with borderline personality disorder. *Journal of Traumatic Stress, 23*(4), 421–429.

Harned, M. S., Rizvi, S. L., & Linehan, M. M. (2010). Impact of co-occurring PTSD on suicidal women with BPD. *American Journal of Psychiatry, 167*(10), 1210–1217.

Hofman, S. G., Sawyer, A. T., Witt, A. A., & Oh, D. (2010). The effect of mindfulness-based therapy on anxiety and depression: A meta-analytic review. *Journal of Consulting and Clinical Psychology, 78*(2), 169–183.

Kabat-Zinn, J., & Kabat-Zinn, M. (1997). *Everyday blessings: The inner work of mindful parenting.* New York: Hyperion.

Katz, L. Y., Cox, B. J., Gunasekara, S., & Miller, A. (2004). Feasibility of dialectical behavior therapy for suicidal adolescent inpatients. *Journal of the American Academy of Child and Adolescent Psychiatry, 43*, 276–282.

Klein, D. A., & Miller, A. (2011). Dialectical behavior therapy for suicidal adolescents with borderline personality disorder. *Child and Adolescent Psychiatric Clinics of North America, 20*, 205–216.

Lang, J. M., Ford, J. D., & Fitzgerald, M. M. (2010). An algorithm for determining use of trauma-focused cognitive-behavioral therapy. *Psychotherapy Theory, Research, Practice, and Training, 47*(4), 554–569.

Linehan, M. M. (1993). *Cognitive-behavioral treatment of borderline personality disorder.* New York: Guilford Press.

Linehan, M. M., Armstrong, H. E., Suarez, A., Allmon, D., & Heard, H. L. (1991). Cognitive-behavioral treatment of chronically parasuicidal borderline patients. *Archives of General Psychiatry, 48*, 1060–1064.

Linehan, M. M., Comtois, K. A., Murray, A. M., Brown, M. Z., Gallop, R. J., Heard, J. L., et al. (2006). Two-year randomized controlled trial and follow-up of dialectical behavior therapy vs. therapy by experts for suicidal behaviors and borderline personality disorder. *Archives of General Psychiatry, 63*, 757–766.

Linehan, M. M., McDavid, J., Brown, M. Z., Sayrs, J. H. R., & Gallop, R. J. (2008). Olanzapine plus dialectical behavior therapy for women with high irritability who meet criteria for borderline personality disorder: A double blind, placebo-controlled pilot study. *Journal of Clinical Psychiatry, 69*, 999–1005.

Lynch, T. R., Morse, J. Q., Mendelson, T., & Robins, C. J. (2003). Dialectical behavior therapy for depressed older adults: A randomized pilot study. *American Journal of Geriatric Psychiatry, 11*(1), 33–45.

Lynch,T. R., Trost, W. T., Salsman, N., & Linehan, M. M. (2007). Dialectical behavior therapy for borderline personality disorder. *Annual Review of Clinical Psychology, 3*, 181–205.

Miller, A. L., Rathus, J. H., & Linehan, M. M. (2007). *Dialectical behavior therapy with suicidal adolescents.* New York: Guilford Press.

Miller, A. L., Wyman, S. E., Glassman, S. L., Huppert, J. D., & Rathus, J. H. (2000). Analysis of behavioral skills utilized by adolescents receiving dialectical behavior therapy. *Cognitive and Behavioral Practice, 7*, 183–187.

Neacsiu, A. D., Rizvi, S. L., & Linehan, M. M. (2010). Dialectical behavior therapy skills use as a mediator and outcome of treatment for borderline personality disorder. *Behavior Research and Therapy, 48*(9), 832–839.

Prinstein, M. J. (2008). Introduction to special section on suicide and nonsuicidal self-injury: A review of unique challenges an important directions for self-injury science. *Journal of Consulting and Clinical Psychology, 76*(1), 1–8.

Rathus, J. H., & Miller, A. L. (2000). Dialectical dilemmas in working with suicidal adolescents. *Cognitive and Behavioral Practice, 7*, 435–445.

Rathus, J. H., & Miller, A. L. (2002). Dialectical behavior therapy adapted for suicidal adolescents. *Suicide and Life-Threatening Behaviors, 32*, 146–157.

Rathus, J. H., & Miller, A. L. (2013). *DBT skills training manual for adolescents with emotional dysregulation.* New York: Guilford Press. (Manuscript in preparation)

Stepp, S. D., Burke, J. D., Hipwell, A. E., & Leober, R. (2012). Trajectories of ADHD and ODD symptoms as precursors of BPD symptoms in adolescent girls. *Journal of Abnormal Child and Adolescent Psychology, 40*(1), 7–20.

Stepp, S. D., Pilkonis, P. A., Hipwell, A. E., Loeber, R., & Stouthamer-Loeber, M. (2010). Stability of borderline personality disorder features in girls. *Journal of Personality Disorders, 24*, 460–472.

Wagner, A. W., Rizvi, S. L., & Harned, M. S. (2007). Applications of DBT to the treatment of complex-trauma-related problems: When one case formulation does not fit all. *Journal of Traumatic Stress, 20*(4), 391–400.

Wilkinson, P., Kelvin, R., Robert, C., Dubicka, B., & Goodyer, I. (2011). Clinical and psychosocial predictors of suicide attempts and nonsuicidal self-injury in the adolescent depression antidepressants and psychotherapy trial. *American Journal of Psychiatry, 168*(5), 495–501.

Zanarini, M. C. (2000). Childhood experiences associated with the development of borderline personality disorder. *Psychiatric Clinics of North America, 23*, 89–101.

PART III

SYSTEMIC APPROACHES TO TREATMENT

CHAPTER 13

The Neurosequential Model of Therapeutics

Bruce D. Perry
Christine L. Dobson

The Neurosequential Model of Therapeutics© (NMT) is a developmentally sensitive and neurobiologically informed approach to clinical problem solving. Although it has been implemented in multiple clinical populations across the full developmental spectrum (infants to adults), this approach was developed, and has been most widely used, with traumatized and maltreated children and youth (e.g., Barfield, Gaskill, Dobson, & Perry, 2011). Its utility is most apparent with the most complex cases of maltreatment and psychological trauma, which are the focus of this chapter.

As has been well documented over the last 20 years, intrauterine substance use, neglect, chaos, attachment disruptions, and traumatic stress all impact the development of the brain and result in complicated and heterogeneous functional presentations in children, youth, and adults. Furthermore, the timing, severity, pattern, and nature of these developmental insults have variable and heterogeneous impact on the developing brain (Perry, 2001, 2002). The result is a complex clinical picture with increased risk of physical health, sensorimotor, self-regulation, relational, cognitive, and a host of other problems (e.g., Felitti et al., 1998; Anda et al., 2006). The current DSM neuropsychiatric labels do not capture this complexity. The development of evidence-based treatments for these complex children and youth has been challenging. The very heterogeneity of their developmental histories and functional presentations impedes the creation of the homogeneous "groups" required for quality outcome or phenomenological research (e.g., Jovanovic & Norrholm, 2011). The clinical challenges are even more daunting. A 15-year-old child may have the self-regulation capacity of a 5-year-old, the social skills of a 3-year-old, and the cognitive organization of a 10-year-old. And, due to the unique genetic, epigenetic, and developmental history of each child, it is very difficult to apply a "one-size-fits-all" treatment approach (Ungar & Perry, 2012). The NMT was developed to help address some of these complexities (Perry, 2006, 2009).

The NMT is not a specific therapeutic technique; it is multidimensional assessment "lens" designed to guide clinical problem solving and outcome monitoring by providing a useful "picture" of the client's current strengths and vulnerabilities in context of his or her developmental history. This neurodevelopmental viewpoint, in turn, allows the clinical team to select and sequence a set of enrichment, educational, and therapeutic interventions to best meet the needs of the client. The NMT draws on a rich evidence base from research in multiple disciplines (e.g., the neurosciences, social sciences, psychology, public health, epidemiology) to create a semistructured and clinically practical way to ensure that the clinical team considers and, to some degree, quantifies crucial elements of the client's developmental history and current functioning. This approach greatly aids the clinician in his or her efforts to practice in an evidence-based, developmentally sensitive, and trauma-informed manner (Brandt, Diel, Feder, & Lillas, 2012). The goal of this semistructured process is to "force" the clinician/clinical team to systematically consider key developmental factors that influence the client's current functioning.

The NMT is meant to complement, not replace, other useful metrics or assessment elements; each organization and clinical team have developed an assessment process; the NMT was designed to complement and, to some degree, provide a neurodevelopmental framework for the data obtained from these various assessments. The functional data for a client gathered in either quantitative (e.g., Weschler Intelligence Scale for Children, Wide Range Achievement Test, Child and Adolescent Functional Assessment Scale, Child and Adolescent Needs and Strengths, Child Behavior Checklist, Trauma Symptom Checklist for Children, Parenting Stress Index) or qualitative (e.g., direct observation, interview, parent/teacher report) ways are organized into a neuroscience-focused "map." This map provides the clinical team with an approximation of the current functional organization of the client's brain.

The ChildTrauma Academy (CTA) has developed a set of manualized elements to facilitate the exporting and use of the NMT. These elements include the NMT clinical practice tools (see below); an NMT certification process (90 hours of didactic and case-based training to ensure exposure to core concepts of traumatology, developmental psychology, neurobiology, and related areas relevant to a developmentally sensitive and trauma-informed approach); an ongoing NMT fidelity process for certified users; and NMT psychoeducational materials and related caregiving and educational components (the Neurosequential Model© in Education: NME; and Neurosequential Model© in Caregiving [NMC]) to facilitate the creation of a developmentally sensitive, trauma-informed clinical setting, home, school, and community (see *www.ChildTrauma.org* for more information on each of these elements of the NMT).

The theoretical background and rationale for the core elements of the NMT are presented elsewhere (see Perry, 2006, 2009; Kleim & Jones, 2008; Ludy-Dobson & Perry, 2010). This chapter illustrates the use of the NMT by presenting a clinical case in which a client had been treated previously in multiple systems. The clinical narrative and accompanying NMT reports illustrate how the clinical team used these "metrics" to develop and implement treatment.

Case Example: James

James is a 10-year-old boy living in a therapeutic foster home. He has no biological siblings and there are two older biological children (of the foster parents) in the home. The foster parents are middle-age, employed, and experienced. They have four biological children (two adults and the two older teens living at home) and have successfully fostered dozens of children. James has been in out-of-home care since age 3. He has lived in this foster home for approximately 2 years.

Developmental History and Initial Presentation

James's mother was an 18-year-old runaway from a foster home. His biological father was a 24-year-old with a history of substance abuse and assaultive behaviors. During the pregnancy James's mother acknowledges episodic binge alcohol and polysubstance use. She received minimal prenatal care, but apparently there were no complications with the birth. For the first 18 months of his life, James lived with his mother in a chaotic and abusive environment apparently permeated by domestic violence, drug use, multiple moves, and profound neglect. At 18 months, he was removed by child protective services after neighbors reported that he was left alone for days on end. He was severely malnourished, had bruises, insect bites, and possibly cigarette burns. He was lethargic, nonreactive, and exhibited profound hypotonia. He was placed in foster care, where he rapidly gained weight, began to show more appropriate social behavior (e.g., verbalization, eye contact), and began to catch up in motor development. He resumed contact with his mother at 24 months. Episodic extreme "tantrums" emerged around that time, appearing to be associated with the preunification supervised visits with his mother. She complied with all elements of the reunification plan, and he was returned to her care at 26 months.

He was once again removed at age 38 months (this time permanently) after he was found wandering the streets at night. He was not toilet trained, had minimal speech, indiscriminate affectionate behaviors and touch defensiveness, and profound primitive self-soothing behaviors such as rocking, head banging, fecal smearing, and hoarding of food. He was placed in a foster home, where he had severe difficulties with attention, sleep, impulsivity, aggression, oversexualized behaviors, speech and language delays, fine motor and large motor coordination, among many other problems. All of these issues resulted in referral for mental health services, where he was diagnosed with attention-deficit/hyperactivity disorder (ADHD) and was placed on psychostimulants. No other therapy or evaluation was provided at that time.

This intervention and the efforts of the first foster family were ineffective. His behaviors ultimately led to a terminated placement. This pattern repeated itself: Over the next several years James had five different placements and two psychiatric hospitalizations prior to entering the home of the current foster family. He was also enrolled, and expelled, from several child care, early childhood, and educational settings. Over this time, he had at least five different assessments and multiple changes in treatment. Two of the clinical settings utilized trauma-focused cognitive-behavioral therapy (TF-CBT); we were unable to determine from the records aspects of fidelity, training, or progression through the TF-CBT protocol at these sites. What was clear, however, is that the impact of the interventions at this time was minimal. His behaviors remained extreme. He exhibited frequent explosive behaviors, particularly when he was told "no" or when he did not get his way. The undersocialized and odd behaviors described above persisted.

Over time, his diagnoses accumulated to include bipolar disorder, oppositional defiant disorder, ADHD, reactive attachment disorder, rule out childhood schizophrenia, rule out autism spectrum disorder, pervasive developmental disorder, intermittent explosive disorder, and, in several of the assessments, posttraumatic stress disorder (PTSD) was added to the other diagnoses. He received multiple medication "trials" and ultimately ended up on Risperdal, Adderall, lithium, and clonidine. No significant enduring improvement in behavior or academic functioning was seen by foster parents, school personnel, or child protective services workers—indeed most of reports described escalation in his aggressiveness and inability to manage his impulsivity. Ultimately, all who worked with James became fatigued, resulting in a series of failed placements.

At age 8½ James was referred to his current foster home. He was placed in a special education classroom in the local public school and was performing at the level of PreK academically. He was referred to a clinical group that this foster family had worked with previously. Clinicians in this group were trained in dialectical behavior therapy (DBT), TF-CBT, parent–child interactive therapy (PCIT), eye movement desensitization and reprocessing (EMDR), and were becoming certified in the NMT. For the first 6 months of treatment, James worked with a clinician who utilized a TF-CBT approach in combination with some behavior modification, psychoeducation for the foster family, and consultation to the school. Several attempts were made to progress to the trauma narrative phase with minimal success. The medication combination (see above) that he was on when he came to the foster home was maintained. He received tutoring and speech and language therapy. After an initial 6-week "honeymoon" following placement, James began to struggle both in school and at home with an escalation of the behaviors described earlier.

NMT Case Consultation

James's case was selected and presented as part of the NMT certification process by a training clinician. The initial NMT Metric Report for James is shown in online Appendix 1 (Figure 13.1 is an excerpt from the appendices; the complete appendices are online at *www.childtrauma.org/images/stories/Articles/PerryDobson_Appendices_2012.pdf*). The first page of the initial NMT Metric Report summarizes the findings of the semistructured developmental history. As outlined in Table 13.1, this process involves quantifying the nature, timing, and severity of adverse experiences as well as relational health factors. As can be seen in the graphs on page 1 of online Appendix 1, estimates of James's developmental adversity and relational health during this time put him in a very high-risk category throughout his development. When there is incomplete historical information, the scoring strategy is for the assessor to use clinical judgment to reconstruct the history but to be conservative so that the reconstruction is, if anything, an underestimate of developmental risk. The brain develops in a use-dependent fashion, essentially as a reflection of the developmental environment; the level of developmental adversity (along with minimal relational or social buffers) that James experienced would predictably alter the developing brain and lead to a complex and clinically confusing presentation. Broad-based functional compromise, of course, was well documented in James's history.

The second page of this initial assessment (see online Appendix 1) shows how James's brain-mediated functioning was organized on the NMT brain map, summarizing his pervasive neurobiological compromise. On the left-hand side of the page are the specific functional areas that are scored and on the right are a series of "maps" that organize these functions at James's age in order to provide a normative benchmark (see also Table 13.1). The resulting "map" is a heuristic construct that is reflective of the actual organization of the brain. The functional scores are color-coded (see key on page 2 of online Appendix 1): pink/red indicating either

CURRENT CNS FUNCTIONALITY

	Time	1-Year	Typical
Brainstem			
1 Cardiovascular/ANS	8	10	12
2 Autonomic Regulation	6	9	12
3 Temperature regulation/Metabolism	9	10	12
4 Extraocular Eye Movements	9	10	12
5 Suck/Swallow/Gag	5	8	12
6 Attention/Tracking	3	6	12
DE/Cerebellum			
7 Feeding/Appetite	7	9	11
8 Sleep	4	8	11
9 Fine Motor Skills	6	8	10
10 Coordination/Large Motor Functioning	6	8	9
11 Dissociative Continuum	4	6	10
12 Arousal Continuum	2	7	10
13 Neuroendocrine/Hypothalamic	8	8	10
14 Primary Sensory Integration	6	8	11
Limbic			
15 Reward	4	6	11
16 Affect Regulation/Mood	4	6	10
17 Attunement/Empathy	4	6	10
18 Psychosexual	4	6	9
19 Relational/Attachment	4	7	9
20 Short-term memory/Learning	7	9	11
Cortex			
21 Somato/Motorsensory Integration	5	7	10
22 Sense Time/Delay Gratification	3	6	8
23 Communication Expressive/Receptive	8	9	11
24 Self-Awareness/Self-Image	4	6	8
25 Speech/Articulation	8	9	10
26 Concrete Cognition	7	8	9
Frontal Cortex			
27 Nonverbal Cognition	6	7	8
28 Modulate Reactivity/Impulsivity	2	4	8
29 Math/Symbolic Cognition	4	5	8
30 Reading/Verbal	4	5	8
31 Abstract/Reflective Cognition	3	5	8
32 Values/Beliefs/Morality	4	5	8
Total	**168**	**231**	**317**

FIGURE 13.1. Change in James's brain-mediated functioning over time.

TABLE 13.1. Elements of the Web-Based NMT Metrics

1. Demographics

2. History—Developmental
   a. Genetic
   b. Epigenetic
   c. Part A. Adverse events measure
      i. Developmental timing
         1. Nature, severity, pattern
   d. Part B. Relational health measure
      i. Developmental timing
         1. Bonding and attachment
         2. Family supports
         3. Community supports

3. Current status
   a. Part C. Central nervous system (CNS) functional status measure
      i. Brainstem
      ii. Diencephalon/cerebellum
      iii. Limbic
      iv. Cortex/frontal cortex
   b. Part D. Relational health measure
      i. Family
      ii. Peers
      iii. School
      iv. Community

4. Recommendations
   a. Therapeutic web
   b. Family
   c. Client
      i. Sensory integration
      ii. Self-regulation
      iii. Relational
      iv. Cognitive

underdeveloped or severely impaired functioning, yellow shades indicating moderate compromise or precursor developmental functioning, and green shades indicating typical and appropriately emerging functional capacity of a young adult. Each client, therefore, is compared against a fully organized young adult *and* age-typical peers.

James's initial brain map scores demonstrated significant and pervasive functional problems; corresponding to these scores there are pink or red boxes in every area of his brain. This is a typical pattern seen in individuals whose extreme and prolonged histories of developmental chaos, neglect, and trauma are similar to what James experienced. What this map suggests is that, despite being 9 years old at the time of his assessment, James had the developmental capabilities—in multiple domains—of a much younger child. On the third page of the initial assessment in online Appendix 1, the degree to which James is behind his same-age peers in four main functional domains (sensory integration, self-regulation, relational, and cognitive) is readily apparent.

One of the most important items on this assessment is the cortical modulation ratio (CMR). This ratio gives a crude indicator of the "strength" of cognitive regulatory capacity relative to the "dysregulation" (i.e., disorganization, underdevelopment, impairment) of lower networks in the brain; in essence, it is an estimate of how hard it is for a client to use cortical (top-down, executive functioning) mechanisms to self-regulate. This factor is related to the executive function and "self-control" indicators (Moffitt et al., 2010; Piquero, Jennings, & Farrington, 2010) known to be predictive of positive outcomes in high-risk children. The higher the CMR value, the "stronger" the cortical mechanisms of self-control. A typical 9-year-old child would have a CMR of 4.7; James's CMR was 0.72 (more typical of an infant; there is only a millisecond between impulse and action, providing an explanation for many of his aggressive, impulsive, and inattentive behaviors). This finding alone can tell a great deal about his previous failure with "evidence-based treatment" provided by good clinicians following appropriate training. He was not, at that point, neurodevelopmentally capable of benefiting from that work. For any cognitive-predominant activity (e.g., routinely following verbal commands from a caregiver, sitting and attending in a classroom, engaging in TF-CBT) to be successful, the CMR needs to be greater than 1.0. And even then, the level of sustained attention will be very brief. The older the child, the greater the expectation that he or she will be capable of sitting and "learning" ("He is, after all, 10 years old"); yet this is a significant challenge for many severely maltreated children such as James. He literally is not biologically able to do the things that are expected of him. The result can be a toxic negative feedback cycle of adults getting frustrated, angry, confused, and demoralized, while James feels stupid, inadequate, misunderstood, rejected, and unloved. All of this just creates more threat, loss, rage, and chaos—reinforcing and adding to his history of developmental adversity.

NMT Recommendations

Central to NMT recommendations is the recognition of the importance of the therapeutic, educational, and enrichment opportunities provided in the broader community, especially school. The power of relationships and the mediation of therapeutic experiences in culturally respectful relational interactions are core elements of the NMT recommendations (Ludy-Dobson & Perry, 2010). Although not a formal wraparound process, the NMT recommendation process starts with a focus on the *therapeutic web:* the collective of healthy, invested adults and peers who provide the relational milieu of the child: The quality and permanence of this relational milieu are two of the most essential elements of successful outcomes (see Mears, Yaffe, & Harris, 2010; Bruns et al., 2010). As seen in online Appendices 2 and 4, various elements of the community, culture, and school are taken into consideration as the clinical team attempts to increase and support healthy relational connections. In the case of James, his school needed support and psychoeducation to create realistic expectations and services to "meet" James where he was at, developmentally.

The next set of recommendations focuses on the family, often the key to the therapeutic approach. In many cases, the parents' histories will mirror the child's developmental history of chaos, threat, trauma, or neglect. When this is the case, the NMT will include the parents and provide recommendations to help address their multiple needs in addition to those of their child. Transgenerational aspects of vulnerability and strength in a family play important roles in the child's educational, enrichment, and therapeutic experiences. When the caregivers and parents are healthy and strong, their capacity to be present, patient, positive, and nurturing is enhanced. When the parents' needs are unmet and their own mental health is compromised as a result, it is unrealistic to ask them to play a central role in the child's healing process. In the case of James, although the foster parents were experienced and nurturing and had previously worked with children who were maltreated, they were not very "trauma-informed" in terms of their responses and interventions. Psychoeducation to help them understand James's specific neurocognitive deficits leading to his difficulty in inhibiting impulses, his need for control, his relational sensitivity (i.e., sensitized to both intimacy and abandonment, making it difficult at times for the foster parents to find the "right" emotional distance), his resultant impaired developmental capabilities, and the need for their own self-care. Further, James had alienated the siblings in the household; they needed to be included in psychoeducational efforts to help them understand James and repair their relationship with him.

The final stage of treatment planning involves the client. Individual recommendations are based upon the client's neurodevelopmental organization. As described in online Appendix 2, the general direction for the selection and sequencing is based upon selecting the lowest "level" of significant impairment and then moving up the neurodevelopmental ladder. The selection and timing of enrichment, educational, and therapeutic experiences are guided by the developmental capabilities and vulnerabilities of the child. The NMT consultation process suggests some, but not all, activities that can provide patterned, repetitive, and rewarding experiences. The goal is to help create therapeutic experiences that are sensitive to developmental status in various domains and to state regulation capacity.

As seen in the recommendations for James, the team felt that his current educational and therapeutic approach was too "top-heavy." At this point in his treatment, James was not capable of benefiting from cognitive-predominant or even typical relational interactions; recall his CMR was less than 1.0. He was too dysregulated. The recommendations (see online Appendix 2, p. 3) suggested suspending tutoring, speech and language therapy, and TF-CBT, and creating an enriched somatosensory diet with a variety of experiences that would plausibly help provide the necessary density of patterned rhythmic experiences required to help create "bottom-up" regulation and reorganization (see Kleim & Jones, 2008; Perry, 2008). The goal is to provide the bottom-up regulation that can allow other relational and cognitive experiences to succeed; the challenge in this case is to make sure that when he is regulated, that the relational and cognitive expectations and opportunities are developmentally appropriate for him (and not selected based on his chronological age).

Reevaluation and Progress

The clinical team shifted their approach with James based upon the NMT assessment. A little over 1 year later, the team repeated the NMT metrics (see Figure 13.1 and online Appendix 3).

The clinical team and foster family acted on most of the key initial recommendations (see online Appendix 4). The results of the multidimensional enrichment, educational, and therapeutic experiences are visible in the change in James's functioning scores from beginning NMT (Figure 13.1, left-hand column) to 1 year later (Figure 13.1, middle column). More importantly, James did not act in ways that disrupted the placement or got him kicked out of school, as had occurred repeatedly in the past. His medications were slowly decreased and ultimately stopped completely. His CMR doubled from 0.7 to 1.4—still not at age level but certainly at a level that would allow him to begin to tolerate and benefit from cognitive-predominant experiences. He was now ready to benefit from tutoring, speech and language interventions, and TF-CBT. The success experienced by the developmentally sensitive teachers, foster parents, and James contributed to a positive and rewarding environment, leading to a shift from the negative, toxic cycle described earlier to a positive healing cycle.

Program Review, Clinical Outcomes, and Research

This is, of course, one client, but he is representative of hundreds of similar "stories" from our NMT-certified clinical partners. A central question from this approach arises: which aspect of this multidimensional approach resulted in the positive outcome? Was it the "in-room" aide? The creation of regulatory time in school? The psychoeducation for the foster family? Stopping the medications? The challenge of tracking outcomes and developing an "evidence base" and outcome studies for the clinical settings using the NMT will have to be differentiated, to some degree, from the application of specific treatments (many of them evidence-based treatments) that end up being recommended by the NMT process. For this reason we have built elements to do this into the NMT Follow-up Recommendations section (see Fidelity and Follow Up columns, online Appendix 4). Multiple projects are underway to examine various aspects of the application of the NMT, and, although NMT is still a "young" approach, the central collection of data using the web-based metric will allow a very rapid accumulation of data from which to learn. We anticipate ongoing modifications and improvements in this approach; the initial clinical outcomes are very promising, as illustrated by James's case.

Of primary interest to our group is whether the brain map (a heuristic construct) is actually reflective of actual brain organization. A comparison of actual neuroimaging using single photon emission computed tomography (SPECT) scanning and independent creation of the NMT brain map is underway. The preliminary analysis is promising; areas of the brain that have abnormal perfusion on the SPECT scan match remarkably well with the areas determined to be abnormal on the NMT Brain Map (preliminary results available from first author).

Conclusion

The NMT offers a cost-effective way to introduce a developmentally sensitive and neurobiology-informed perspective into clinical settings. The capacity to utilize this approach in public systems means that large numbers of children with complex issues can be evaluated with relatively high fidelity. This will allow the creation of more homogeneous groups to study the clinical phenomenology and neurobiology associated with maltreatment. Currently there are more than 4,000 children, youth, and adults in the NMT clinical dataset. Over 50 organizations are using this approach as part of their standard clinical practice. More than 100 individuals and sites are currently being trained. The projected number of NMT-assessed individuals will approach 15,000 in the next 2 years. As with any approach, there are shortcomings—most notably, the need for training in the core concepts, the challenge of fidelity, and the lack of available resources to follow through with the NMT-derived key recommendations. We believe that these are outweighed by the capacity to track outcomes, ensure acceptable fidelity, and help create a developmentally sensitive, trauma-informed lens through which to understand children with complex issues and their families.

References

Anda, R. F., Felitti, R. F., Walker, J., Whitfield, C., Bremner, D. J., Perry, B. D., et al. (2006). The enduring effects of childhood abuse and related experiences. *European Archives of Psychiatric and Clinical Neuroscience, 256*(3), 174–186.

Barfield, S., Gaskill, R., Dobson, C., & Perry, B. D. (2012). Neurosequential Model of Therapeutics© in a therapeutic preschool: Implications for work with children with complex neuropsychiatric problems. *International Journal of Play Therapy, 21*(1), 30–44.

Brandt, K., Diel, J., Feder, J., & Lillas, C. (2012). A problem in our field. *Journal of Zero to Three, 32*(4), 42–45.

Bruns, E. J., Walker, J. S., Zabel, M., Matarese, M., Estep, K., Harburger, D., et al. (2010). Intervening in the lives of youth with complex behavioral health challenges and their families: The role of the wraparound process. *American Journal of Community Psychology, 46*, 314–331.

Felitti, V. J., Anda, R. F., Nordenberg, D., Williamson, D. F., Spitz, A. M., Edwards, V., et al. (1998). Relationship of childhood abuse and household dysfunction to many of the leading causes of death in adults: Adverse Childhood Experiences Study. *American Journal of Preventive Medicine, 14*, 245–258.

Jovanovic, T., & Norrholm, S. D. (2011). Neural mechanisms in fear inhibition in PTSD. *Frontiers in Behavioral Neuroscience, 44*, 1–8.

Kleim, J. A., & Jones, T. A. (2008) Principles of experience-dependent neural plasticity: Implications for rehabilitation after brain damage. *Journal of Speech, Language, and Hearing Research, 51*, S225–S239.

Ludy-Dobson, C., & Perry, B. D. (2010). The role of healthy relational interactions in buffering the impact of childhood trauma. In E. Gil (Ed.), *Working with children to heal interpersonal trauma* (pp 26–44). New York: Guilford Press.

Mears, S. L., Yaffe, J., & Harris, N. J. (2009). Evaluation of wraparound services for severely emotionally disturbed youths. *Research on Social Work Practice, 19*, 678–685.

Moffitt, T. E., Arseneault, L., Belsky, D., Dickson, N., Hancox, R. J., Harrington, H., et al. (2010). A gradient of childhood self-control predicts health, wealth and public safety. *PNAS Early Edition*. Available online at *www.pnas.org/cgi/doi/10.1073/pnas.1010076108.*

Perry, B. D. (2001). The neuroarcheology of childhood maltreatment: The neurodevelopmental costs of adverse childhood events. In K. Franey, R. Geffner, & R. Falconer (Eds.), *The cost of maltreatment: Who pays? We all do* (pp. 15–37). San Diego: Family Violence and Sexual Assault Institute.

Perry, B. D. (2002). Childhood experience and the expression of genetic potential: What childhood neglect tells us about nature and nurture. *Brain and Mind, 3*, 79–100.

Perry, B. D. (2006). The Neurosequential Model of Therapeutics: Applying principles of neuroscience to clinical work with traumatized and maltreated children. In N. B. Webb (Ed.), *Working with traumatized youth in child welfare* (pp. 27–52). New York: Guilford Press.

Perry, B. D. (2008). Child maltreatment: The role of abuse and neglect in developmental psychopathology. In T. P. Beauchaine & S. P. Hinshaw (Eds.), *Textbook of child and adolescent psychopathology* (pp. 93–128). New York: Wiley.

Perry, B. D. (2009). Examining child maltreatment through a neurodevelopmental lens: Clinical application of the Neurosequential Model of Therapeutics. *Journal of Loss and Trauma, 14*, 240–255.

Piquero, A. R., Jennings, W. G., & Farrington, D. P. (2010). On the malleability of self-control: Theoretical and policy implications regarding a general theory of crime. *Justice Quarterly, 27*(6), 803–834.

Ungar, M., & Perry, B. D. (2012). Trauma and resilience In R. Alaggia & C. Vine (Eds.), *Cruel but not unusual: Violence in Canadian families* (pp. 119–143). Waterloo, Ontario, Canada: WLU Press.

CHAPTER 14

Developmental Trauma Therapy Models

Julian D. Ford
Margaret E. Blaustein
Mandy Habib
Richard Kagan

Children who are victimized by sexual, physical, or emotional maltreatment or violence must cope not only with fear but also with the disruption or interruption of normal development. Often the challenge is further complicated by the loss of, or abandonment by, primary caregivers who are impaired (e.g., by mental health or substance use problems), neglectful, or victims themselves of past or current traumatic maltreatment or violence that interferes with their ability to parent successfully (Charuvastra & Cloitre, 2008). Such "developmentally adverse interpersonal traumas" (Ford, 2005, p. 410) place children at risk not only for anxiety or affective disorders (e.g., posttraumatic stress disorder [PTSD]) but also for a wide range of lifelong externalizing and physical health disorders due to deficits in core self-regulatory capacities (e.g., emotion dysregulation, dissociation, physical illness, social withdrawal, aggression; Cloitre, Stovall-McClough, Zorbas, & Charuvastra, 2008; D'Andrea, Ford, Stolbach, Spinazzola, & van der Kolk, 2012; Felitti et al., 1998; Koenen, 2006).

The combination of traumatic victimization and disrupted attachment bonding has been hypothesized to constitute a complex form of psychological trauma (Cook et al., 2005) that is particularly detrimental to biopsychosocial health and development in childhood, adolescence, and across the lifespan (Charney, 2004; Finkelhor, Ormrod, & Turner, 2007; van der Kolk, Roth, Pelcovitz, Sunday, & Spinazzola, 2005). In neurobiological terms, this trauma seems to be a consequence of a shift from a brain (and body) focused on *learning* to a brain (and body) focused on *survival* (Ford, 2009) for the child and the child's primary relationships. Exploration and learning to acquire new knowledge are normative in childhood and adolescence (Andersen, 2003; Eisenberg et al., 1995; Kagan, 2001; Lewis, 2005). By contrast, vigilance and self-protective adaptations designed to promote *survival* involve very different patterns of brain activation that facilitate rapid automatic adjustments to avert harm and mobilize or diminish arousal (e.g., brainstem, midbrain, amygdala; Neumeister, Henry, & Krystal, 2007; Teicher et al., 2003) instead of neural connections among areas of the brain that are involved in complex learning and adaptation (e.g., anterior and posterior cingulate, insula, medial and dorsolateral prefrontal cortex, hippocampus; Lanius et al., 2010; Matsumoto, Suzuki, & Tanaka, 2003; May et al., 2004; Milad et al., 2007; Rauch, Shin, & Phelps, 2006). A survival-focused brain appears to automatically defend against external threats, but in so doing, can overutilize crucial bodily systems that are essential to prevent exhaustion, injury, or illness ("allostasis"; Friedman & McEwen, 2004) and to promote learning and relatedness (e.g., reward seeking, distress tolerance, emotion modulation, problem solving, autobiographical memory).

When psychological trauma disrupts or interrupts early life development, the resultant survival-based patterns of brain activation and associated ways of perceiving, feeling, thinking, interacting, and defining one's self or identity can be can be extremely difficult to alter. These children often are diagnosed with severe internalizing disorders (e.g., bipolar disorder, reactive attachment disorder, dissociative disorders, anorexia, psychosis), externalizing disorders (e.g., intermittent explosive disorder, oppositional defiant disorder, substance abuse), and personality disorders (e.g., borderline traits) (Ford, Connor, & Hawke, 2009). This combination of anxiety, affective, somatic, behavioral, and interpersonal impairments originally was characterized as a juvenile variant of bipolar disorder, but has been shown empirically to be better described and treated as a "dysregulation" syndrome (Althoff, Ayer, Rettew, & Hudziak, 2011). Prospective research has demonstrated that these dysregulated children tend to have severe PTSD symptoms (Ayer et al., 2009) and that they are at risk for severe problems with psychosocial self-regulation in adulthood (Althoff, Verhulst, Rettew, & Hudziak, & van der Ende, 2010).

Therefore, a new psychiatric diagnosis has been proposed (though not included in DSM-5) for dysregulated traumatized children; developmental trauma disorder (DTD; van der Kolk, 2005). DTD requires a history of exposure to traumatic maltreatment or violence and fundamental disruption of attachment bonding with primary caregivers. DTD's symptom are forms of dysregulation and persistently altered beliefs and expectancies in the affective, somatic, cognitive, behavioral, interpersonal, and self/identity domains. One of the criteria required to demonstrate the clinical utility (First et al., 2003) of a new diagnosis is empirical evidence that existing treatments have limited efficacy for the syndrome. Children and adolescents who have been maltreated certainly can benefit from a variety of existing psychotherapies, with two important caveats. First, a systematic review of treatment outcomes for sexually abused children concluded that PTSD symptom reduction and overall psychosocial adjustment are strongly enhanced by a range of therapeutic interventions—but that problems with disruptive behavior, social competence, sexualized behavior, coping with stress, self-appraisal, and emotion regulation were at best moderately improved (Harvey & Taylor, 2010). Second, studies testing the efficacy of the best-validated treatment for childhood PTSD, with children with histories of sexual abuse, polyvictimization, and traumatic loss, have found the therapy (trauma-focused cognitive behavior therapy [TF-CBT]) to have limited efficacy with children and adolescents who have severe problems with anger, aggression, and impulsivity (Cohen, Berliner, & Mannarino, 2010). Thus, there appears to be a need for adaptations of the existing therapies (see Cohen, Mannarino, Kliethermes, & Murray, 2012) or the development of novel treatments for children with DTD-like problems.

A related criterion for clinical utility of a diagnosis is whether the symptoms provide a rational basis for new approaches to treatment. This is the case with regard to DTD, and in fact several novel therapeutic interventions have been developed, manualized, and are being tested in both scientific clinical trials and field study evaluations (Ford & Cloitre, 2009). This chapter provides an introduction to four therapy models designated as evidence-based or promising by the National Child Traumatic Stress Network (NCTSN; *www.nctsnet.org*) specifically to enable children and youth with histories of developmentally adverse interpersonal (complex) trauma to regain (or acquire for the first time) the ability to self-regulate across several biopsychosocial domains.

Trauma Affect Regulation: Guide for Education and Therapy

Trauma Affect Regulation: Guide for Education and Therapy (TARGET©) was designed and empirically validated originally as a therapy for adults with complex PTSD (Ford, Steinberg, & Zhang, 2011); it has been adapted for children and adolescents with complex trauma histories and DTD-like impairments. TARGET is manualized as a relatively brief (i.e., 10–12 sessions) one-to-one or group psychotherapy, but also has been adapted for more extended treatment and to be delivered as a family (Ford & Saltzman, 2009) or milieu (e.g., residential or inpatient; Ford & Hawke, 2012) psychotherapy.

TARGET begins with psychoeducation about the DTD symptoms that occur as the result of a shift in the brain's interconnections between an "alarm center" (i.e., a colloquial description of the amygdala and its afferent inputs and efferent outputs) and information retrieval ("filing") and executive ("thinking center") systems (i.e., a colloquial description of the hippocampus and the medial and dorsolateral prefrontal cortex and their interconnections with areas throughout the brain). This biological model provides a destigmatizing rationale for overcoming DTD by learning skills to strengthen the "filing" and "thinking" centers, to not just turn down but reset the brain's "alarm"—that is, to shift from a hypervigilant preoccupation with survival to a focus on enhancing personal control through exploration and learning.

TARGET then engages the youth in learning a seven-step sequence for focused thinking that draws on skills taught in cognitive-behavioral therapy, mindfulness and meditative therapies, and experiential psychotherapies. The goal is not to modify the youth's thinking but to demonstrate to each client how he or she is capable of intentionally using the ability to think systematically and clearly in order to achieve a balanced emotional state—that is, moderate arousal, engagement, and hopefulness, as opposed to emotional states involving excessive arousal or dissociation, detachment or preoccupation, and shame, hostility, or hopelessness that predominate in DTD. The focusing skills are summarized in an easily learned acronym, "FREEDOM": Focusing the mind on one thought that the client chooses based on his or her core values and hopes; Recognizing current triggers for "alarm" reactions; distinguishing alarm-driven ("reactive") versus adaptive ("main") Emotions, thoughts (Evaluations), goal Definitions, and behavioral Options; and dedicating self to Make a positive contribution to the world by gaining control of alarm reactions.

The FREEDOM steps are learned and practiced incrementally through dialogue with a therapist or counselor, or in guided interactions in a therapy group or a milieu program. This learning process involves the application of cognitive-behavioral therapy techniques, including observational learning via modeling, opportunities for guided practice with coaching and self-monitoring, and individualized applications in the youth's natural environment to promote generalization and refine the application of skills. The client is given a structured FREEDOM practice exercise template with which to review recent or historical experiences, either with the clinician or independently, between or following therapy sessions. The practice exercise is designed to enable clients to distinguish alarm reactions from focused self-regulation as a way to enhance their ability to use their innate skills for focused self-regulation while experiencing DTD or PTSD symptoms. The goal is not to eliminate symptoms (which may, paradoxically, increase in severity during this time) but to encourage mindful awareness and acceptance (Hayes, Luoma, Bond, Masuda, & Lillis, 2006) by self-monitoring them, recognizing their adaptive value, and choosing to focus on and utilize more self-congruent emotions, thoughts, goals, actions, and criteria for self-evaluation.

TARGET also has a creative arts activity designed to enhance positive and negative emotion recognition skills by having participants create personalized "lifelines" via collage, drawing, poetry, and writing. The lifeline provides a way to apply the FREEDOM steps to constructing a life narrative that includes traumatic and stressful events but does not involve repeated retelling of them. TARGET does not require trauma memory processing, but instead engages youth in a process of learning how to systematically reconstruct narratives describing current or past stressful events. The intervention's premise is that knowing how to reconstruct memories that are predominantly dysphoric, fragmented, and incomplete, in order to make them more emotionally and cognitively coherent and complete, will enhance the client's ability to regulate distressing emotions related either to past traumas or current stressful life events. Some children and adolescents spontaneously apply the FREEDOM skills to constructing a narrative of specific past traumatic events, whereas others choose instead to use the skills to enhance their sense of mastery of current events and symptoms.

One randomized clinical trial with girls involved in delinquency and two field trials with adolescents in juvenile justice residential programs have provided evidence of TARGET's effectiveness with children and adolescents ages 11–18 years old. In the randomized clinical trial study, TARGET delivered as a one-to-one therapy was more effective than a relational therapy in reducing PTSD (intrusive reexperiencing and avoidance) and anxiety symptoms and improving posttraumatic cognitions and emotion regulation (Ford, Steinberg, Hawke, Levine, & Zhang, 2012). The relational therapy was an active intervention rather than a minimal contact control condition, as evidenced by its superiority to TARGET in reducing girls' self-reported anger and increasing their sense of hope. In the two quasi-experimental design juvenile justice field trial studies, TARGET was delivered as a group and milieu intervention, and was found to be associated with greater reductions in violent incidents and punitive disciplinary sanctions (e.g., restraints, seclusion; Ford & Hawke, 2012; Marrow, Knudsen, Olafson, & Becker, 2012), reductions in recidivism (Ford & Hawke, 2012), reductions in depression and anxiety (Marrow et al., 2012), and improvements in sense of hope and engagement in rehabilitation (Marrow et al., 2012), than matched comparison groups receiving services as usual. Thus, TARGET shows promise with complexly traumatized youth as a one-to-one, group, and milieu therapy model.

Attachment, Self-Regulation, and Competency

The Attachment, Self-Regulation, and Competency (ARC) treatment model (Kinniburgh, Blaustein, Spinazzola, & van der Kolk, 2005; Blaustein &

Kinniburgh, 2010) is a components-based framework of intervention for youth who have experienced complex trauma and for the systems of care (familial and structural) surrounding these youth. The framework resulted from efforts to identify, define, and describe core components addressed in the treatment of complex trauma in children, and to build a flexible, adaptable organizing structure for clinical and nonclinical providers. Nine primary treatment targets are identified within three primary domains. A tenth target incorporates the nine core goals in the integration of traumatic experience. Each target is further broken down into key subskills, which can be addressed through an array of intervention strategies.

The *attachment domain* focuses on the importance of building safe, trauma-informed caregiving systems for youth who have experienced trauma in order to better support these children and adolescents in meeting developmental and treatment goals. Central to the interventions within this domain is the awareness that trauma-impacted children and families find themselves in many different systems—for instance, the family, educational systems, treatment systems, and the community. As such, the targets of intervention may be primary caregivers—that is, biological, foster, and adoptive parents—but may also (or instead) be other caregiving systems, such as treatment providers, residential staff, schools, and child welfare personnel. Four primary targets of intervention are specified. *Caregiver management of affect* emphasizes the key role of supporting caregivers in understanding and addressing their own emotional responses through psychoeducation, self-awareness, and building coping strategies and concrete supports. *Attunement* focuses on increasing the ability of the caregiver(s) to accurately read and respond to child behaviors, emotions, and needs, and emphasizes the role of psychoeducation about trauma and its impacts. *Consistent response* supports the development of predictable, safe responses to children's behavior that increase, rather than decrease, felt safety and often involves the integration of caregiver affect management and attunement along with concrete skill building in trauma-sensitive behavioral strategies. Finally, *routines and rituals* supports and strengthens those patterns of experience that provide predictability and rhythm and connect the child/family to themselves (routines) and to their community (rituals) over time.

The *self-regulation* domain targets the dysregulation of self and internal experience that often occurs following complex trauma exposure, with the primary goal of supporting children in safely and effectively managing their experience on multiple levels—behavioral, emotional, physiological, and relational. Three key targets are addressed. *Affect identification* specifies skills for supporting children in building self-awareness, including the capacity to identify and discriminate internal emotional and physiological states. *Modulation* emphasizes identifying and building strategies to support youth in maintaining arousal states that are both *comfortable* and *effective* (i.e., appropriate to the circumstances). Finally, *expression* supports youth in building skills and tolerance for effectively sharing internal experience with others.

The *competency* domain provides a basis for addressing two core targets that have been linked to resilience in stress-impacted youth in a developmentally appropriate way. *Executive functions* targets the ability, at an age-appropriate level, to identify problems and goals, inhibit reactive responses, identify alternatives, and implement solutions. *Self and identity* supports the building of a sense of self that is coherent across time, experience, and affective state, which incorporates positive and unique elements, and which includes a future template.

The tenth target, *trauma experience integration* (TEI), describes a framework for applying the nine primary targets to the active exploration, integration, and processing of historical experiences and of fragmented self-states. For instance, attunement skills support caregivers' accurate understanding of trauma-related behaviors and responses. Affect identification and modulation skills are essential for supporting the child in exploring current experience. Executive function skills are used to support a self-reflective process and identify functions of behavior and sense of self/ identity as a way to anchor the child in the rationale for doing the work and for creating future goals.

The ARC framework has been applied to guide treatment, refine systems, and train clinicians in numerous service settings, including outpatient mental health centers, inpatient programs, residential treatment centers, schools, juvenile justice facilities, and child welfare systems. In a study with young child welfare–involved children, treatment using the ARC framework was followed by reduced self-reported behavioral symptoms and favorable rates of permanency after 1 year in placement as compared with state averages (92% vs. Alaska state average of 40%) (Arvidson et al., 2011). In another study with adoptive children and families, pre–post analyses demonstrated that clinicians rated children who completed a 16-week ARC-based treatment as showing reductions in PTSD symptoms. Children and their parents reported reductions in problem behavioral symptoms. Mothers reported increased adaptive skills, and both parents reported reduced distress (Blaustein, Kinniburgh, Abot, Peterson, & Spinazzola, 2012). Program evaluation data collected by the NCTSN showed that children receiving ARC-based services demonstrated reductions in behavior problems and posttraumatic stress symptoms comparable to those for children receiving TF-CBT (ICF Macro, 2010). Field study results also support ARC's effectiveness in residential settings. In three programs utilizing the ARC treatment framework as a guide for clinical and systems initiatives as well as staff training, there was a 45–68% reduction in restraints utilized by staff as an intervention; notably, this contrasted with increases in restraints during that same time period in similar programs within the same system (Kinniburgh, Hodgdon, Gabowitz, Blsustein, & Spinazzola, in press). Youth in these programs self-reported reduced behavioral and PTSD symptoms during the project period. Taken together, these results are supportive of the utility of ARC as a flexibly applied, components-based framework for youth who have experienced complex trauma.

Structured Psychotherapy for Adolescents Responding to Chronic Stress

Structured Psychotherapy for Adolescents Responding to Chronic Stress (SPARCS) is a structured, phase-oriented, 16-session group intervention that was specifically designed for use with adolescents with complex trauma histories who continue to live in chaotic (and oftentimes violent) environments and have a range of social, emotional, and behavioral difficulties (*http://sparcstraining.com/index.php*). SPARCS involves cognitive and behavioral techniques, skills, and concepts adapted from dialectical behavior therapy for adolescents (see DeRosa & Rathus, Chapter 12, this volume), TARGET (described above), and trauma and grief component therapy for adolescents (Layne et al., 2008). Each SPARCS session is an hour in length and can be delivered weekly or biweekly. Although participants do not formally construct a trauma narrative, they discuss ways that traumatic experiences have shaped their expectations of others and their understanding of the world. The SPARCS curriculum underscores developmental tasks unique to this age group and capitalizes on adolescents' burgeoning sense of independence, peer connection, and increased capacity to consider abstract concepts such as justice and loyalty in their decision making. The curriculum and the training use a strength-based perspective in conceptualizing the impairments with which many traumatized teens struggle. For example, behaviors typically labeled as "bad" (e.g., drinking, fighting, avoiding), are framed as efforts by the youth to survive and cope with difficult situations.

The four C's (described below) represent the overarching goals of SPARCS, promoting resilience through the development and strengthening of existing important self-regulatory, problem-solving, and communication skills. Through a combination of role plays, *in vivo* practice, and colorful take-home worksheets, adolescents practice four core skills that correspond to each of the C's outlined below (for a more detailed review of the skills, see Habib et al., 2012).

The four C's consist of (1) Cultivating awareness (of self and others) through the use of *mindfulness* to become aware of internal emotional, cognitive, and physiological experiences and their relationship to external contextual factors (e.g., the look on someone's face, tone of voice, stressful environmental surroundings) that may be operating as triggers or trauma reminders; (2) Coping effectively by self-identifying *MUPS* (coping strategies such as substance use or self-harm that work in the short term but Mess you UP in the long run) and through the use of short- and long-term coping and problem-solving skills (*distress tolerance* skills and the *LET 'M GO* steps, respectively); (3) Connecting with others by using the *MAKE A LINK* communication skills; and (4) Creating meaning by helping adolescents recognize the values and beliefs (e.g., loyalty, respect, independence) that drive their thoughts, feelings, and ultimately behaviors, and assisting them in making decisions that reflect those values. Youth practice these skills using role plays, experiential activities, group discussion, and extra-session practice assignments designed to promote self-regulation in the "here and now."

The curriculum is manual-guided. Each session builds on concepts and skills introduced in preceding sections. The treatment begins with psychoeducation regarding the effects of stress and trauma on the mind, body, and emotions, and draws a distinction between low-magnitude versus high-magnitude stressors. Adolescents learn to understand their reactions through a trauma lens and to recognize intense emotions and extreme behaviors as necessary adaptations they have made in order to survive. Interpersonal violence, particularly at the hands of someone who is trusted, instills deep and lasting mistrust and hypervigilance in relationships. For adolescents who have experienced abuse or witnessed domestic violence, even minor stressors or seemingly innocuous interactions with others can serve as trauma reminders and trigger intense emotional and behavioral responses. Additionally, basic cognitive and physiological self-regulatory skills adapted from dialectical behavior therapy (DBT) are taught from the beginning and practiced in later sessions in order to help the youth slow down and establish an emotional, behavioral, and cognitive foundation that optimizes learning and skill mastery. The DBT distress tolerance skills of "distract" and "self-soothe" are taught to strengthen coping resources, followed by sessions on problem solving and communication. The final sessions include activities and worksheets that promote exploration of adolescents' self-perception and identity and generate discussion of future goals, views of the world and others, and sense of hopefulness.

The SPARCS curriculum is implemented with extensive training, a detailed manual for use by clinicians (DeRosa & Pelcovitz, 2008), and colorful workbooks that include in-session handouts as well as practice worksheets for use by group members between sessions *(http://sparcstraining.com/index.php)*. Adaptations of SPARCS include an individual therapy version for adolescents, a version for children ages 6–11, and a brief (five or six session) "skills-training only" version that can be delivered by peer leaders (SPARCS-I, SPARCS- Juniors, and SPARCS-ST).

The intervention and training program was created, tested, refined, and finalized in collaboration with community partners in a variety of settings across the country. Pilot testing has indicated that adolescents receiving SPARCS—including those in outpatient, school, residential, and juvenile justice settings—report improvements on measures of emotional distress, posttraumatic stress symptoms, interpersonal relations, physical complaints, conduct problems, and inattention/hyperactivity (Habib et al., 2012; *http://sparcstraining.com/index.pjp*). In a pilot program conducted by the Illinois Department of Children and Family Services, adolescents in foster care receiving SPARCS were half as likely to run away and one-fourth less likely to be arrested or hospitalized than youth in a comparison group, and also were less likely to drop out of treatment (*http://sparcstraining.com/index.pjp*; Weiner, Schneider, & Lyons, 2009).

Upon beginning SPARCS, one adolescent casually informed the clinician that, "I am bipolar and 'crazy.'" After two sessions, he said, with a look of dawning incredulity, "Do you think that maybe I'm so aggressive because of everything I've gone through? And maybe that's why I smoke [marijuana] so much?" That his past experiences impacted his current functioning and that he was not what he was diagnosed had not occurred to him until he received SPARCS. Halfway through the SPARCS sessions, his symptoms were noticeably reduced, he was using more adaptive and mindful coping tactics, and he no longer identified himself as "bipolar" or "crazy." This adolescent's response illustrates the potential that SPARCS provides to help adolescents recover from complex trauma.

Real Life Heroes

Real Life Heroes (Kagan, 2004, 2007a, 2007b) was developed as an integrated trauma and resiliency-centered framework for latency-age children with complex trauma histories. The model is designed to help practitioners in child welfare programs engage children, families, and systems of care using trauma-informed services, including children who lack stable relationships with caregivers and children referred for high-risk behaviors. Real Life Heroes provides tools to reframe referrals based on pathologies and blame into a shared "journey," a "pathway" to healing and recovery focused on restoring (or building) emotionally supportive enduring relationships and promoting development of affect regulation skills for children and caregivers. The model uses the metaphor of the heroic quest and engages caregivers and a collaborative team of caring adults working together with an integrated trauma and resiliency-informed framework to help children with complex trauma. Creative arts and shared life story work provides a means for children and caregivers to develop the safety and attunement needed for reintegration of traumatic memories in the context of increased security and affect regulation.

Real Life Heroes focuses on three primary components for strengthening resiliency: collaboration (caregivers and practitioners working together), commitment (emotionally supportive and enduring relationships), and courage (restoring hope, trust, and confidence). An activity-based workbook helps to engage the children and promote the safety needed in sessions for them to work with practitioners and caregivers to build the skills and interpersonal resources needed to reintegrate painful memories and to foster healing after serial traumatic experiences. Learning about heroes includes sharing stories of how family members and people of the child's ethnic heritage have learned from and overcome hard times. With these stories of caring and overcoming as a foundation, children are encouraged to develop their own strengths and resources.

In each session children learn to recognize physical clues to their emotions and stress reactions and how to express these safely. Sessions include use of a thermometer to share feelings of stress, self-control, madness, sadness, gladness, and safety. The use of magic tricks and centering activities engage children in learning and practicing skills, developing feelings of mastery, and reducing stress. The workbook helps children and caregivers share experiences and develop affect regulation skills via art, rhythm, music, and movement. Practitioners help children make their drawings into "three-chapter stories" with a beginning, middle, and end so that children learn they can *move through* both good times, and later "tough times," and make things better in their lives instead of feeling helpless, stuck, or overwhelmed. Stories enhance children's feelings of pride, which counter the shame resulting often from years of experiencing neglect, losses, emotional/physical/sexual abuse, and family violence.

Chapter by chapter, practitioners can help children and families strengthen skills and resources to reduce the power of the "monsters" (including multiple and serial traumas) that have afflicted their past and shaped high-risk and other problem behaviors as indicators of distress. Shared activities help children grow stronger than their fears and change old ways of coping that, more often than not, got them into more trouble. The workbook helps children change how they see themselves from feeling hurt, unwanted, damaged, or hopeless to feeling that they can *move through* these feelings and the traumas of the past to experience security with emotionally supportive adults committed to helping children.

Real Life Heroes chapters match the phase-based components outlined by best-practice guidelines (Ford & Cloitre, 2009). Core components include strategies and step-by-step procedures and worksheets outlined in the *Practitioner's Manual* and training curricula to ensure (1) safety for the child and the child's family (psychological, physical, and emotional); (2) strengths- and relationships-focused assessments and service planning; (3) self-regulation development in all phases of treatment for both the child and caregivers; (4) trauma memory reintegration matched to the child and caregiver's capacity that incorporates components from several PTSD treatments for children; and (5) prevention and management of disruptions of primary relationships and crises, including trauma reactions using "personal power plans." Interventions and activities are prioritized based on the child's current affect regulation and the strength and availability of emotionally supportive and enduring relationships.

Real Life Heroes has been successfully pilot-tested in home-based and placement child welfare services (Kagan, Douglas, Hornik, & Kratz, 2008) and utilized in a wide range of child and family service agencies in the United States and Canada. The HEROES Project, a community practice site of the NCTSN funded by the Substance Abuse and Mental Health Services

Administration, is currently evaluating an integrated cross-systems, collaborative intervention for eight child and family service programs centered on use of Real Life Heroes, child–parent psychotherapy (see Klatzkin, Lieberman, & Van Horn, Chapter 16, this volume) for ages 0–5, and NCTSN curricula to resource parents, residential counselors, intensive in-home workers, and child protective service workers to provide service teams with a common trauma- and resiliency-informed framework for assessments, service planning, prioritization, session activities, fidelity, and session-by-session and 3-month evaluation measures. Preliminary results for Real Life Heroes demonstrated significant reductions in caregiver and child ratings of traumatic stress symptoms and behavioral problems, along with significant increases in children's perceptions of increased social support.

Conclusion

TARGET, ARC, SPARCS, and Real Life Heroes represent a next generation of models for psychotherapy with children and adolescents who have experienced complex trauma. Although each model addresses the stress reactivity, avoidance, emotional numbing, and hypervigilance that characterize PTSD in children and adolescents, they differ from established pediatric PTSD psychotherapies such as TF-CBT (Kliethermes, Nanney, Cohen, & Mannarino, Chapter 10, this volume) in several ways (Ford & Cloitre, 2009). Most importantly, these therapies emphasize providing traumatized youth with an understanding of how a wide range of emotional, behavioral, relational, learning, and health problems can be understood as—and resolved by learning how to modify—the adaptations that the body and mind make in order to endure and survive traumatic stressors (Ford, 2005, 2009). Each therapy offers a relational foundation informed by attachment research and theory, and teaches skills to help the youth and their caregivers and adult mentors/role models recognize stress reactions and self-regulate their bodies, emotions, thinking, and behavior. Correspondingly, the therapies do not require detailed disclosure and processing of specific traumatic events by the youth client, as is the case in PTSD-focused therapies such as TF-CBT. They do, however, provide a structure for the youth and caregiver to create coherent narratives describing their lives both in the recent past and over their entire life course—for example, the hero's journey in Real Life Heroes or the lifeline in TARGET. As youth and caregivers experience their often surprising abilities to make sense of stressful events or the larger chronology of their lives, the new narrative creation skills can be applied to processing specific trauma memories. Thus, developmental trauma-focused therapies and PTSD-focused therapies are potentially highly complementary, and are already being utilized in a sequential manner by trauma-informed clinicians and programs; for example, with youth who are difficult to engage initially due to oppositional defiance (Cohen et al., 2010), TARGET has been used as a foundation for subsequent TF-CBT trauma processing.

The developmental trauma focus is represented by all of the therapies described in other chapters in this book, including several that are explicitly designed to address the developmental disruptions caused by early life interpersonal trauma (e.g., child–parent psychotherapy, Klatzkin, Lieberman, & Van Horn, Chapter 16; integrated treatment of complex trauma, Lanktree & Briere, Chapter 8; trauma systems therapy, Navalta, Brown, Nisewaner, Ellis, & Saxe, Chapter 18, this volume). However, the therapies described in this chapter represent an attempt to translate the complexity of psychotherapy with complexly traumatized children and adolescents into behaviorally specific and precisely sequenced treatment curricula and manuals. Permitting substantial clinical judgment and flexibility in implementing the manualized therapy procedures (see DeRosa, Amaya-Jackson, & Layne, Chapter 6, this volume), these models are readily teachable to, and replicable by, not only clinicians but also by clinically guided youth services providers (e.g., case managers, residential treatment staff, juvenile detention officers; e.g., Ford & Blaustein, in press). As such, they represent a vehicle not only for individual or group therapy but also for systemic therapeutic intervention (Ford & Blaustein, in press) with family systems (Ford & Saltzman, 2009), large child and family services organizations (as described in greater detail in the Sanctuary model; Bloom, Chapter 15, this volume), and community organizational systems (as described more fully in the trauma systems therapy model; Navalta et al., Chapter 18, this volume).

The developmental trauma-focused psychotherapies described in this chapter also highlight an important principle of clinical and scientific innovation. Although each model is distinct and disseminated as a singular package by its developers (with detailed workbooks, clinician/leader training and manuals, and protocols for monitoring fidelity, quality, and outcomes), they represent the result of a creative process of cross-pollination. TARGET, ARC, SPARCS, and Real Life Heroes came into being and were developed and refined over the past 15 years by a group of colleagues (including this chapter's coauthors and their collaborators) who not only shared a vision of translating the science of complex trauma into effective interventions, but moreover, generously shared their clinical insights and tools to facilitate the concurrent synergistic development of all four models. The intervention models also benefited greatly from key concepts and components shared, equally generously, by the developers of many of the therapeutic models described in other chapters in this book. Thus, instead of being the product of fierce competition among rivals, these developmental trauma-focused interventions have grown as the result of a different kind of competition: a striving among co-creators to support one another in achieving the best possible array of therapeutic services for complex trauma survivors. The developmental trajectory of these therapy models offers heartening proof that innovation in clinical practice and science can indeed mirror the collaborative ethos that is a fundamental guiding principle of these models in their work with complex trauma survivors.

References

Althoff, R. R., Ayer, L. A., Rettew, D. C., & Hudziak, J. J. (2011). Assessment of dysregulated children using the Child Behavior Checklist: A receiver operating characteristic curve analysis. *Psychological Assessment, 22*(3), 609–617.

Althoff, R. R., Verhulst, F. C., Rettew, D. C., Hudziak, J. J., & van der Ende, J. (2010). Adult outcomes of childhood dysregulation: A 14-year follow-up study. *Journal of the American Academy of Child and Adolescent Psychiatry, 49*(11), 1105–1116.

Andersen, S. (2003). Trajectories of brain development. *Neuroscience and Biobehavioral Reviews, 27,* 3–18.

Arvidson, J., Kinniburgh, K., Howard, K., Spinazzola, J., Strothers, H., Evans, M., et al. (2011). Treatment of complex trauma in young children: Developmental and cultural considerations in application of the ARC intervention model. *Journal of Child and Adolescent Trauma, 4*(1), 34–51.

Ayer, L., Althoff, R., Ivanova, M., Rettew, D., Waxler, E., Sulman, J., et al. (2009). Child Behavior Checklist Juvenile Bipolar Disorder (CBCL-JBD) and CBCL Posttraumatic Stress Problems (CBCL-PTSP) scales are measures of a single dysregulatory syndrome. *Journal of Child Psychology and Psychiatry, 50,* 1291–1300.

Blaustein, M., & Kinniburgh, K. (2010). *Treating traumatic stress in children and adolescents: How to foster resilience through attachment, self-regulation, and competency.* New York: Guilford Press.

Blaustein, M., Kinniburgh, K., Abot, D., Peterson, M., & Spinazzola, J. (2012). *Applications of the ARC framework to intervention with post-adoptive children and families.* Boston: Justice Resource Institute.

Charney, D. S. (2004). Psychobiological mechanisms of resilience and vulnerability. *American Journal of Psychiatry, 161,* 195–216.

Charuvastra, A., & Cloitre, M. (2008). Social bonds and posttraumatic stress disorder. *Annual Review of Psychology, 59,* 301–328.

Cloitre, M., Stolbach, B. C., Herman, J. L., Kolk, B. V., Pynoos, R., Wang, J., et al. (2009). A developmental approach to complex PTSD: Childhood and adult cumulative trauma as predictors of symptom complexity. *Journal of Traumatic Stress, 22,* 399–404.

Cloitre, M., Stovall-McClough, C., Zorbas, P., & Charuvastra, A. (2008). Attachment organization, emotion regulation, and expectations of support in a clinical sample of women with childhood abuse histories. *Journal of Traumatic Stress, 21*(3), 282–289.

Cohen, J., Berliner, L., & Mannarino, A. (2010). Trauma-focused CBT for children with co-occurring trauma and behavior problems. *Child Abuse and Neglect, 34,* 215–224.

Cohen, J. A., Mannarino, A. P., Kliethermes, M., & Murray, L. A. (2012). Trauma-focused CBT for youth with complex trauma. *Child Abuse and Neglect, 36,* 528–541.

Cook, A., Spinazzola, J., Ford, J. D., Lanktree, C., Blaustein, M., Cloitre, M., et al. (2005). Complex trauma in children and adolescents. *Psychiatric Annals, 35,* 390–398.

D'Andrea, W., Ford, J. D., Stolbach, B., Spinazzola, J., & van der Kolk, B. A. (2012). Understanding interpersonal trauma in children: Why we need a developmentally appropriate trauma diagnosis. *American Journal of Orthopsychiatry, 82,* 187–200.

DeRosa, R., & Pelcovitz, D. (2008). Group treatment for chronically traumatized adolescents: Igniting SPARCS of change. In D. Brom, R. Pat-Horenczyk, & J. Ford (Eds.), *Treating traumatized children: Risk, resilience, and recovery* (pp. 225–239). London: Routledge.

Eisenberg, N., Fabes, R. A., Murphy, B., Maszk, P., Smith, M., & Karbon, M. (1995). The role of emotionality and regulation in children's social functioning: A longitudinal study. *Child Development, 66,* 1360–1384.

Felitti, V., Anda, R., Nordenberg, D., Williamson, D., Spitz, A., Edwards, V., et al. (1998). Relationship of childhood abuse and household dysfunction to many of the leading causes of death in adults. *American Journal of Preventive Medicine, 14,* 245–258.

Finkelhor, D., Ormrod, R., & Turner, H. (2007). Poly-victimization: A neglected component in child victimization. *Child Abuse and Neglect, 31,* 7–26.

First, M., Pincus, H., Levine, J., Williams, J., Ustun, B., & Peele, R. (2003). Clinical utility as a criterion for revising psychiatric diagnoses. *American Journal of Psychiatry, 161,* 946–954.

Ford, J. D. (2005). Treatment implications of altered neurobiology, affect regulation, and information processing following child maltreatment: *Psychiatric Annals, 35,* 410–419.

Ford, J. D. (2009). Neurobiological and developmental research: Clinical implications. In C. Courtois & J. D. Ford (Eds.), *Treating complex traumatic stress disorders: An evidence-based guide* (pp. 31–58). New York: Guilford Press.

Ford, J. D., & Blaustein, M. E. (in press). Systemic self-regulation: A framework for trauma-informed services in residential juvenile justice programs. *Journal of Family Violence.*

Ford, J. D., & Cloitre, M. (2009). Best practices in psychotherapy for children and adolescents. In C. Courtois & J. D. Ford (Eds.), *Treating complex traumatic stress disorders: An evidence-based guide* (pp. 59–81). New York: Guilford Press.

Ford, J. D., Connor, D. F., & Hawke, J. (2009). Complex trauma among psychiatrically impaired children. *Journal of Clinical Psychiatry, 70,* 1155–1163.

Ford, J. D., & Hawke, J. (2012). Trauma affect regulation psychoeducation group and milieu intervention outcomes in juvenile detention facilities. *Journal of Aggression, Maltreatment, and Trauma, 21,* 365–384.

Ford, J. D., & Saltzman, W. (2009). Family therapy. In C. Courtois & J. D. Ford (Eds.), *Treating complex traumatic stress disorders: An evidence-based guide* (pp. 391–414). New York: Guilford Press.

Ford, J. D., Steinberg, K., Hawke, J., Levine, J., & Zhang, W. (2012). Randomized trial comparison of emotion regulation and relational psychotherapies for PTSD with girls involved in delinquency. *Journal of Clinical Child and Adolescent Psychology, 41,* 27–37.

Ford, J. D., Steinberg, K., & Zhang, W. (2011). A randomized clinical trial comparing affect regulation and social problem-solving psychotherapies for mothers with victimization-related PTSD. *Behavior Therapy, 42,* 561–578.

Friedman, M. J., & McEwen, B. (2004). Posttraumatic stress disorder, allostatic load, and medical illness. In P. Schnurr & B. L. Green (Ed.), *Physical health consequences of exposure to extreme stress* (pp. 157–188). Washington, DC: American Psychological Association.

Harvey, S. T., & Taylor, J. E. (2010). A meta-analysis of the effects of psychotherapy with sexually abused children and adolescents. *Clinical Psychology Review, 30*(5), 517–535.

Hayes, S., Luoma, J., Bond, F., Masuda, A., & Lillis, J. (2006). Acceptance and commitment therapy: Model, processes and outcomes. *Behaviour Research and Therapy, 44,* 1–25.

ICF Macro. (2010, December). *Evaluation of the National Child Traumatic Stress*

Initiative: FY 2010 Annual Progress Report, Executive Summary. Retrieved from www.icfi.com/insights/projects/health/national-child-traumatic-stress-initiative

Kagan, J. (2001). Emotional development and psychiatry. *Biological Psychiatry, 49,* 973–979.

Kagan, R. (2004). *Rebuilding attachments with traumatized children: Healing from losses, violence, abuse, and neglect.* Binghamton, NY: Haworth Press.

Kagan, R. (2007a). *Real Life Heroes: A life storybook for children* (2nd ed.). Binghamton, NY: Haworth Press.

Kagan, R. (2007b). *Real life heroes: Practitioner's manual.* Binghamton, NY: Haworth Press.

Kagan, R., Douglas, A., Hornik, J., & Kratz, S. (2008). Real Life Heroes pilot study: Evaluation of a treatment model for children with traumatic stress. *Journal of Child and Adolescent Trauma, 1*(1), 5–22.

Kinniburgh, K. J., Blaustein, M., Spinazzola, J., & van der Kolk, B. A. (2005). Attachment, self-regulation, and competency. *Psychiatric Annals, 35*(5), 424–430.

Kinniburgh, K., Hodgdon, H., Gabowitz, D., Blaustein, M., & Spinazzola, J. (in press). Development and implementation of trauma-focused programming in residential schools using the ARC framework. *Journal of Family Violence.*

Koenen, K. (2006). Developmental epidemiology of PTSD: Self-regulation as a core mechanism. *Annals of the New York Academy of Sciences, 1071,* 255–266.

Lanius, R. A., Bluhm, R. L., Coupland, N. J., Hegadoren, K. M., Rowe, B., Theberge, J., et al. (2010). Default mode network connectivity as a predictor of post-traumatic stress disorder symptom severity in acutely traumatized subjects. *Acta Psychiatrica Scandinavica, 121,* 33–40.

Layne, C., Beck, C., Rimmasch, H., Southwick, J., Moreno, M., & Hobfoll, S. (2008). Promoting "resilient" posttraumatic adjustment in childhood and beyond. In D. Brom, R. Pat-Horenczyk, & J. D. Ford (Eds.), *Treating traumatized children: Risk, resilience, and recovery* (pp. 13–47). London: Routledge.

Lewis, M. D. (2005). Self-organizing individual differences in brain development. *Developmental Review, 25,* 252–277.

Marrow, M., Knudsen, K., Olafson, E., & Bucher, S. (2012). The value of implementing TARGET within a trauma-informed juvenile justice setting. *Journal of Child and Adolescent Trauma, 5,* 257–270.

Matsumoto, K., Suzuki, W., & Tanaka, K. (2003). Neuronal correlates of goal-based motor selection in the prefrontal cortex. *Science, 301,* 229–232.

May, J. C., Delgado, M., Dahl, R., Stenger, A., Ryan, N., Fiez, J., et al. (2004). Event-related magnetic resonance imaging of reward-related brain circuitry in children and adolescents. *Biological Psychiatry, 55,* 359–366.

Milad, M. R., Wright, C. I., Orr, S. P., Pitman, R. K., Quirk, G. J., & Rauch, S. L. (2007). Recall of fear extinction in humans activates the ventromedial prefrontal cortex and hippocampus in concert. *Biological Psychiatry, 62,* 446–454.

Neumeister, A., Henry, S., & Krystal, J. (2007). Neurocircuitry and neuroplasticity in PTSD. In M. J. Friedman, T. M. Keane, & P. Resick (Eds.), *Handbook of PTSD* (pp. 151–165). New York: Guilford Press.

Rauch, S., Shin, L., & Phelps, E. (2006). Neurocircuitry models of posttraumatic stress disorder and extinction: Human neuroimaging research—past, present, and future. *Biological Psychiatry, 60,* 376–382.

Teicher, M., Andersen, S., Polcari, A., Anderson, C., Navalta, C., & Kim, D. (2003). Neurobiological consequences of early stress and childhood maltreatment. *Neuroscience and Biobehavioral Reviews, 27,* 33–44.

van der Kolk, B. (2005). Developmental trauma disorder. *Psychiatric Annals, 35,* 439–448.

van der Kolk, B., Roth, S., Pelcovitz, D., Sunday, S., & Spinazzola, J. (2005). Disorders of extreme stress. *Journal of Traumatic Stress, 18,* 389–399.

CHAPTER 15

The Sanctuary Model

Sandra L. Bloom

The challenges that children in intensive therapeutic treatment are up against are complex and often originated in exposure to multiple forms of adversity. In brief, these children have (1) difficulty with maintaining safety in interpersonal relationships largely due to disrupted attachment experiences and the erosion of trust that accompanies such experiences; (2) significant challenges in adequately managing distressing emotions in ways that are not self-destructive, including exercising the capacities for self-discipline, self-control, and willpower; (3) cognitive problems, particularly when stress occurs and the development of essential cortical functions has not gone smoothly; (4) problems with open and direct communication at home and at school that pose significant challenges because they frequently communicate through behavior, not directly, openly, or in words; (5) feelings of helplessness and powerlessness in the face of a world that they perceive as unjust and cruel, and as a result, may be repeatedly bullied or become bullies themselves; (6) no clear sense of social responsibility even into adulthood, and their moral development may have been affected by disrupted attachment experiences and inadequate role models; (7) likely experienced significant loss while lacking the capacity to grieve secondary to the emotional management problems; (8) a tendency to repeat the experiences that are a part of their past; and (9) often a lack of any hope that the future will be any better than the past, while their emotional and cognitive challenges interfere with the capacity to plan ahead and tolerate delayed gratification.

All of this means that, in the context of the treatment/intervention setting, much is demanded of managers, therapists, caregivers, and educators. We must teach, role model and support the development of (1) safety skills and significant improvements in the capacity for interpersonal trust; (2) emotional management skills, including self-control, self-discipline, and the exercise of will power; (3) cognitive skills, including the ability to identify triggers and problematic patterns while still being able to think in the presence of strong emotion; (4) communication skills that include rehearsals in what to say and how to say it; (5) participatory and leadership skills; (6) judgment skills, including socially acceptable and fair behavioral schemas; and (7) skills to manage grief and plan for the future. This work is complex and interactive, demanding much of those who work to change the developmental trajectories of children and adolescents suffering from complex posttraumatic problems.

What characteristics best describe people who are able to do this challenging work? They need to be secure, reasonably healthy adults, who have good emotional management skills themselves. They must be intellectually and emotionally intelligent—and the latter is probably even more important than the former. They need to be able to actively teach new skills and routines while serving as role models for what they are teaching. There are constant demands on them for patience and for empathy, so they must be able to endure intense emotional challenge. As they balance the demands of work and home, managers and supervisors, children/clients and their own families, they must be self-disciplined, self-controlled, and never abuse their own personal power.

Given this description, it becomes easier to understand why, as a society and in particular in its mental health and social service systems, we are facing a workforce crisis. As a national report has stated, "A growing proportion of the U.S. workforce will have been raised in disadvantaged environments that are associated with relatively high proportions of individuals with diminished cognitive and social skills" (Knudsen, Heckman, Cameron, & Shonkoff, 2006, p. 10155). Given the rates of exposure to childhood adversity in the general population, staff members at all levels of social service and other mental health organizations are likely to have their own past histories of experiences that are not entirely dissimilar to the people they are supposed to help, and they may have unresolved interpersonal challenges that are also not dissimilar (Felitti & Anda, 2010). In a recent survey of a residential treatment setting for children, almost three-quarters of staff respondents to the Adverse Childhood Experiences (ACE) questionnaire had an ACE score of at least 1 and 16% had an ACE score of 4 or more (Esaki & Larkin, 2011), making this issue a significant part of the workforce crisis.

Additional factors play an important role in this crisis. Extraordinary demands are placed upon social service workers who are paid low salaries and whose organizations receive inadequate funding. The job complexity and ambiguity is high whereas the payoff is low, particularly for those in any type of institutional setting where the least educated, trained, and supervised staff spend the most time with profoundly injured children. And these workers are not in environments that are safe. Forty-eight percent of all nonfatal injuries from occupational assaults and violent acts occur in health care and social services (Occupational Safety and Health Administration, 2004). In fact, after law enforcement, persons employed in the mental health sector have the highest rates of all occupations of being victimized while at work or on duty (Bureau of Justice Statistics, 2001). Actual rates of violence expose the problems with physical safety, but there are other safety issues as well that can be thought of as threats to psychological, social, and moral safety.

Thus, although working with traumatized children can be stressful, the main causes of workplace stress cannot be laid at the feet of the children and their families: "The main sources of stress for workers are the ways in which organizations operate and the nature of the relationships that people experience within the work setting" (Bloom & Farragher, 2010, p. 70). This is not an individual problem but a social one, partly due to controllable but severe dysfunctions within those organizations and largely related to inadequate and unscientific paradigms for intervening in the lives of traumatized people, families, and communities.

Managing Organizational Culture

The Sanctuary Model is designed to address these dilemmas by intervening at the level of organizational culture in order to change the habits and routines of everyone in the organization and the organization as a whole. The Sanctuary Model is an evidence-supported, theory-based, developmentally grounded, and trauma-informed methodology for helping all members of staff and whole organizations to become healthier while achieving better outcomes for the populations they serve. The Sanctuary Model is firmly rooted in 18th and 19th century Quaker philosophy and its practical application as "Moral Treatment," an early attempt to apply principles of relational nonviolence to the treatment of the mentally ill, with dramatically good results (Bloom & Farragher, 2013). Two other important historical movements occurred following the devastation of World War II that have influenced the development of the Sanctuary Model: the democratic therapeutic community movement (Whiteley, 2004) and the human rights movement, particularly in reference to the universal human reactions to overwhelming stress (Bloom, 2000). The Sanctuary Model programs were originally developed from 1980 to 2001 in a short-term, acute inpatient psychiatric setting for adults who were traumatized as children (Bloom,

1997, 2013). The Sanctuary Model is currently being used as a systematic organizational change process for over 250 human service delivery systems around the country and internationally, many of them serving children and adolescents.

A computer metaphor is most useful in conveying the significance of this model. An operating system in a computer is the master program that controls the computer's basic functions and allows other programs to run on the computer if they are compatible with the operating system. As our understanding of trauma survivors has grown, we recognize that exposure to severe and overwhelming trauma, particularly when it begins in childhood, disrupts the individuals' normal development of brain and mind—their "operating system"—resulting in profound "software" problems, as described above, and a personality that has become "trauma-organized" (Bloom & Farragher, 2010).

Similarly, organizational culture represents the operating system for an organization. Every organization has a culture that represents long-held organizational patterns, routines, and habits that, although remembered and taught to every new employee, are largely unconscious and automatic, as most habits are. The nature of the organizational culture largely determines whether or not the organization is able to fulfill its mission and reach its stated goals. Organizational culture may or may not be aligned with the actual values and mission that the organization claims to follow (Schein, 1999). Alignment of values is usually seen as management-driven, if it is referred to at all, and mental health and social service organizations are at a distinct disadvantage in this regard.

Within social services and mental health organizations, there is no universal requirement for anything that resembles management training. CEOs and CFOs may have had training in their background if the organization is large and especially if they came up through the ranks of some other business sector. They are also more likely to have MBAs or some administrative degree that at least academically qualifies them for the job of managing other people. But the key middle managers who actually set in motion the routines that guide daily interactions with staff, children, and families usually are promoted from within the organization or at least from within the social service, education, and social work professions. The training these professionals typically receive is whatever they experienced being managed by other people in similar circumstances—beginning, of course, with their own parents.

Contrast this process with an organization such as Starbucks, where even a newly hired high school dropout working as a barista in the first year will spend at least 50 hours in Starbucks' classrooms, and dozens more at home with Starbucks' workbooks and talking to the assigned Starbucks mentor. Or consider the Container Store, where employees receive more than 185 hours of training in their first year alone. They are taught to recognize what to do when confronted with an angry coworker or an overwhelmed customer, and they rehearse routines for calming shoppers or defusing a confrontation (Duhigg, 2012).

Not so for staff in our caregiving institutions who must engage in the emotional labor of spending 8–12 hours a day trying to help some of the most wounded, suffering, and sometimes dangerous children and adults on the planet to heal and recover from the adversity that life has dealt them. This startling contrast sums up what is a social, political, and economic problem, not a professional one. Starbucks is selling coffee; the company is enormously profitable, and its management realizes that continuing profitability has as much to do with the good service of employees as it does with the quality of their brew. We, on the other hand, are trying to develop and change minds and rewire brains, and our society has not yet awakened to the fact that not changing those brains is costing our society uncounted billions of dollars every year. The Centers for Disease Control and Prevention estimate that child abuse and neglect alone cost us $124 *billion* a year (Fang, Brown, Florence, & Mercy, 2012).

Compound the lack of adequate education, preparation, and training with breaches in basic safety; diminished funding; an unstable reimbursement system; social devaluation of caregiving work; and an inadequate theoretical framework for delivering services—and we end up with hauntingly parallel processes wherein symptomatic behavior is replicated at every level—client, staff, management, organization (Alderfer & Smith, 1982). The fundamental rationale for the Sanctuary Model is to create parallel processes of recovery by radically altering the operating system for organizations as a whole and for everyone who has contact with that organization. That means intervening at the level of organizational culture in order to change the habits and routines of everyone in the organization as well as the organization as a whole.

Key Features of the Sanctuary Model

The Sanctuary Model is structured around a philosophy of belief and practice that shifts organizations' existing ways of operating in approaching the treatment of traumatized children and families. To make such a shift, organizations must identify the habits and routines that are not compatible with developmentally grounded, trauma-informed care, and develop new and more useful habits and strategies. Organizational change of this sort requires radical alterations in the basic mental models upon which interventions have traditionally been based; without such change, treatment is bound to fall short of full recovery or to fail entirely. Mental models exist at the level of very basic assumptions, far below conscious awareness and everyday function, yet they guide and determine what individuals can and cannot think about and act upon (Senge et al., 2000). An explicit change in mental models must occur in the leaders of an organization and the staff in order to change their implicit models, and then to teach these these new mental models to the children and their families.

The term *creating Sanctuary* refers to the shared experience of creating and maintaining physical, psychological, social, and moral safety within a social environment—any social environment, but especially one directed toward mental health treatment—and thus reducing systemic violence. The process of creating Sanctuary begins with getting everyone on the same page—eliciting, sharing, arguing about, and finally agreeing on the basic values, beliefs, guiding principles and philosophical principles that are to shape attitudes, decisions, problem solving, conflict resolution, and behavior (Bloom & Farragher, 2013). The Sanctuary Model is built upon four pillars that are described below: Trauma Theory, the Sanctuary Commitments, S.E.L.F., and the Sanctuary Toolkit.

Trauma Theory

Although the impact of overwhelmingly horrific experiences—natural or humanmade—has been recognized throughout history, the modern scientific study of trauma originated in the disasters, terror, and wars of the 20th century (Bloom, 2000). Trauma Theory has challenged and undercut many "sacred cows" involving centuries of reductionism best characterized for those of us in mental health by either "mindless" or "brainless" psychiatry (Eisenberg, 1986). It has demonstrated, among other things, the interconnected and interdependent nature of human biology, psychology, sociology, and morality

As the study of psychological trauma has developed, much has been learned about the entire stress continuum and the extent to which stress, particularly repetitive conditions over the course of childhood, can impact normal development (usually, if not always, adversely). Along with the expanding field of interpersonal neuroscience we are learning how limited our freedom really is, since so much of behavior once learned becomes automatic and runs outside of conscious awareness. As it turns out, what we call "free will" is not nearly as free as we would like to believe it is (Gazzaniga, 2011). At the same time, much is being learned about how the social milieu can influence the brain, now known to be more malleable and "plastic" than was once assumed, and how important belief, faith, meaning, and purpose are in changing the brain (Duhigg, 2012).

In the Sanctuary Model, everyone in an organization needs to have a clear understanding about how toxic stress and trauma have affected the children served, and often the staff as well. Furthermore, it is vital that everyone recognizes that unacknowledged and unaddressed stress responses can result in problematic and unhealthy behaviors in both clients and staff. This understanding can be liberating and can lead to major changes in attitudes and behavior. One comprehensive training manual and accompanying training materials on the definitions and impact of traumatic stress on human development are provided for all of the clinical staff who have direct contact with children and families and another for all of the indirect care staff (i.e., administrative assistants, finance officers, maintenance and food service staff, and all the other people who are necessary to keep an organization functioning) *(Sanctuary Indirect Care and Direct Care Staff Training Manual)*.

The Sanctuary Commitments

The seven Sanctuary Commitments represent the guiding principles for implementation of the Sanctuary Model, the basic structural elements of its "operating system." Each of the commitments supports trauma recovery goals for children, families, staff, and the organization as a whole. The commitments are designed to create a parallel process that provides support for the organization and its staff at the same time as they provide an environment of recovery. Other than the newer scientific findings regarding stress, trauma, and attachment, these commitments represent universal principles typical of all human rights cultures. They become the norms that structure the organizational culture and make it easier for organizational leaders to consciously and deliberately apply the principles to whatever they do.

For the organizational climate to be ethically consistent, the Sanctuary Commitments need to be embraced by the board of directors and senior leadership, conveyed throughout the organization, through middle management, to the direct care and support staff and ultimately to the children and families. Often, when organization leaders hear the seven commitments, they assume that the commitments already guide their organizational culture. In many cases this is at least partially true since it is likely that there are many divergent views of these commitments and what they mean and how to actualize them in everyday interactions.

The change process, however, can be frightening for organizational leaders, and they rightfully perceive significant risk in opening themselves up to criticism when they attempt to level hierarchies and share power. The gains can be substantial, but a leader only finds that out after learning how to tolerate the anxiety and uncertainty that inevitably accompanies real change. It should also be noted that change does not occur just because a leader wants it to. Leaders may be willing to share power with others, but this does not necessarily mean that those others are always willing to assume power and the responsibility that comes with it. Although staff and clients may indicate that they want a greater voice, creating the conditions in which they have one is not always welcomed. It is easy to stay in or slide back to a familiar and comfortable nonparticipatory arrangement.

The challenge in the Sanctuary Model is to establish and maintain a value-based system, even in the face of what are extraordinary ethical dilemmas, the kinds of dilemmas that human service delivery professionals encounter every day (Bloom & Farragher, 2010). All sorts of tensions exist within any meaningful value system. The Sanctuary Commitments are trauma-informed objectives that apply to children and their families, staff, and the organization as a whole. They are not cure-alls. Inevitable conflicts, unintended consequences, and unforeseeable circumstances will need to be resolved each day in each program, requiring judgment and flexibility. Organizational processes are needed that provide enough structure to be able to respond flexibly in ways that support the emergence of innovative solutions to complex problems. The seven Sanctuary Commitments are described in fuller detail in Bloom and Farragher (2013) and are summarized in Figure 15.1 (Bloom & Farragher, 2010).

S.E.L.F.: A Compass for the Recovery Process

S.E.L.F. is an acronym that represents the four key interactive aspects of recovery from bad experiences. S.E.L.F. provides a nonlinear, cognitive-behavioral therapeutic approach for creating new, developmentally grounded, trauma-informed routines for facilitating change, regardless of whether these routines involve individual children, families, staff problems, or the organization as a whole.

S.E.L.F. is a compass that allows the exploration of four key domains of healing:

1. *Safety:* attaining physical, psychological, social, and moral safety in self, relationships, and environment.
2. *Emotional management:* identifying various emotions and their levels of intensity and modulating emotions in response to memories, persons, events.
3. *Loss:* feeling grief and dealing with personal losses while recognizing that all change involves loss.
4. *Future:* trying out new roles and ways of relating and behaving as a "survivor/thriver" to ensure personal, professional, and organizational safety, to find meaning, to make more viable life choices, and to help others. A focus on the future compels imaginative planning and to think ahead in ways that may have previously been precluded by ongoing posttraumatic symptoms.

While using S.E.L.F., the children, their families, and staff are able to embrace a shared, nontechnical language that is neither blaming nor judgmental. It allows all to put the larger recovery process in perspective, recognizing that safety issues may crop up repeatedly as the child wrestles with painful feelings and memories. Accessible language demystifies what sometimes is experienced as confusing and even insulting clinical or psychological jargon that can confound children, families, and even staff.

GROWTH AND CHANGE
- All change means loss but human intention can change the future

DEMOCRACY
- Complex problems require complex responses

NONVIOLENCE
- Physical, psychological, social, moral safety

EMOTIONAL INTELLIGENCE
- Human behavior makes sense if we have information

SOCIAL LEARNING
- Mistakes happen and we must learn from them

OPEN COMMUNICATION
- Information is the flow of life so communication must be open and direct

SOCIAL RESPONSIBILITY
- Social justice is the key to a peaceful, nonviolent society

FIGURE 15.1. The Sanctuary Commitments.

In the Sanctuary Model, S.E.L.F. is used as a habit-changing tool for many different organizational and treatment tasks. When faced with the complex problems that are typical of the children and families served, it is easy for a helper to lose his or her way, to focus on what is the most frightening or the easiest to understand and manage, rather than on what may be the true, underlying stumbling block. Similarly, clients are most likely to pay attention to whatever problems are causing the most pain in the present, even though, from a helper's point of view, what they are doing or not doing will likely cause them greater suffering in the long term.

As a result, it is easy for staff and children to get stuck on safety issues. When someone is doing something that is obviously dangerous, it is hard *not* to focus entirely on that danger. But an exclusive focus on physical safety may lead nowhere if underlying issues are not identified and addressed. S.E.L.F. functions as a kind of compass to get participants out of the maze of confusing symptoms. By using these four apparently simple concepts that actually are like the cardinal points of a compass, helpers and children can rapidly organize problems into categories of *safety, emotions, loss,* and *future,* which then can lead to a more complex treatment or service plan. It has the added value of conveying an implicit message that it is possible to change what has previously seemed insurmountable by "chunking out" the chaos of people's lives into more manageable bits—without losing sight of the complexity of the challenges.

But S.E.L.F. is not only applied to the children and their families. In parallel, these compass points represent problems that arise within the treatment or service setting between staff and children, among members of staff, and between line and support staff and administrators. Applied to such issues as change management, staff splitting, poor morale, rule infraction, administrative withdrawal and helplessness, misguided leadership, and collective disturbance, S.E.L.F. can also assist a stressed organization to conceptualize its own present dilemma and move into a better future through a course of complex decision making and conflict resolution. To do so, an organization must envision the *future* it wants to actualize, wrestle with the inevitable barriers to change that are related to *loss*, develop skills to manage the individual and interpersonal *emotions* and multiple conflicts surrounding change, while calculating the possible present and potential *safety* issues in making change, but also in *not* making change.

The Sanctuary Toolkit

The Sanctuary Toolkit includes a range of practical, routine skills that enables individuals and organizations to develop new habits and deal with difficult situations more effectively, build community, develop a deeper understanding of the effects of adversity and trauma, and build a common language and knowledge base. Community meetings and universal safety plans promote a focus on social responsibility, democracy, and nonviolence on a routine, daily basis. The Sanctuary Toolkit "rewires" the organization and, in doing so, opens up new pathways for communal problem solving.

Many of our tools are organized around S.E.L.F.; we teach S.E.L.F.-based treatment planning, psychoeducation, team meetings, and organizational assessment, and we use S.E.L.F. to structure red flag reviews (i.e., emergency team meetings called to deal with an urgent concern). The model helps staff, children, and parents to maintain focus while providing a shared language and meaning system for everyone, regardless of their training, experience, or education. It also helps staff members to see the parallels between what the children and their families have experienced and what is going on with the staff and the organization and to intervene when the unfolding of a collective disturbance is noticed. This bidirectional focus helps everyone to see the interactive and interdependent nature of their shared lives.

Implementing the Sanctuary Model

The Sanctuary Institute

The *Sanctuary Institute* is a five-day intensive training experience on the Sanctuary Model. Teams of five to eight people, from various levels of the organization, come together to learn from our faculty, who are colleagues from other organizations implementing Sanctuary. Together teams begin to create a shared vision of the kind of organization they want to create. These teams will eventually become the Sanctuary Steering Committee for their organization. The training experience usually involves staff from several organizations, and generally these organizations are very different in terms of size, scope, region and mission. This diversity helps to provide a rich learning experience for the participants.

During the training, the steering committee engages in prolonged facilitated dialogue that serves to surface the major strengths, vulnerabilities, and conflicts within the organization. By looking at shared assumptions, goals, and existing practice, staff members from various levels of the organization are required to share in an analysis of their own structure and functioning, often asking themselves and each other provocative questions that have never been overtly asked. Many of these questions have not been raised because participants have never felt safe enough to speak their minds or their hearts, even after many years of working together. Although the continual focus is on the fundamental question of "Are we safe?," participants quickly learn that in the Sanctuary Model, being *safe* means being willing to take risks by being willing to say what needs to be said and hear what needs to be heard. *Safety is vital but* being safe *does not necessarily mean being comfortable.*

Participants look at the change process itself and are asked to anticipate the inevitable resistance to change that is a fact of life in every organization. They look at management styles, the way decisions are made and conflicts resolved. In the process of these discussions, they learn what it means for leaders, staff, children, and families to engage in more democratic processes in terms of the simultaneous increase in rights and responsibilities. They evaluate the existing policies and procedures that apply to staff, children, and families and ask whether or not they are effective in achieving their shared goals. They are asked to learn about and become thoroughly familiar with the psychobiology of trauma and disrupted attachment and the multiple ways that posttraumatic stress disorder (PTSD), complex PTSD, and other trauma-related disorders present in the children, adults, and families with which they work. They are challenged to begin thinking about the implications of that knowledge for treatment. They also learn how high levels of stress in the organization can impact relationships, emotions, and decision making at every level of the organization. They develop an understanding of the S.E.L.F. as a tool for organizing treatment. They learn about vicarious trauma, traumatic reenactment, and the importance of understanding themselves and providing support for each other, along with the concept of posttraumatic growth. They are introduced to the various components of the Sanctuary Toolkit and the role the toolkit plays in changing organizational habits.

The Sanctuary Steering Committee members are instructed to go back to their organization and create a Core Team—a larger, multidisciplinary team that expands its reach into the entire organization. It is this Core Team that will activate the entire system. The Sanctuary Core Team should have representatives from every level of the organization to ensure that a "voice" from every sector is heard. It is vital that all key organizational leaders become actively involved in the process of change and participate in this Core Team. The Core Team is armed with a *Sanctuary Direct Care Staff Training Manual*, a *Sanctuary Indirect Staff Training Manual*, a *Sanctuary Implementation Manual*, several psychoeducational curricula, and ongoing consultation and technical assistance from Sanctuary faculty members. The process of Sanctuary Implementation extends over 3 years and aims toward Sanctuary Certification. Organizational change takes several years to really get traction and then continues—hopefully—throughout the life of the organization. The objective of the implementation and technical assistance is to nudge an organization closer and closer to the "edge of chaos" where creative, self-organizing change occurs, without destabilizing it to such a point that it becomes dangerously chaotic.

The responsibility of Sanctuary Core Team members is to actively represent and communicate with their constituents and to become trainers and cheerleaders for the entire organization. The Core Team works out team guidelines and expectations of involvement for individual team members as well as a meeting schedule and decides on safety rules for the constructive operation of the team itself. The Core Team is ultimately responsible for the development of an implementation process aimed at including the entire organization in the change process that involves teaching everyone about the Sanctuary Commitments, Attachment Theory, Trauma Theory, S.E.L.F., and the Sanctuary Toolkit. The Core Team facilitates the development of educational programs for direct care staff as well as indirect care staff who work in human resource, finance, facilities management, food service, and administration. It is likely that Core Team members will facilitate changes in admissions, interviewing of new staff, orientation programs, supervisory practices, as well as training and education policies. They oversee a plan for greater client participation in planning and implementation of their own service plan and figure out how they are going to engage a wider network of their stakeholders in the community in the Sanctuary change process. The ultimate goal is to take meaningful steps to change the organization's culture and engage as many community members as possible in the process.

As discussions are taking place in the Core Team, participating staff begin to make small but significant changes. Members take risks with each other and try new methods of engagement and conflict resolution. They feed these innovations and their results back into the process discussions. The Core Team must always maintain a balance between *process* and *product*. It is not enough to talk about how things will change; there must also be actual changes in the way business is conducted. The Core Team members therefore not only plan together how best to share what they are learning with the larger organization but also decide how to integrate the Sanctuary Toolkit into the day-to-day operation of the organization, how to evaluate how well these initiatives are taking hold in the organization, and how to train all agency personnel and children in the Sanctuary principles.

The work of the Core Team is facilitated by a combination of trainings and consultations provided by faculty at the Sanctuary Institute who move an organization through a series of steps to align the practices, attitudes, and philosophies of an organization toward a trauma-informed perspective. As this happens, more democratic, participatory processes begin to emerge. These processes are critical because they are most likely to lend themselves to the solution of very complex problems while improving staff morale, providing checks and balances to abuses of power, opening up the community to new sources of information, and achieving better outcomes with the children.

From the outset of implementation the Core Team members must decide on indicators they want to use to evaluate their program in an ongoing way—their Sanctuary Program Evaluation Plan. The indicators should be observable and measurable and consistent with standards established by Sanctuary leaders. There should be a regular process of evaluation and review that involves all Core Team members. It is vital to create a thorough method for reviewing problems and failures and establishing remedial courses of action. But likewise there must be methods for reviewing and capturing successes.

The impact of creating a developmentally grounded, trauma-informed culture using the Sanctuary Model should be observable and measurable, often by paying special attention to areas that are already being measured in the organization. The expected outcomes include less physical, verbal, emotional violence, including (but not limited to) reduced/eliminated seclusion and restraint; systemwide understanding of complex biopsychosocial and developmental impact of trauma and abuse and what that means for the service environment; less victim blaming; less punitive and judgmental responses; clearer, more consistent boundaries on the part of staff, higher expectations, better linkage between rights and responsibilities; earlier identification of and confrontation with abusive use of power in all of its forms; improved ability to articulate goals and create strategies for change; expanded understanding and awareness of reenactment behavior, resistance to change, and how to achieve a different outcome; more democratic environment at all levels; more diversified leadership and embedding of leadership skills in all staff; and, most important, better outcomes for children, staff, and the organization.

The Sanctuary Network

The Sanctuary Institute is the gateway to the Sanctuary Network, a community of organizations dedicated to the implementation of developmentally grounded, trauma-informed services. All members are committed to the belief that we can do better for our clients and our colleagues as well as our society if we can accept that the people we serve are not sick or bad, but injured, and that the services we provide must provide hope, promote growth, and inspire change.

As of the beginning of 2012, the Sanctuary Institute has trained over 250 organizations worldwide. These include adult inpatient psychiatric and substance abuse facilities, domestic violence shelters, residential programs and group homes for children, schools and educational programs, juvenile justice facilities, and large programs that have a wide variety of inpatient, outpatient, partial, community-based, and residential programs. The Sanctuary Network has grown into a community of organizations helping each other to become more trauma-informed and to improve services and outcomes. The Sanctuary Network sponsors an annual conference that features innovations in practice. The network also disseminates new materials to its members, has a website, and holds regular webinars and other opportunities for members to share and learn. With greater geographic spread, local networks are beginning to form as well.

Sanctuary Certification

Sanctuary® is a registered trademark and the right to use the Sanctuary name in relation to a psychological model or program is contingent on engagement in the certified training program and an agreement to participate in an ongoing, peer-review certification process. The Sanctuary certification process is designed to promote, sustain, and strengthen an organization's commitment to the maintenance of a healthier, developmentally grounded, trauma-informed culture for all stakeholders. Programs usually seek Sanctuary Certification in the 2- to 3-year period after participation in the Sanctuary Institute. Research is under way in the hope of moving the Sanctuary Model from an "evidence-supported" to an "evidence-based" approach.

Certification is a symbol that an organization provides a higher level of care, a trauma-sensitive environment for children and their families, and a better environment for staff who provide care. This process affirms an organizational commitment to ensure fidelity to the Sanctuary Model and meet the standard of providing a safe, secure, and developmentally appropriate environment in which children and staff will recover and thrive. Agencies that meet the Sanctuary Standards can expect to experience improved treatment outcomes, enhanced staff communication, reductions in violence and critical incidents, increased job satisfaction, lower rates of staff turnover, and better leadership.

When an organization becomes a certified Sanctuary organization, there is an agreement that it will maintain its practice in accordance with the tenets of Sanctuary, utilize the S.E.L.F. framework for Sanctuary practice, maintain Sanctuary training, expand the scope of developmentally grounded and trauma-informed and trauma-specific clinical treatment, and routinely recertify the staff and the organization. Certified Sanctuary organizations also agree to follow and maintain the Sanctuary Certification Standards postcertification between surveys.

Sanctuary Model Outcomes

To date, one controlled, randomized trial of the implementation of the Sanctuary Model in children's residential settings has been conducted. The model was piloted in four residential units that self-selected to participate in the initial phase of the project; then four additional residential treatment units were randomly assigned to implement the Sanctuary Model the following fall. Eight other units that provided the standard residential treatment program served as the control group. Changes in the therapeutic communities and in youth were assessed every 3–6 months. To summarize the results of the randomized control study, from baseline to 6 months, there were changes in staff attitudes and perceptions in five domains of organizational culture among those who received the Sanctuary Model training:

- *Support:* how much children help and support each other; how supportive staff is toward the children
- *Spontaneity:* how much the program encourages the open expression of feelings by children and staff
- *Autonomy:* how self-sufficient and independent staff perceive the children to be in making their own decisions
- *Personal problem orientation:* the extent to which children seek to understand their feelings and personal problems
- *Safety:* the extent to which staff feel they can challenge their peers and supervisors, can express opinions in staff meetings, are not blamed for problems, and have clear guidelines for dealing with children who are aggressive.

Changes in the children were just beginning to unfold as the study ended, including a decrease in children's conflict-escalating communication and increases in their positive management of tension (Rivard et al., 2004). In a quasi-experimental study of residential programs for children using the Sanctuary Model, there were similar positive changes in organizational culture, whereas comparable programs not using the Sanctuary Model did not report those improvements (McSparren & Motley, 2010).

The first seven child-serving facilities that participated in the 5-day training that begins the process of Sanctuary implementation were evaluated for changes in their rates of restraints and holds. Three programs exhibited over an 80% decrease in the number of restraints, two had over a 40% drop, one exhibited a 13% decrease, and one had a 6% drop. A subsequent 3-year study of child organizations using the Sanctuary Model showed an average of 52% reductions in physical restraints after the first year of implementation (Banks & Vargas, 2009c). Within the first six years of implementation in the Andrus Center residential program and school, there was a 90% decrease in critical incidents with a 54% increase in the average number of students served (Banks & Vargas, 2009a).

Working with schools is part of the Sanctuary Institute focus. In one school for emotionally disturbed children that has become certified in the Sanctuary Model, after 2 years of implementation, 64% of the students achieved realistic or ambitious rates of reading improvement. In addition, 99% of the children were promoted to the next grade. There was a 41% reduction in the number of children requiring inpatient psychiatric hospitalization and a 25% reduction in days children spent in inpatient hospitalization. The same school enjoyed a 56% placement rate in public and private school programs once the students graduated (Banks & Vargas, 2009b).

As part of the Pennsylvania Department of Public Welfare's (DPW) efforts to reduce and eliminate restraints in children's treatment settings, DPW entered into a partnership with the Sanctuary Institute to bring the Sanctuary Model to Pennsylvania in 2007. The University of Pittsburgh worked with Pennsylvania's DPW, the Sanctuary Institute, and 30 participating provider residential sites to conduct an open evaluation of the implementation of the model. Annual surveys were conducted from 2008 to 2010. The evaluation of the implementation of the Sanctuary Model in residential facilities found that greater implementation was associated with a number of positive outcomes: lower staff stress and higher staff morale, increased feelings of job competence and proficiency, and a greater investment in the individuals served. The implementation of the Sanctuary Model was also significantly associated with improved organizational culture and climate and a substantial decrease in the reported use of restraints by many sites (Stein, Kogan, Magee, & Hindes, 2011).

Additionally, an analysis of service utilization in the DPW project from 2007 to 2009 of children discharged from Sanctuary Model residential treatment facilities (RTFs), versus other RTFs, was conducted by Community Care Behavioral Health. It demonstrated that although both groups had a similar average (mean) length of stay in 2007, by 2009 Sanctuary Model RTF providers had (1) a substantially shorter length of stay and a somewhat greater decrease in median length of stay; (2) a substantial increase in the percentage of discharged youth who received outpatient services in the 3 months following discharge; and (3) a lower increase in the percentage of children readmitted to RTFs in the 90 days following discharge (Community Care Behavioral Health, 2011). As the authors of the report wrote,

> The implementation of the Sanctuary Model in residential facilities in Pennsylvania appears to have had a positive impact, with the greatest benefits being seen by residents and staff of those sites who were most successful in implementing the full Sanctuary Model. The positive outcomes associated with implementing the Sanctuary Model have occurred at a time of uncertainty and programmatic and staffing change in many facilities, which speaks to the dedication of all involved in the implementation of Sanctuary. At the same time, the variation observed in implementation does

suggest an opportunity to consider strategies to support future implementation efforts, as well as the need for providing continued support to sites that have implemented Sanctuary to ensure sustained positive outcomes. (Stein et al., 2011, p. 7).

Conclusion

The Sanctuary Model is a blueprint for clinical and organizational change, which at its core promotes safety and recovery from adversity through the active creation of a trauma-informed community. A recognition that trauma is pervasive in the experience of human beings forms the basis for the Sanctuary Model's focus not only on the people who seek treatment but equally on the people and systems who provide that treatment. This chapter has provided a description of the Sanctuary Model, an evidence-supported, developmentally grounded, trauma-informed intervention for an entire organization.

References

Alderfer, C. P., & Smith, K. K. (1982). Studying intergroup relations embedded in organizations. *Administrative Science Quarterly, 27*(1), 35.

Banks, J. A., & Vargas, L. A. (2009a). *Sanctuary at Andrus Children's Center.* Yonkers, NY: Andrus Center for Learning and Innovation. Available at *www.sanctuaryweb.com/PDFs_new/Banks%20and%20Vargas%20Sanctuary%20at%20 Andrus.pdf.*

Banks, J. A., & Vargas, L. A. (2009b). Sanctuary in schools: Preliminary child and organizational outcomes. *Available at www.sanctuaryweb.com/PDFs_new/ Banks%20and%20Vargas%20Sanctuary%20in%20Schools.pdf.*

Banks, J. A., & Vargas, L. A. (2009c). *Contributors to restraints and holds in organizations using the Sanctuary Model.* Yonkers, NY: Andrus Center for Learning and Innovation. Available at *www.sanctuaryweb.com/PDFs_new/Banks%20 and%20Vargas%20Contributors%20to%20Restraints%20and%20Holds.pdf.*

Bloom, S. L. (1997). *Creating sanctuary: Toward the evolution of sane societies.* New York: Routledge.

Bloom, S. L. (2000). Our hearts and our hopes are turned to peace: Origins of the ISTSS. In A. Shalev, R. Yehuda, & A. S. McFarlane (Eds.), *International handbook of human response trauma* (pp. 27–50). New York: Plenum Press.

Bloom, S. L. (2013). *Creating Sanctuary: Toward the evolution of sane societies* (2nd ed.). New York: Routledge.

Bloom, S. L., & Farragher, B. (2010). *Destroying sanctuary: The crisis in human service delivery systems.* New York: Oxford University Press.

Bloom, S. L., & Farragher, B. (2013). *Restoring sanctuary: Transform your organization and change the world.* New York: Oxford University Press.

Bureau of Justice Statistics. (2001). Violence in the workplace, 1993–99: Bureau of Justice Statistics Special Report. Washington, DC: Bureau of Statistics, U.S. Department of Justice. Available at *http://bjs.ojp.usdoj.gov/content/pub/pdf/vw99.pdf.*

Community Care Behavioral Health. (2011). Assessing the implementation of a residential facility organizational change model: Pennsylvania's implementation of the Sanctuary Model. Available at *www.ccbh.com/pdfs/articles/Sanctuary_Model_3Pager_20110715.pdf.*

Duhigg, C. (2012). *The power of habit: Why we do what we do in life and business.* New York: Random House.

Eisenberg, L. (1986). Mindlessness and brainlessness in psychiatry. *British Journal of Psychiatry, 148,* 497–508.

Esaki, N., & Larkin, H. (2011). *Prevalence of adverse childhood experiences (ACEs) among child service providers.* Unpublished data available through *nesaki@jdam. org.*

Fang, X., Brown, D. S., Florence, C. S., & Mercy, J. A. (2012). The economic burden of child maltreatment in the United States and implications for prevention. *Child Abuse and Neglect, 36*(2), 156–165.

Felitti, V. J., & Anda, R. F. (2010). The relationship of adverse childhood experiences to adult medical disease, psychiatric disorders, and sexual behavior: Implications for healthcare. In R. Lanius & E. Vermetten (Eds.), *The hidden epidemic: The impact of early life trauma on health and disease* (pp. 77–87). New York: Cambridge University Press.

Gazzaniga, M. (2011). *Who's in charge?: Free will and the science of the brain.* New York: HarperCollins.

Knudsen, E. I., Heckman, J. J., Cameron, J. L., & Shonkoff, J. P. (2006). Economic, neurobiological, and behavioral perspectives on building America's future workforce. *Proceedings of the National Academy of Science, 103*(27), 10155–10162.

McSparren, W., & Motley, D. (2010). How to improve the process of change. *Nonprofit World, 28*(6), 14–15.

Occupational Safety and Health Administration. (2004). *Guidelines for Preventing Workplace Violence for Health Care & Social Service Workers.* Washington, DC: U.S. Department of Labor.

Rivard, J. C., McCorkle, D., Duncan, M. E., Pasquale, L. E., Bloom, S. L., & Abramovitz, R. (2004). Implementing a trauma recovery framework for youths in residential treatment. *Child and Adolescent Social Work Journal, 21*(5), 529–550.

Schein, E. H. (1999). *The corporate culture: A survival guide—sense and nonsense about culture change.* San Francisco: Jossey Bass.

Senge, P., Cambron-McCabe, N., Lucas, T., Smith, B., Dutton, J., & Kleiner, A. (2000). *Schools that learn: A fifth discipline fieldbook for educators, parents, and everyone who cares about education.* New York: Doubleday.

Stein, B. D., Kogan, J. N., Magee, E., & Hindes, K. (2011, September 29). *Sanctuary Survey Final State Report* (unpublished data).

Whiteley, S. (2004). The evolution of the therapeutic community. *Psychiatric Quarterly, 75*(3), 233–248.

CHAPTER 16

Child–Parent Psychotherapy and Historical Trauma

Amy Klatzkin
Alicia F. Lieberman
Patricia Van Horn

> The past is never dead. It's not even past.
> —WILLIAM FAULKNER

Historical trauma has a profound impact on the psychological functioning of individuals and, like interpersonal trauma, gets transmitted from generation to generation. Maria Yellow Horse Brave Heart (2010) defines historical trauma as "cumulative emotional and psychological wounding over the lifespan and across generations, emanating from massive group trauma" (p. 2). Traumatic historical events with long-term psychological consequences include collective catastrophes such as war, famine, and forced colonization as well as intracountry genocide in the absence of war (e.g., Cambodia in the 1970s, Rwanda in the 1990s). Racial, gender, and religious oppression may also lead to historical trauma, as evidenced, for example, by the legacies of slavery, the Holocaust, massacres of Native Americans, the removal of Native American children from their families and communities for placement in boarding schools, and culturally or politically sanctioned discriminatory practices such as female infant abandonment (Brave Heart, 1999, 2010; Johnson, 1996). Tracing current individual and interpersonal conflicts to their possible roots in historical trauma can have significant beneficial effects, creating understanding and compassion in the parent generation for the grandparent generation and freeing the parent generation from the mindless repetition of the past in the present with the child.

The impact of historical trauma across generations is particularly relevant when its effects filter down from the broader social–cultural–political arena into the lives of young children and their parents. In early childhood, a traumatic stressor can be defined as an unpredictable, uncontrollable external event that threatens the physical or psychological integrity of the child and induces overwhelming fear, horror, or helplessness (Zero to Three, 2005). Exposure to a traumatic event, whether direct (as in physical or sexual abuse) or indirect (as a witness to violence, war, or natural disaster), puts a young child at risk of serious mental health problems, such as posttraumatic stress disorder (PTSD), conduct disorder, anxiety, and depression, and may disrupt not only the child's developmental momentum but also the safety and security of the child–parent relationship (Lieberman & Van Horn, 2005). In the moment of trauma, children are flooded with negative affect so intense that it often exceeds their developmental capacity to self-regulate (see Schore, Chapter 1, this volume). If the parent is unable to protect the child from this overwhelming distress, the traumatic event shatters the child's internal working model of the parent as a secure base and protective shield (Bowlby, 1969/1982; Freud, 1920/1959). It also changes the child's worldview. Before the trauma, the child may view the world as a sufficiently predictable, sufficiently benevolent place and people as generally trustworthy. Afterward, negative attributions and mental representations may consistently displace the child's previous expectations of care and safety (Janoff-Bulmann, 1992).

Although any trauma in early childhood may interfere with normal biopsychosocial development, complex forms such as historical trauma and other chronic types of victimization disrupt development more than an isolated traumatic event (Lieberman, Chu, Van Horn, & Harris, 2011). The child's functioning may be impaired across multiple domains, affecting attachment, self-concept, cognition, and regulation of affect and behavior (Cook et al., 2005). Because infants and young children depend on their primary caregivers for safety and co-regulation of physical and emotional states, the risk of developmental disturbances increases when a caregiver is also the source of danger (Freud, 1926/1959; Main & Hesse, 1990).

Trauma in early childhood not only may alter the child's general beliefs about self and the world, but more specifically may damage the relationship between a securely attached child and an attuned parent. The parent may form distorted negative attributions of the child, and the child and parent may develop mutual adverse expectations of each other (Pynoos, 1997). If, before the trauma, the quality of attachment was insecure and parental attunement intermittent, the relationship may deteriorate further under the stress of the traumatic event, leading to internalizing problems such as anxiety, depression, avoidance, somatization, and emotional withdrawal and/

or to externalizing problems in the form of aggressive or self-endangering behaviors. The child may also lose trust in bodily sensations, leading to increased arousal in the form of sleep problems, nightmares, hypervigilance, and distractibility. He or she may regress to an earlier stage of development, losing skills that had been mastered. When the parent has also experienced trauma—as is often the case with historical trauma, which affects entire communities and societies—the child's problems are compounded by the parent's impaired affect regulation, negative attributions, and confusion about what is safe and what is dangerous. These effects may persist long after the traumatic event ends, particularly when either member of the dyad is triggered by a traumatic reminder or secondary adversity. Often parent and child become traumatic reminders for each other (Pynoos, 1997). Therefore, in addition to broad-based interventions designed to help entire societies recover from traumatic historical events, it is crucial to provide therapeutic assistance to the individual children and families whose most basic relationships (e.g., the parent–child dyad) have been altered by historical trauma.

Child–Parent Psychotherapy for Traumatized Children

This chapter describes child–parent psychotherapy (CPP) as a treatment model for traumatized children and presents a case in which the exploration of interpersonal trauma opened the door to understanding the impact of historical trauma on four generations of an immigrant family. CPP is an evidence-based, manualized dyadic treatment model for children in the first 6 years of life who have experienced, or are at risk of, mental health problems because of adverse life circumstances or traumatic events (Lieberman & Van Horn, 2009). With its foundations in psychoanalysis and attachment theory (Fraiberg, Adelson, & Shapiro, 1975; Bowlby, 1969/1982), CPP uses a multitheoretical approach—developmentally informed, culturally attuned, and trauma focused—to change maladaptive interactions and distorted perceptions with the goal of promoting safety and trust in the child–parent relationship. CPP provides a clinical model for treating trauma-related disturbances in the child's developmental course and mental health and in the quality of the parent–child relationship (Lieberman & Van Horn, 2008).

The process of CPP involves helping the parent and child learn to play together and supporting the parent in witnessing the child's play, particularly when the child reenacts violent events or engages in disturbing, repetitive symbolic play. At times the therapist takes the stance of an observer to "watch, wait, and wonder" with the parent about the child's play (Johnson, Dowling, & Wesner, 1980; Wesner, Johnson, & Dowling, 1962). At other times the therapist becomes the translator of experience and feelings or thinks together with the parent about the meaning of the child's behavior. If deemed appropriate, the therapist may suggest cognitive-behavioral strategies, mindfulness practices, or other interventions to help the dyad regulate affect and behavior while continuing to explore the subjective meaning for the child and the parent of thoughts, feelings, and maladaptive responses associated with the trauma. Knowing that parent and child may experience the same event differently and have different emotional responses, the child–parent psychotherapist endeavors to hold the perspectives of both members of the dyad, helping the parent understand the child's internal world and helping both child and parent understand each other's perspectives, motivations, behaviors, and emotional states.

Restoring safety in the environment and in the parent–child relationship is the first goal of treatment and the cornerstone of all other therapeutic goals. If necessary, the child–parent psychotherapist assists the parent in securing basic needs, such as safe living conditions and adequate clothing, household supplies, and nourishment. Within the framework of increased environmental safety, the clinician then works with the dyad to promote affect regulation, restore trust in bodily sensations, and foster reciprocity in the parent–child relationship. By providing developmental guidance to explain and normalize the traumatic response, the therapist helps the parent understand the child's behavior as an effort to self-protect and works with the parent to promote more accurate reality testing and more realistic responses to threat. These skills in turn increase the parent's capacity to provide a secure base and reengage the child in learning in order to restore developmental progress. Ultimately the therapist and parent co-create a narrative with the child that places the traumatic event firmly in the past so that parent and child can dependably distinguish between remembering the trauma and reliving it (Lieberman & Van Horn, 2005).

Because the locus of healing in CPP is the child–parent relationship, whatever the therapist can do to support the parent is intended as a means to support the child as well. If the situation warrants, the child–parent psychotherapist provides crisis intervention and concrete assistance with problems of daily living. Often the most pressing need at the outset of treatment is to establish physical safety by helping the parent create a safety plan and by promoting the parent's ability to act as a protective shield (Lieberman & Van Horn, 2005, 2008).

Key forces that shape the parent's perspective include cultural background, attachment status, and trauma history (Ghosh Ippen, 2009). For this reason CPP assesses the parent's as well as the child's history and current functioning. The child–parent psychotherapist needs to understand the complexity of the traumatic experience for child and parent (single or recurrent events, range of events), its context (familial, societal, historical, and cultural), and its repercussions in the present and in the past. The initial assessment aims to identify traumatic reminders and secondary adversities, such as increased susceptibility to dysregulation of thoughts, feelings, or behavior and decreased capacity to cope and problem solve. The comprehensive assessment of the parent's trauma history enables the therapist to help the parent anticipate and cope with traumatic reminders that may arise from the child's play—reminders that may trigger the parent's response to traumas experienced in his or her childhood as well as in adulthood and that may then be projected onto, and enacted with, the child.

Drawing on its foundation in infant–parent psychotherapy, CPP looks for "ghosts in the nursery" to understand how the past influences the present (Fraiberg et al., 1975). Ghosts are said to arise when parents unconsciously reenact the maladaptive parenting behaviors they experienced as children. Unresolved conflicts, losses, trauma, and negative parenting styles can be transmitted from generation to generation, as when an abused child becomes an abusive parent, the child of an alcoholic becomes or marries an alcoholic, or the daughter of a violent father marries a violent man. Yet ghosts do not always commandeer the infant–parent relationship. They may be transient, arising only under certain stressful circumstances, or banished altogether when the compelling reality of the baby makes an emotional claim on the mother that helps her keep unresolved early conflicts from contaminating their relationship (Fraiberg, 1980). A history of abuse in the parents' past does not doom them to repeat it. For some parents, the memory of childhood fear and pain allows them to see their own child as a new beginning, a chance to set things right. For others, helping them remember how it felt to be the helpless and terrified child—in other words, reconnecting narrative memory to affect—may empower them to parent their own children differently.

In a parallel exploration of protective factors, strengths, and wellness, CPP also looks for "angels in the nursery" by facilitating the retrieval of loving and supportive memories, recognizing the positive influences of benevolent relationships, and promoting identification with the protector (Lieberman, Padrón, Van Horn, & Harris, 2005, p. 507). Just as ghosts can hide from conscious awareness, so too can angels. A skilled therapist can support parents as they search for angels even in dark places. For example, a parent who did not experience her own mother as protective may come to understand her mother's behavior as an *attempt* to protect her and benefit in the present from recognizing that previously misunderstood intent. When a parent cannot retrieve any benevolent memories, therapy can provide a corrective experience that serves to create new experiences of safety, love, and support in both the parent–child relationship and the therapeutic relationship.

Drawing on the Clients' Sociocultural and Historical Context in CPP

Although trauma affects people of all races, ethnicities, and cultures, of all sexual orientations, and at all socioeconomic levels, the way people typically respond to and understand traumatic experiences may vary widely among different groups and subgroups. Cultural competency and "contextually congruent interventions" are therefore critical to working with diverse populations (Brown, 2008; Ghosh Ippen, 2009). Yet therapists cannot be competent in all the cultures their clients represent or accurately predict a particular family's variations from cultural norms. While it is the therapist's responsibility to develop cross-cultural competence and seek consultation as needed, the parent may be the best guide to how the family actually lives the culture.

Using CPP as a conceptual clinical framework, Ghosh Ippen (2009) encourages clinicians to "focus not only on culture but also on the family's history, current situation, and future goals" (p. 107). With immigrant parents, clinicians tend to look at the family's history of immigration and adaptation to the new country and at the events in the country of origin that led directly to the decision to emigrate. It is possible, however, to gain greater insight by widening the focus beyond the family to include external historical events and indirect experiences that act as traumatic stressors on individuals. In addition, extending the time line back several generations before immigration may reveal cumulative communal trauma—such as a history of gender, racial, religious, or political oppression in the family's country of origin—that continues to affect family members in the present. The following case study shows how opening a dialogue about historical trauma can lead to contextually congruent interventions and the co-creation of a multigenerational trauma narrative that assists the healing process.

A CPP Case Involving the Intergenerational Transmission of Traumatic Stress

A Mother and Daughter Begin Therapy

When Rose Liu and her 4-year-old daughter, Sophia Zhang, were referred to a clinic for CPP, Sophia's symptoms were typical for a young child who had witnessed domestic violence: separation anxiety, explosive anger, aggression, oppositional behavior, withdrawal, sleep problems, and somatic complaints. Sophia's externalizing behaviors clashed with the cultural expectations of her immigrant Chinese parents and grandparents, increasing intrafamilial conflict. The therapist assigned to the case, a European American woman about 10 years younger than Rose, knew she would need to understand the family's response to Sophia's behavior in order to identify culturally competent interventions.

In the intake assessment, Rose told the therapist that she was having a hard time coping with Sophia's outbursts. "We used to be so close," Rose said, "but now she's always angry, and she even hits me. Chinese children do not hit their parents. My parents criticize me for her behavior, but I don't know how to stop it." The therapist empathized with Rose's pain and frustration and reassured her that CPP focuses on healing the parent—child relationship as well as improving behavior. Restoring safety and security in the relationship would be the first goal of treatment.

In addition to exploring Rose's concerns about her daughter, the therapist assessed for trauma in the recent and more distant past. Rose disclosed a history of domestic violence that began when Sophia was about 2 years old. On multiple occasions Sophia's father, Ming Zhang, had abused Rose emotionally and physically (choking, pushing, slapping, hitting) in front of Sophia and her 7-year-old brother, Brandon. Eighteen months earlier Sophia and Brandon were in their father's car when the police pulled them over and arrested Ming for driving under the influence of alcohol and child endangerment. The children saw policemen handcuff their father and take him away in a police car. They were then driven in a separate patrol car to a police station, where Rose picked them up.

Although the parents had joint legal custody, Rose had had sole physical custody since Ming's arrest. Rose, who worked full time as a pharmacist, moved to a new apartment and filed for divorce. Ming spent 3 months in jail and lived in a residential treatment center after his release. Rose reported that he had lost his job with the U.S. Postal Service and was currently unemployed, depressed, and anxious. The paternal grandparents supervised the children's Sunday visits with their father. When interviewed about her own history, Rose reported that she too had witnessed domestic violence (DV) as a child, and her parents continued to have violent arguments. Rose believed that her grandparents on both sides also had a history of DV, and there was a family history of anxiety as well.

Both Rose and Ming were born in 1967 and grew up in Taiyuan, the capital of Shanxi province in northern China. They married in their hometown in 1991 and two years later emigrated to the United States, together with both sets of parents. Brandon and Sophia were born in the United States. Rose, Ming, and the children spoke Mandarin and English at home; the grandparents spoke only Mandarin. Despite frequent loud arguments among the adults, the extended family members remained close, lived in the same neighborhood, and often shared meals. Before the children started preschool, Rose's parents took care of them during the week, and they continued to provide child care as needed. Rose believed that the children had witnessed violent arguments between the maternal grandparents while in their care, though they did not speak about that.

After assessing for trauma, the therapist used a structured interview to discover "angels in the nursery" and other protective factors in Rose's past to reinforce their positive influence and provide a source of internalized support. Rose's most important angel was her maternal grandmother, with whom she lived for 3 years in the 1970s. Rose started university in her hometown in 1984 and developed a close relationship with one of her professors, who encouraged Rose's interest in biochemistry and became a lifelong mentor and friend. Although Rose's grandmother died before the family emigrated and her professor still lived in Taiyuan, Rose felt that both were still present in her life. She hoped she could raise her daughter to be kind, loving, and funny like her grandmother and as smart and academically successful as her professor.

Rose and Sophia attended 19 sessions of CPP over a period of 6 months, during which time many of Sophia's problematic behaviors subsided. She no longer behaved aggressively at home or at preschool. She developed an extensive emotional vocabulary and could usually use it to tell her mother how she was feeling before she became dysregulated. She daydreamed much less at school. At home she was generally compliant, and Rose felt that their close relationship had been restored. Although playing together had initially been difficult for this dyad, they now looked forward to playing with dolls, working on puzzles, and drawing together during sessions.

As they approached the end of their work together, Rose, Sophia, and the therapist co-created a narrative that recapitulated, acknowledged, and made sense of the frightening events she had witnessed, from her repeated exposure to DV to the terrifying day her father was arrested, her separation from him while he was in jail, and her continuing wish that her parents would get back together. Sophia could now express "two different feelings at the very same time," as one of her favorite books put it. She loved and missed her dad while also fearing that he might become violent again.

Sophia still sometimes had unexplained stomachaches, and once in a while she resisted going to preschool, saying that she'd rather stay home and play with Mama. Rose considered these to be small issues compared with the long list of behavioral symptoms with which they began. In a collateral session, Rose and the therapist agreed that it was time to begin termination. Posttreatment assessment measures, however, indicated that both Sophia and Rose still had high levels of anxiety consistent with PTSD. The therapist discussed the problem with her supervisor; both were surprised by the results. They agreed that the dyad would benefit from continuing treatment focused specifically on the anxiety. Rose concurred.

Treatment Resumes with a New Therapist

At this point the original therapist's internship came to an end, and the case was transferred to another clinician (AK), a European American woman about 10 years older than Rose. On meeting Rose and Sophia, the new therapist immediately noticed the anxious quality of their speech. Both spoke with rapid-fire intensity, and Sophia interspersed her words with frequent gasping breaths. If Rose's affect intensified, Sophia's would quickly match it. Mother and daughter were clearly attuned to each other, but that connection appeared to reinforce and amplify the dyad's anxiety. The new therapist hypothesized that lowering the mother's anxiety would also lower the daughter's.

Like many preschoolers, Sophia was afraid of monsters and of the dark, but she had other fears as well. For example, she was afraid of hotel rooms, especially in the mountains. "And the chair," Sophia said, "the chair that moves by itself! You have to get on and shut the door." Rose explained that she meant pulling down the bar on the ski lift. The therapist assured Sophia that lots of people are scared of those moving chairs. "She doesn't want to go anywhere," Rose said. "She's afraid of everywhere but home, and even at home she still sleeps with me and touches me all night. If I move away from her when I'm sleeping, she wakes up." The therapist said it sounded like Sophia's fears were getting in the way of enjoying life and trying new things, and they were also interfering with both Rose's and Sophia's well-being. Rose agreed.

In a collateral session, Rose confided that she herself had always been anxious, even as a child, and she worried that she had passed this trait along to her daughter. "My brother and my parents are even more anxious than I am," she reported. "It must be genetic. My brother has four dead-bolts on his front door and heavy curtains on the windows. He doesn't even live in a dangerous neighborhood." The therapist assured Rose that even if there was a genetic component to Sophia's anxiety, there was much they could do to reduce its impact on her life at home and at school. She described how Rose and Sophia mirrored each other's emotional states, so that when one began to worry, the other would quickly join in, setting off a negative feedback loop. If Rose got individual or group therapy for her anxiety, the therapist suggested, Sophia would likely benefit as well. Rose never rejected the suggestion outright, but she also didn't act on it, so the therapist revised her approach. Instead of targeting the mother's anxiety so the mother could lower the daughter's, the therapist could address the child's anxiety directly, and perhaps the mother would benefit too. It was worth a shot.

Learning to Slow Down and Breathe

At the next session, the therapist introduced a new game, the slow race, which they could play on their way to the toy cabinet. "You're really good at being fast," she told Sophia, "so we don't need to practice that. In the slow race the slowest person wins. Who can be slowest to walk around the carpet?" Sophia tried a few slow steps but couldn't tolerate it long and broke into a run. Rose stood up and said she wanted to do the slow race with Sophia. This time Sophia made it all the way around the carpet moving slowly. She then selected a puzzle from the toy cabinet and began talking about it in her breathless, pressured way. The therapist brought Sophia's attention to the gasping breathing and said gently, "You have time to say what you want and *then* breathe." Sophia thought for a moment and then replied, "I feel like I *can't* breathe." "Is that why you stop in the middle of what you're saying, to take another breath?" the therapist asked. Sophia nodded. The therapist said, "I'm guessing that if you slow down, your breath will last longer. You're very good at breathing. You can trust your breath." Sophia tried speaking a little more slowly and said a whole sentence without gasping. Then she invited her mother to join her on the floor with the puzzle.

From this point on, the therapist began incorporating simple body awareness and mindfulness exercises from *The Mindful Child* (Greenland, 2010) as well as suggestions from participants in Susan Kaiser Greenland's online community, Mindfulness Together *(http://innerkids.ning.com)*. At the beginning of each child–parent therapy session they would all do a starfish stretch (Greenland, 2010), 10 jumping jacks moving and breathing in sync, pinwheel breathing, or the slow race. The therapist used a glitter ball as a metaphor for a mind swirling with worries compared with a quiet mind (with the glitter settled on the bottom). She introduced the idea that people are much more than their thoughts and that they can learn to observe their thoughts without necessarily reacting to them or acting on them. She also explained to Sophia that minds and bodies are linked: "If your breathing is anxious, it can make you feel anxious, and if you feel anxious, you start breathing that way."

After practicing the mindfulness activities for about a month, Rose observed that Sophia was moving more calmly and speaking more fluidly at home as well as in sessions. Her comment opened a port of entry to talk about what the therapist was seeing in Rose—how much calmer she seemed, how her shoulders were relaxed, her speech was slower, and her affect less intense. "I'm learning," she said. "The exercises have been good for me. I can see that when I'm calm, it's easier for Sophia to be calm. It's really working."

A Port of Entry to the Past

Like many Chinese American children, Sophia attended Chinese School in the afternoons. Lunar New Year was fast approaching, and Sophia's class was going to sing and dance at the school's celebration. After performing one of the songs in session, Sophia asked the therapist, "Have you ever been to China?" As it happened, the therapist had taught at a university in north China for two years during the 1980s, but she had not disclosed that. Out of respect for the child, however, she answered the question honestly. Rose and Sophia asked many questions, and when the therapist told them where she had lived and when, Rose exclaimed, "I started university in Taiyuan in 1984!" The therapist had lived in the capital city of a neighboring province and had taught students the same age as Rose.

The therapist's disclosure of her experience in China opened the first historical port of entry, as Rose described her life during the months leading up to her college graduation in 1989. On the national stage that spring, student activists across China launched a pro-democracy movement that ultimately attracted more than a million protesters from all walks of life, triggering a power struggle in the Communist Party leadership at the highest levels (Richelson & Evans, 1999). The largest demonstrations took place in the heart of the nation's capital, Tiananmen Square in Beijing, the site of a brutal crackdown on June 4, 1989, when the army entered the city and attacked protesters (Richelson & Evans, 1999).

In the provincial capital of Taiyuan, Rose knew little about the democracy movement. Her parents made sure of that. During the spring of 1989 they repeatedly took her to the hospital. Rose couldn't figure out why her parents thought she was sick; she began to wonder if there wasn't something terribly wrong with her—so terrible that no one would name it. Suddenly in the middle of June the trips to the hospital ceased. No one told her why, and she did not ask. No one ever mentioned her "illness" again. Rose was hugely disappointed when college graduation ceremonies were canceled—in fact, all large public gatherings were forbidden at that time—and baffled when she heard that graduating seniors would have to sign a statement attesting that they had not participated in demonstrations.

Looking back, Rose now realized how worried her parents must have been. They had lived through the Cultural Revolution (1966–1976)—a decade of chaos, repression, and violence (Lü, 1994–1995)—and were terrified of getting in trouble. During the Cultural Revolution children were encouraged to listen in on their parents' conversations and report any "counterrevolutionary" content. Such reports, even from a young child, could lead to public "struggle sessions," brutal punishments, and even expulsion to reform-through-labor camps (Kleinman & Kleinman, 1994). Rose's parents learned to keep silent about anything even remotely related to politics. When they heard about the demonstrations in 1989, they decided it would be safer for Rose to be in the hospital with an imaginary ailment than to risk her involvement in the democracy movement. They never explained what they were doing, and Rose didn't ask. "I was just a little girl during the Cultural Revolution," Rose explained. "I don't remember much about it except that everyone was anxious and scared all the time—for years! But no one ever explained what they were scared of."

"When you think about the Cultural Revolution and 1989," the therapist said, "both were traumatic events on many levels, from the personal to the political." Rose agreed that during the Cultural Revolution the whole country was traumatized for a decade. They talked about the intergenerational transmission of trauma, how traumatized parents implant their own emotional responses and any resultant instability in their children, and how children internalize the parents' stress and social mistrust. "Yes!" Rose said excitedly. "My brother won't open his curtains. He never wants anyone to see inside. During the Cultural Revolution, it was dangerous. But he was just a kid then too. He must have gotten that fear from my parents." "Grandma told us not to open the curtains this morning," Sophia added. Rose replied, "They're still scared, Sophia, even though the things that made them afraid happened a long time ago back in China." Rose said she remembered after June 4, 1989, seeing people who had been arrested for participating in the demonstrations paraded through town on open-backed trucks, crackling loudspeakers broadcasting their crimes. "Half of everyone's head was shaved," she said, "and they had big signs around their necks. They looked so scared."

"You can see how your brother inherited your parents' trauma," said the therapist, "and you've experienced your own too—the aftermath of 1989, the domestic violence between your parents and with your husband. I think in coming here you are trying to prevent the transmission of your and your parents' trauma to Sophia. And it's working. As you lower your anxiety, hers lowers too." The therapist recounted ways in which Rose was selecting what of her history and culture she wanted to pass on to Sophia and what she wanted to change for her—how she was taking steps to ensure that her daughter inherited the best of both cultures and to give her daughter the secure and carefree childhood she wished she had had.

Sophia had always enjoyed her mother's stories of her childhood in China, although she had never heard stories like these. Periodically the therapist would rephrase Rose's comments for Sophia—for example, "Mama is telling me that things were very scary in China when she was a little girl." Because the therapist was familiar with modern Chinese history, Rose did not need to explain the Cultural Revolution or the pro-democracy movement of 1989; she talked only about her personal experiences during those times, and she did so with remarkable equilibrium. In fact, she modeled what Siegel (2007) calls a FACES state: "flexible, adaptive, coherent, energized, and stable" (p. 78). Sophia, who worked on art projects during those sessions, mirrored her mother's affect. The therapist felt optimistic about this dyad's ability to reduce their anxiety to within the normal range.

One Port of Entry Opens Another: Tracking Trauma through Four Generations

In a collateral meeting with Rose a week before Sophia's fifth birthday, the therapist explored the impact of historical trauma on Rose's family as a way to understand and normalize the high level of anxiety afflicting generation after generation. Twentieth-century Chinese history comprised decades of traumatic political events that could easily have exacerbated a genetic predisposition to anxiety disorders. The therapist began by drawing out more of Rose's memories of early childhood. Born in December 1967, she was nearly 9 by the time the Cultural Revolution finally ended. In an article titled "How Bodies Remember," Arthur Kleinman and Joan Kleinman (1994) describe the traumatic social upheaval of that period:

> Between 1966 and 1976 China experienced a decade of brutal political turmoil. . . . Tens of millions of people were affected by criticism, physical assault, suicide, and murder. . . . Literally hundreds of millions were caught up in the whirlwind of accusation, counteraccusation, self-criticism, and criticism of others. The ancient spine of Chinese society, the bureaucratic order,

dislocated; factions fought each other . . . ; families were broken; systems of communication, transportation, justice, public safety, health, and welfare fragmented. Parents were attacked by children; teachers were assaulted by students; Red Guards—adolescent and young adult revolutionaries—broke into homes, looted their contents, beat their occupants, and destroyed precious objects such as ancestral tablets, heirlooms, and books. (p. 713)

Rose's mother was pregnant with Rose for most of 1967 (see Figure 16.1), one of the most violent and chaotic years of the Cultural Revolution (MacFarquhar & Schoenhals, 2006). Rose and the therapist discussed the events of that year and thought together about the potential impact of the sociopolitical environment of fear and violence on her mother and the developing fetus. The therapist guessed that Rose had been "bathed in cortisol" *in utero*. Rose stated that her brother, who was 5 when Rose was born, had terrifying memories from that time. The family lived in a work unit between two munitions factories allied with different factions of Red Guards that fought pitched battles in the street. He remembers the family escaping in the back of a truck as bullets flew around them.

When Rose was 5 all the schools near her home were still closed, so her mother enrolled her in a school in the rural village where her maternal grandmother lived. Although life in the impoverished Shanxi countryside was harsh, under her grandmother's roof Rose felt especially loved, understood, and safe. Walking through the fields from her grandmother's house to the school felt almost magical, especially in the springtime when the fruit trees blossomed. Rose lived with her grandmother for 3 years and to this day can recall in vivid detail the sights, sounds, and smells of village life. Her grandmother was her "angel in the nursery," and the 3 years she lived with her in the midst of the Cultural Revolution were Rose's angel years.

Winding back the clock another generation, Rose and the therapist created a time line of historical events experienced by four generations of her family over 100 years, showing a clear positive trend toward less trauma, despite the DV in Rose's marriage (see Figure 16.2). In creating this visual presentation of traumatic historical events, the therapist intended to instill hope that the family history of high anxiety was not just a genetic predisposition about which they could do nothing. Given decade upon decade of historical trauma, it made sense that any family propensity toward anxiety might be exacerbated by external events such as those noted in Figure 16.2. Seeing that Sophia had not experienced any political or social trauma, Rose began to feel hopeful that she could change the family pattern. Hope reduced Rose's anxiety—and in turn, Sophia's as well.

Connecting Past and Present: Co-Constructing an Intergenerational Trauma Narrative with a 5-Year-Old

It was now time to revise and expand the trauma narrative that Rose and the first CPP therapist had co-created with Sophia to make sense of the

1966	*From 1966 to 1969 tens of millions of Chinese suffer violent persecution; more than half a million die.*
May–August	In a bid to regain control of the Communist Party, Mao Zedong launches the Great Proletarian Cultural Revolution.
	Student insurrection begins at Beijing University and quickly spreads across the country.
August–November	With Mao's approval, radical students become Red Guards, the new vanguard of the revolution. They quickly gain power and split into factions, terrorizing ordinary citizens. For 2 years they rampage out of control.
	Mao closes universities and schools and condemns all forms of religion.
1967	
January	Red Guards overthrow provincial leaders.
March	*Rose's mother becomes pregnant.*
July–August	Insurrections erupt across the country. Red Guards rule through violence, intimidation, and chaos. Millions of innocent people are "struggled against" because of their class background, publicly humiliated in mass rallies, and shipped off to remote work camps for "reeducation." Executions and suicides abound. Mass purges continue for years.
	Rival factions of Red Guards fight each other. Tens of thousands of people take part in pitched battles in the streets.
	Mao enlists the People's Liberation Army (PLA) to bring order. There are numerous bloody clashes between the PLA and Red Guard factions.
December	*Rose is born. Her parents give her a revolutionary name, Hong (Red).*
1968	
July	The PLA takes control of government offices, schools, and factories, breaking the power of the Red Guards.
December	Mao dismantles the Red Guards by sending millions of young people to the countryside "to learn from the peasants."
	Urban youth continue to be sent off to the countryside for a decade, finally being permitted to return to the cities in the late 1970s.
1969–1975	Although the Cultural Revolution continues under Mao's leadership, political stability is gradually restored.
	Universities begin to reopen (1970–1974).
1976	
July	A 7.8 earthquake devastates North China, killing a quarter of a million people. The epicenter is in the province directly east of Rose's. Millions sleep outside for months in fear of aftershocks and collapsing buildings.
September	Mao Zedong dies.

FIGURE 16.1. The sociopolitical context of Rose's life in China: From Cultural Revolution to emigration. Sources of data: FitzGerald (1968); Gold (1984); Kleinman and Kleinman (1994); Lü (1994–1995); MacFarquhar (n.d.); MacFarquhar and Schoenhals (2006); Nathan (1989); and Richelson and Evans (1999).

October	Armed forces arrest Mao's wife and her radical associates. The Cultural Revolution finally ends, but in interior provinces such as Rose's, the aftermath of fear and political uncertainty lasts well into the 1980s.
. . .	
1980–1981	China begins "opening to the outside world."
1983	Anti-Spiritual Pollution Campaign: Many fear that the Cultural Revolution might return, but the campaign fizzles out, economic liberalization picks up, and opening accelerates.
1984	*Rose begins university.*
1987	Anti-Bourgeois Liberalization Campaign: Despite some purges, the campaign is widely disregarded, prompting the "bourgeois liberal" astrophysicist Fang Lizhi to state, "No one is afraid of anyone anymore."
1989	Democracy Movement begins at Beijing University and quickly spreads. By late spring mass demonstrations take place all over the country.
April–May	Students take over Tiananmen Square in Beijing, call for a general strike, demand democratic reform. More than 1,000 students begin a hunger strike in Tiananmen Square. Protests are televised nationwide.
	The PLA enters Beijing and then withdraws.
June 4–5	Troops approach Tiananmen Square in tanks and open fire. Estimates of deaths range from the official 241 to 1,000 or more.
July	*Rose graduates university.*
	University graduation ceremonies canceled nationwide to prevent large gatherings of students.
1991	*Rose Liu marries Ming Zhang.*
1993	*Rose and family emigrate to the United States.*

FIGURE 16.1. (*continued*)

frightening and confusing experiences she had endured, from the DV to her father's arrest and imprisonment to her unrealizable dream that the family would all live together again. The new narrative mentioned that terrible things had happened to the family in China long before Sophia was born and also addressed the family history of domestic violence not only between Sophia's parents, but also between her maternal grandparents and great-grandparents. As a metaphor for the intergenerational transmission of trauma, they talked about the "box of terrible things" that is passed from parent to child, child to grandchild, and gets bigger and heavier if you don't open it up and talk about what's inside. Because Rose and Sophia could talk about their extended family's box of terrible things without getting triggered, they were now able to remember bad experiences from the past without feeling as if they were reliving them. In addition, they could identify good things—the "angels in the nursery"—that had helped each generation survive even in extreme adversity.

Historical events		Rose's grandparents	Rose's parents	Rose	Sophia
1900s	Qing dynasty on its knees, dominated and humiliated by Western powers; Boxer Rebellion leads to armed conflict between rebels and Western forces				
1910s	Collapse of Qing dynasty, Republican Revolution, warlord era begins, World War I, May 4th Movement				
1920s	Warlord era, 1925–1927 Revolution, Civil War				
1930s	Civil War, depression, Japanese invasion (20 million Chinese die)				
1937–1945	Japanese occupation, Anti-Japanese War/World War II, Civil War				
1945–1949	Civil War				
1949	Communist triumph (positive or negative depending on family's class status)				
1958–1961	Great Leap Forward: massive famine, 30 million die				
1966–1976	Cultural Revolution: more than half a million die, millions more forcibly displaced				
1976	Tangshan earthquake (7.8): a quarter of a million die				
1989	Students launch Democracy Movement, leading to nationwide mass demonstrations; Beijing massacre of June 4: hundreds, possibly thousands, die				
Intrafamilial stressors					
1993	Emigration to the United States				
	Domestic violence				

FIGURE 16.2. Four generations of historical trauma and domestic violence. Sources of data: Bowblis (2000); MacFarquhar (n.d.); MacFarquhar and Schoenhals (2006); and Spence and Chin (1996).

The summer before Sophia started kindergarten, Rose and the therapist agreed on a schedule for termination and began to do posttreatment assessment measures. Although the Child Behavior Checklist (CBCL) still indicated elevated anxiety, the levels were significantly lower than in the original assessment, and the Trauma Symptom Checklist for Young Children (TSCYC)—designed specifically to assess trauma-related symptoms in children ages 3–12—showed no elevations at all. In other words, Sophia's PTSD was itself a thing of the past. Most strikingly, her scores on the Wechsler Preschool and Primary Scale of Intelligence (WPPSI II) showed remarkable improvements—verbal and global language scores increased from average to high-average, full scale from average to superior, and performance from average to very superior—suggesting that trauma symptoms had interfered with cognitive functioning at intake (Gil, Calev, Greenberg, Kugelmass, & Lerer, 1990; Samuelson & Cashman, 2009; Mueller-Pfeiffer et al., 2010).

Conclusion

To support families struggling with the intergenerational transmission of historical trauma, the clinician needs both to assess for it and to address it in treatment planning. Although the therapists treating Rose and Sophia followed an extensive assessment protocol at intake that inquired about parents' life stressors, including exposure to war and terrorism, there was no systematic assessment for other types of cumulative historical trauma. Political trauma such as the decade-long Cultural Revolution would have gone unmentioned had the second therapist not been familiar with 20th-century Chinese history and explored with Rose how those events had affected her and her family. Cultural competence alone does not open that dialogue.

A clinician can become sufficiently conversant with historical trauma that may have affected a client or his or her family in past generations if the clinical history taking includes a careful review of the sociopolitical as well as cultural history of the client's family in past generations, along with more traditional assessment foci such as the family's history of medical and mental health problems. Often a simple Internet search can locate a summary of major historical events anywhere in the world. If a client's family emigrated from Iran, for example, the therapist could find a link to the BBC's "chronology of key events" in Iranian history from C.E. 224–2011 in less than a minute *(http://news.bbc.co.uk/2/hi/middle_east/country_profiles/806268.stm)*. The therapist might then inquire whether family members were affected by, or involved in, the pro-democracy protests of 1999, the Iran–Iraq War of 1980–1988, the overthrow of the Shah in 1979, or repression by the secret police before or after the emergence of the Islamic state. Sometimes an online search retrieves an extensive literature on survivors and descendants of historical trauma. The requisite clinical skill here is not knowing the history per se, but rather figuring out what questions to ask.

Carol Kidron (2003) proposed that if PTSD

> allows the invasive past of the trauma survivor to be perpetually present, then the more recent construct of intergenerationally transmitted PTSD has extended the temporal range between the traumatic founding event and its sequelae. It is this temporal extension, which enables descendants to embody and commemorate a distant traumatic past. (p. 538)

With historical trauma that afflicted entire nations, races, genders, or peoples, the therapist needs both cultural competence and an awareness of history in order to develop what Ghosh Ippen (2009) describes as "contextually congruent interventions . . . that guide family members in a way that is responsive to where they are, where they've come from, and where they hope to go" (p. 116). Ultimately, the parent holds the key to understanding how historical trauma plays out in the present for the dyad in the therapy room. The onus is on the therapist to open the dialogue and help the parent find that key.

References

Bowblis, J. (2000). China in the 20th century. In *King's College History Department*. Retrieved from *http://departments.kings.edu/history/20c/china.html*.

Bowlby, J. (1982). *Attachment and loss: Vol. 1. Attachment* (2nd ed.). New York: Basic Books. (Original work published 1969)

Brave Heart, M. Y. H. (1999). *Oyate ptayela:* Rebuilding the Lakota Nation through addressing historical trauma among Lakota parents. *Journal of Human Behavior in the Social Environment, 2*(1–2), 109–126.

Brave Heart, M. Y. H. (2010). *Culturally congruent assessment and intervention with indigenous peoples of the Americas*. Retrieved from *http://hsc.unm.edu/som/psychiatry/crcbh/docs/Archive/11-09-10.CulturallyCongruentAssessment.pdf*.

Brown, L. S. (2008). *Cultural competence in trauma practice: Beyond the flashback*. Washington, DC: American Psychological Association.

Cook, A., Spinazzola, J., Ford, J. D., Lanktree, C., Blaustein, M., Cloitre, M., et al. (2005). Complex trauma in children and adolescents. *Psychiatric Annals, 35*(5), 390–398.

FitzGerald, C. P. (1968). Reflections on the Cultural Revolution in China. *Pacific Affairs, 41*(1), 51–59.

Fraiberg, S. (1980). *Clinical studies in infant mental health*. New York: Basic Books.

Fraiberg, S., Adelson, E., & Shapiro, V. (1975). Ghosts in the nursery: A psychoanalytic approach to the problems of impaired infant–mother relationships. *Journal of the American Academy of Child Psychiatry, 14,* 387–421.

Freud, S. (1959). Beyond the pleasure principle. In J. Strachey (Ed. & Trans.), *The standard edition of the complete psychological works of Sigmund Freud* (Vol. 19, pp. 1–30). London: Hogarth Press. (Original work published 1920)

Freud, S. (1959). Inhibitions, symptoms and anxiety. In J. Strachey (Ed. & Trans.), *The standard edition of the complete psychological works of Sigmund Freud* (Vol. 20, pp. 75–175). London: Hogarth Press. (Original work published 1926)

Ghosh Ippen, C. M. (2009). The sociocultural context of infant mental health: Toward contextually congruent interventions. In C. H. Zeanah, Jr. (Ed.), *Handbook of infant mental health* (3rd ed., pp. 104–119). New York: Guilford Press.

Gil, T., Calev, A., Greenberg, D., Kugelmass, S., & Lerer, B. (1990). Cognitive functioning in post traumatic stress disorder. *Journal of Traumatic Stress, 3*(1), 29–45.

Gold, T. B. (1984). "Just in time!": China battles spiritual pollution on the eve of 1984. *Asian Survey, 24*(9), 947–974.

Greenland, S. K. (2010). *The mindful child: How to help your kid manage stress and become happier, kinder, and more compassionate.* New York: Free Press.

Janoff-Bulmann, R. (1992). *Shattered assumptions: Towards a new psychology of trauma.* New York: Free Press.

Johnson, F. K., Dowling, J., & Wesner, D. (1980). Notes on infant psychotherapy. *Infant Mental Health Journal, 1,* 19–33.

Johnson, K. (1996). The politics of the revival of female infant abandonment in China, with special reference to Hunan. *Population and Development Review, 22*(1), 77–98.

Kidron, C. A. (2003). Surviving a distant past: A case study of the cultural construction of trauma descendant identity. *Ethos, 31*(4), 513–544.

Kleinman, A., & Kleinman, J. (1994). How bodies remember: Social memory and bodily experience of criticism, resistance, and delegitimation following China's Cultural Revolution. *New Literary History, 25,* 708–23.

Lieberman, A. F., Chu, A., Van Horn, P., & Harris, W. W. (2011). Trauma in early childhood: Empirical evidence and clinical implications. *Development and Psychopathology, 23,* 397–410.

Lieberman, A. F., Padrón, E., Van Horn, P., & Harris, W. W. (2005). Angels in the nursery: The intergenerational transmission of benevolent parental influences. *Infant Mental Health Journal, 26*(6), 504–520.

Lieberman, A. F., & Van Horn, P. (2005). *"Don't hit my mommy!": A manual for child–parent psychotherapy with young witnesses of family violence.* Washington, DC: Zero to Three: National Center for Infants, Toddlers, and Families.

Lieberman, A. F., & Van Horn, P. (2008). *Psychotherapy with infants and young children: Repairing the effects of stress and trauma on early attachment.* New York: Guilford Press.

Lieberman, A. F., & Van Horn, P. (2009). Child–parent psychotherapy: A developmental approach in infancy and early childhood. In C. H. Zeanah, Jr. (Ed.), *Handbook of infant mental health* (3rd ed., pp. 439–449). New York: Guilford Press.

Lü, X. (1994–1995). A step toward understanding popular violence in China's Cultural Revolution. *Pacific Affairs, 67*(4), 533–563.

MacFarquhar, R. (n.d.). 20th century Chinese timeline. In *Perspectives on China with Harvard Professor Roderick MacFarquhar.* Retrieved April 23, 2012, from *http:// athome.harvard.edu/programs/macfarquhar/macfarquhar_timelineset.html.*

MacFarquhar, R., & Schoenhals, M. (2006). *Mao's last revolution.* Cambridge, MA: Belknap Press.

Main, M., & Hesse, E. (1990). Parents' unresolved traumatic experiences are related to infant disorganized attachment status: Is frightened and/or frightening parental behavior the linking mechanism? In M. T. Greenberg, D. Cicchetti, & E. M. Cummings (Eds.), *Atttachment in the preschool years: Theory, research, and interventions* (pp. 161–182). Chicago: University of Chicago Press.

Mueller-Pfeiffer, C., Martin-Soelch, C., Blair, J. R., Carnier, A., Kaiser, N., Rufer, M., et al. (2010). Impact of emotion on cognition in trauma survivors: What is the role of posttraumatic stress disorder? *Journal of Affective Disorders, 123*(1–2), 287–292.

Nathan, A. J. (1989). Chinese democracy in 1989: Continuity and change. *Problems of Communism, 38,* 16.

Pynoos, R. S. (1997, February). *The transgenerational repercussions of traumatic expectations.* Paper presented at the Southern Florida Psychiatric Society/University of Miami School of Medicine, Miami, FL.

Richelson, J. T., & Evans, M. L. (1999). *Tiananmen Square, 1989: The declassified history.* National Security Archive electronic briefing book 16. Retrieved from *http://www.gwu.edu/~nsarchiv/NSAEBB/NSAEBB16/documents/index.html.*

Samuelson, K., & Cashman, C. (2009). Effects of intimate partner violence and maternal posttraumatic stress symptoms on children's emotional and behavioral functioning. In R. Geffner, D. Griffin, & J. Lewis (Eds.), *Children exposed to violence: Current issues, interventions and research* (pp. 132–146). New York: Routledge.

Siegel, D. J. (2007). *The mindful brain: Reflection and attunement in the cultivation of well-being.* New York: Norton.

Spence, J. D., & Chin, A. (1996). *The Chinese century: A photographic history of the last hundred years.* New York: Random House.

Wesner, D., Johnson F., & Dowling, J. (1962). What is maternal–infant intervention?: The role of infant psychotherapy. *Psychiatry, 45,* 307–315.

Zero to Three. (2005). *Diagnostic classification of mental health and developmental disorders of infancy and early childhood, revised (DC:0–3R).* Washington, DC: Author.

CHAPTER 17

Parent–Child Interaction Therapy

Anthony J. Urquiza
Susan Timmer

When examining the application of Parent–Child Interaction Therapy (PCIT) to traumatized children, one might legitimately ask, "In what ways would a behaviorally oriented, evidence-based, parenting program benefit a child who has a history of being traumatized?" On the following pages, we describe ways in which PCIT can benefit certain types of children and families who have experienced trauma—especially when the children exhibit significant behavioral disruption. We also provide a description of a "typical" case of a young, severely traumatized boy, which shows that a young child's recovery from exposure to a serious traumatic event is facilitated by including a parent or caregiver as a positive and supportive resilience resource.

Traumatized Children Have Behavioral Problems

It is often difficult to detect the effects of trauma in young children, because they do not recognize or cannot articulate the connection between the traumatic event and how they feel and behave (i.e., traumatic symptoms) due to their developmental immaturity and limitations (e.g., expressive language ability, social cognition, intellectual functioning). Common problems for which some traumatized children are referred to treatment include disruptive, defiant, verbally and physically (and sometimes sexually) aggressive behavior and oppositional behavior. The experience of being victimized (i.e., being abused) and being exposed to violence (i.e., domestic or community violence) are significant predictors of aggressive, noncompliant, defiant behavior in children (e.g., Brown, 2005; Cohen, 2003; Milner, 2000). This pattern of disruptive child behavior appears to stem from a combination of parents' frequent modeling of aggressive and hostile behavior (that might also be exhibited in the community) and the child's own angry emotional responses and resulting oppositional behavior tied to being raised in such coercive, hostile, and unsafe environments.

One characteristic of many violent families that contributes to children's disruptive behavior problems is the absence of positive, warm, and nurturing parenting (Fantuzzo et al., 1991). When traumatized children live in families with chaotic lifestyles, in which consistent and positive parent–child relationships are infrequent or nearly nonexistent, their behavioral problems may be less related to their trauma than to the overall chaotic and dysfunctional lifestyle in which they are being raised. The population of children that has disruptive behavioral problems resulting from inconsistent and poor parenting is the group for whom some type of intensive parenting intervention may be most effective (Kaminski, Valle, Filene, & Boyle, 2008), although it should be understood that this type of intervention may not *directly* address the cognitions and affects related to the child's trauma.

Dyadic Interventions with Young, Traumatized Children

Younger and older children respond differently to trauma, with younger children appearing to be more responsive to the stability (or lack of stability) of parental functioning and older children less likely to be as adversely impacted by parent instability (Scheeringa & Zeanah, 2001). In particular, younger children (i.e., toddlers, preschool-age, and early elementary-age children) are highly responsive to parent cues of affective stability and response and to the instability and distress created by adverse family events (e.g., incest/sexual abuse, interpersonal violence), often because their means of coping are still co-regulated by the parent (Chu & Lieberman, 2010; Fogel, Garvey, Hsu, & West-Stroming, 2006; see also Aidenander, Chapter 3, this volume). In contrast, older children (i.e., middle childhood, adolescents, teens) tend to rely more on their own coping skills and cognitions, may be more independent from distress experienced by a parent figure and may develop other sources of support (e.g., peers, teachers, extended kin) (Werner, 1995). Because of these factors, approaches to treatment including both the parent and child are likely to be more effective when they include beginning treatment at an earlier age (Runyon, Deblinger, Ryan, & Thakkar-Kolar, 2004).

PCIT and Traumatized Children

PCIT is a 14- to 20-week, manualized intervention founded on social learning and attachment theories. PCIT is designed for children between 2 and 7 years of age with externalizing behavior problems. The underlying model of change is similar to that of other parent-training programs, asserting that by providing parents with behavior modification skills, they become the agents of change in reducing their child's behavior problems, which in turn promotes more positive parenting. PCIT incorporates both parent and child in the treatment sessions and uses live, individualized therapist coaching for an idiographic (i.e., individualized) approach to changing the dysfunctional parent–child relationship.

PCIT is conducted in two phases. First, the therapist focuses on enhancing the parent–child relationship (child-directed interaction [CDI]), and the second on improving the child's compliance with the behavioral limits and expectations established by the parent (parent-directed interaction [PDI]). Both phases of treatment begin with an hour of didactic training, followed by sessions in which the therapist coaches the parent during play with the child. From an observation room behind a two-way mirror, via a "bug-in-the-ear" receiver that the parent wears, the therapist provides the parent with feedback on his or her use of the skills. Parents are taught and practice specific skills of communication and behavior management with their children. In addition to practicing these skills during clinic sessions, parents are asked to practice with their children at home for 5 minutes every day.

In CDI (typically 7–10 sessions), parents are coached to follow their children's lead in play by describing their activities, reflecting their appropriate verbalizations, and praising their positive behaviors. By the end of CDI, parents generally have shifted from rarely noticing their children's positive behavior to more consistently attending to, praising, and reinforcing appropriate behavior. When caregivers master the skills taught in CDI by demonstrating that they can give behavior descriptions (e.g., "You are building a tall tower"), reflections (i.e., repeating back or paraphrasing the child's words), and praises (e.g., "Thank you for playing so gently with these toys"), with few instances of asking a question or giving a command and no instances of criticizing their child during a 5-minute assessment, they move to the second phase of treatment.

In PDI (typically 7–10 sessions) therapists train parents to give only essential directions and commands and to make them clear and direct, maximizing chances for cooperation and compliance by the child. Parents participating in PCIT learn a specific method of using time-out for dealing with noncompliance. Parents also may be taught "hands-off" strategies (e.g., removal of privileges) if indicated. These strategies are designed to provide caregivers with tools for managing their children's behavior while helping them to avoid using physical power and to focus instead on using positive incentives and promoting children's emotional regulation. Mastery of behavior management skills during PDI is achieved when therapists observe that caregivers are able to use the behavior management strategies without being coached and when parents report that they are able to use the strategies safely and effectively with their child.

PCIT for traumatized children uses the same basic structure while incorporating best practices for helping parents and children cope with the emotional aftermath of trauma. For example, we often ask the parents to practice and model anxiety and stress reduction strategies, such as deep breathing and counting to 10, particularly to enhance children's frustration tolerance. We also coach parents on how to to respond to traumatic play and any mention of a traumatizing event or situation during their coaching session.

PCIT is an assessment-driven treatment. Prior to treatment and upon graduation, parents complete a battery of standardized assessments, including the following measures: Child Behavior Checklist (CBCL, 1½–5 years; Achenbach & Rescorla, 2000) and the Eyberg Child Behavior Inventory (ECBI; Eyberg & Pincus, 1999), two standardized measures of the severity of children's behavior problems; the Trauma Symptom Checklist for Young Children (TSCYC; Briere et al., 2001), a measure of the severity of children's trauma symptoms; the Brief Symptom Inventory (BSI; Derogatis, 1993), a self-report measure of the parent's psychological symptoms; and the short form of the Parenting Stress Index (PSI; Abidin, 1995), a measure of the severity of three sources of stress in the parent role: parental distress, dysfunction in the parent–child relationship, and difficult child behavior.

In addition, the therapist conducts a behavioral assessment pre- and posttreatment, observing the dyad as they play together in three semistructured activities, using the Dyadic Parent–Child Coding System-III (DPICS-III; Eyberg, Nelson, Duke, & Boggs, 2005), a microanalytic coding system, designed by Eyberg and her colleagues (2005) to categorize parent verbalizations in parent–child interactions. The three play situations vary in the amount of control the parent is asked to use. In the first situation CDI, the parent is asked to follow the child's lead in play; parents are told to let the child pick an activity and to play along. In the PDI, parents are instructed to pick an activity and have the child play with the parent according to the parent's rules. In the third and final situation, the parent is directed to have the child to "clean up" without the parent's assistance. For research purposes, we also use a global assessment of the quality of the caregiver–child relationship, the Emotional Availability Scales (EAS, 3rd ed.; Biringen, 2000), to illustrate the quality of change in the parent–child relationship from pre- to posttreatment. The EAS consists of four scales measuring aspects of the parent's behavior toward the child and two scales measuring qualities of the child's behavior toward the parent.

In addition to assessing the parent and child behavior in the DPICS sessions, the therapist uses the first 5 minutes of each weekly treatment session to observe the parent–child interactions in child-directed play. The therapist remains silent during this time, coding the parent verbalizations.

A number of studies demonstrate the efficacy of PCIT for reducing child behavior problems, with positive effects maintained for up to 6 years posttreatment (Hood & Eyberg, 2003). Several studies have also demonstrated the effectiveness of PCIT for traumatized children (e.g., Timmer, Urquiza, Zebell, & McGrath, 2005; Timmer, Ware, Zebell, & Urquiza, 2008), including evidence that young traumatized children have reduced traumatic stress symptoms as a result (Mannarino, Lieberman, Urquiza, & Cohen, 2010). This finding—that participation in a behavioral, intensive parenting program related to a reduction of traumatic stress symptoms— may be initially puzzling to some. However, there are several reasons why traumatized young children would benefit from PCIT.

1. *Management of disruptive behavior.* Some traumatized young children come from chaotic and dysfunctional families and are consistently exposed to poor and inconsistent parenting, leading them to exhibit defiant, oppositional, and aggressive behavior. This behavioral profile qualifies them as an appropriate match for PCIT. There are also indications that externalizing behavior problems may directly result from exposure to a traumatic event (Valentino, Berkowitz, & Stover, 2010). It should therefore not be a surprise that helping parents manage their child's disruptive behavior in a positive, consistent, and firm manner—a primary objective of PCIT—should give the child much-needed support and can result in decreased trauma symptoms.

2. *Child's improved relationship security and stability with the primary caregiver.* Helping parents by enabling and supporting a more positive and supportive parent–child relationship is another primary objective of PCIT (Eyberg, 2004). One of the avenues to recovery from child trauma involves eliciting support from important caregivers. That is, supportive parenting is associated with positive child outcomes in many domains (Greenberg, 1999; Kim et al., 2003)—especially when a child is required to deal with some type of adverse experience. Therefore, it is essential to sustain a positive parent–child relationship and parental support in order to optimize the child's ability to deal with any adverse or traumatic experience. One benefit of PCIT is that by teaching parents how to use the PRIDE skills (parenting skills promoted within the first portion of PCIT: praise, reflection, imitation, description, and enthusiasm) in their interactions with their children, warmth and positive affiliation increase, strengthening the parent–child relationship. Throughout the course of PCIT, coaches

focus on helping parents to recognize and attend to their children's positive behavior by describing and praising it. At the same time, parents are taught to ignore minor negative and inappropriate behaviors so that they can maintain a warm and supportive relationship with their children.

3. *Parents as therapists: Supporting parent–child communication.* Although there are many perspectives on what exactly constitutes psychotherapy, there is a rich literature describing the benefits of parents functioning in a supportive, therapeutic-like role with their children (see Guerney, 2000; Hutton, 2004). The central aspects of this type of filial therapy relationship include the following: (1) a positive relationship between a child and parent; (2) focus on development of appropriate and safe expression/communication; and (3) the use of play as a central theme (Urquiza, Zebell, & Blacker, 2009). With PCIT, parents are instructed in how to engage their children in positive and collaborative play (especially in the first component of PCIT). As a result, there is typically a warmer and more supportive and affectionate relationship between the parent and child. Similarly, the focus on safe and effective communication is a central tenet of PCIT. Parents are directed to communicate issues of safety, concern for the child's well-being, and positive regard for all appropriate and nonaggressive interactions. Because both parents and children generally perceive play activities as positive and enjoyable, sharing positive play experiences in a PCIT session strengthens the communication within the dyad and helps rebuild a relationship history that is, overall, more positive and strengthening.

4. *Management of the traumatized child's affect.* Traumatized young children often have difficulty managing their feelings in emotionally difficult situations (Graham-Bermann & Levendosky, 1998). At the same time young children have underdeveloped coping skills and a limited understanding of the traumatic experience they have endured (Eigsti & Cicchetti, 2004). These developmental limitations can hinder therapeutic efforts to directly address the trauma and its symptoms and to help children understand their responses (especially their feelings) to their trauma. PCIT provides a means to directly address many of the feelings that a child experiences—especially feelings associated with loss of safety, fear, avoidance, and insecurity. In the PCIT for traumatized children protocol (PCIT Training Center, 2012), therapists are instructed to help parents identify a child's thoughts, feelings, and behaviors. Should a child experience some type of unpleasant affect, especially an affect related to feelings of anger, frustration, and fear, parents are coached to recognize and describe these feelings to the child. As children have the experience of the feeling paired with the label presented by parents, they begin to identify and understand the meaning of the distressing affect, which is one of the first steps to being able to discuss and manage these feelings. As children continue to understand these feelings, then parents can assist them in learning to implement

some strategies to manage these feelings (e.g., deep breathing, counting, progressive relaxation).

5. *Decreasing child behavioral problems may increase parental capacities.* For relationship-based interventions to be effective, the caregiver must be able to participate by implementing the skills learned or the ideas discussed during therapy sessions. When primary caregivers have other sources of stress and are trying to cope with the effects of their own traumatic experiences, these problems may not only contribute to children's mental health problems by dampening parents' warmth and sensitivity and interfering with effective parenting (Lovejoy, Graczyk, O'Hare, & Neuman, 2000), but also may disrupt treatment effectiveness (Stevens, Ammerman, Putnam, & Van Ginkel, 2002). Symptoms of posttraumatic stress, such as depression, fatigue, dissociation, and poor concentration, can interfere with the acquisition of parenting skills (Reyno & McGrath, 2006). Furthermore, parental depression increases the likelihood of early treatment termination (Kazdin, 2000). However, research has shown that if traumatized parents can overcome their tendencies to drop out of treatment and are motivated to participate in a relationship-based approach, their own psychological symptoms can be relieved (Timmer et al., 2011). In PCIT for traumatized children, parents are taught how to cope with the emotions that often accompany their children's disruptive behavior by using anxiety reduction skills such as deep breathing and counting silently. They are coached to observe, notice, and react to their children's positive behavior; they are coached to show warmth, enthusiasm, and enjoyment in their interactions with their children. When traumatized parents repeatedly perform these positive and adaptive behaviors throughout the course of PCIT, it is thought that these adaptive responses may begin to generalize or "spill over" to other parts of their lives, replacing maladaptive responses (Timmer et al., 2011).

A Case Study of PCIT with a Traumatized Child

The family in treatment was a 27-year-old mother and her 4-year-old son, Aiden (pseudonym). The mother was married but had been separated from her husband, the boy's biological father, for approximately 2 years. The family was referred to the CAARE Diagnostic and Treatment Center at the University of Davis Medical Center by their child protective services (CPS) social worker because of the child's extremely aggressive verbal and physical behavior toward his mother, including temper tantrums, destructiveness, and impulsive behavior. The referral also noted that the child displayed separation anxiety, crying uncontrollably whenever the mother left him.

The therapist saw the mother and Aiden for 34 PCIT sessions in the clinic: 2 assessment sessions, 2 teaching sessions, and 30 coaching sessions (more than the typical 14–20 sessions). In addition to these in-clinic PCIT sessions, the mother intermittently received her own individual therapy. Toward the end of treatment, the family received in-home support services (4 sessions) to help the mother generalize her PCIT skills.

Aiden lived with his mother and 6-year-old brother and visited with his father on weekends at the home of his paternal grandmother. Aiden's mother and father had a history of domestic violence dating back to the beginning of their relationship, which was approximately 10 years. The most recent incident of extreme violence took place approximately a year before their referral to PCIT, when Aiden was 3 years of age. The mother had arranged to pick up the children after the father's visitation in the parking lot of a grocery store. While the mother was trying to get Aiden out of his car seat, she and the father's girlfriend began exchanging insults, which escalated into scratching and hair pulling. The father, who had been putting the brother into the mother's vehicle, pulled the mother out of his car and held her while the girlfriend physically assaulted the mother, then pushed her back into his car and continued to kick and punch her in front of Aiden. Bystanders called the police and emergency medical services.

In the initial clinical interview, the mother reported that Aiden had been aggressive, destructive, defiant, and impulsive "for years." She believed that the child's behavioral problems resulted from his witnessing domestic violence. However, it should be noted that in addition to being exposed to violence between his parents, Aiden was also exposed to his mother's mental health problems. In a court report dated nine months earlier, Aiden's mother told a social worker that she had received a diagnosis of severe depression and had been taking antidepressant medication. It is suspected that the mother was experiencing depressive symptoms throughout A's life. It is also likely that the mother was experiencing symptoms of posttraumatic stress related to her history of domestic violence. At the time she brought Aiden for PCIT services, she was not receiving any counseling, nor was she taking medication. The mother denied any drug or alcohol abuse.

Aiden's mother had not yet enrolled him in preschool, but was planning to have him enter school the upcoming fall. The mother reported some psychosocial support from family and friends.

In the initial clinical interview, the mother reported that Aiden often cried and refused to leave her, suggesting some separation anxiety, and noted her difficulty managing his aggression, defiance, and oppositional behavior. Because Aiden's behavior showed some features of oppositional defiant disorder, but the source of his disruptive behaviors was unclear, the therapist gave Aiden the diagnosis of disruptive behavior disorder not otherwise specified. The therapist considered the source of his disruptive behavior to be anxiety, posttraumatic stress, and distress possibly resulting from seeing his mother assaulted, the long exposure to his parents' violent relationship, or a yet-to-be-determined cause (e.g., biological, neurological).

Course of Treatment in PCIT

Aiden's intake assessment was conducted in the beginning of June, 2010. The mother agreed with the therapist's suggestion that PCIT would fit their needs, and weekly sessions were scheduled. After the therapist conducted a teaching session, informing the mother about the skills she would need and what to expect from treatment, coaching sessions began. At the beginning of each session, the therapist talked briefly with the mother, asking how Aiden had behaved since she had last seen her and how the mother was doing. During the third session, the mother complained about feeling stressed and depressed by financial difficulties. She also said that her children were more difficult to manage. The therapist referred the mother for her own counseling, suggesting that if she had some support it might be easier for her to make progress in PCIT. Two weeks later, the mother reported that her depressive symptoms were worsening, but that she had an appointment with her physician in 2 weeks for evaluation for antidepressant medication. According to the children's social worker, a few days later (just before the sixth coaching session), the mother phoned the social worker and told her that she was too depressed and overwhelmed to take care of her children. The children told the social worker that their mother was drinking a lot and wouldn't get out of bed. The social worker decided to remove the children from the mother's custody temporarily and place them in their father's home. Anticipating that the Aiden might have a difficult time with the custody change, the PCIT therapist set up an appointment with the father and Aiden for an assessment to determine whether he and Aiden would benefit from PCIT. The father reported that Aiden got angry and argued with him when he set limits, but did not report any serious problems managing his behavior. The observational assessment showed that the father had a fairly controlling style, but played easily with Aiden and had no difficulty obtaining compliance. The therapist and father decided that Aiden did not require PCIT services at that time.

A little more than a month later, Aiden and his mother began coming for PCIT again (without the older brother). At this time the mother had 2 days of visitation a week with her children and had obtained a prescription from a physician and been taking antidepressants for about a month, though she had not received psychotherapy. The mother reported some decrease in depressive symptoms and stated that she was taking her medication. She and the therapist/coach reviewed the mother's progress in treatment and what she still needed to accomplish. They also reviewed the child's treatment needs and goals.

Aiden and his mother made unsteady progress over the next month. At times, she seemed focused and able to use her PCIT skills, reporting better and calmer behavior in her son. At other times, she reported that Aiden kicked and hit her. At these times she also seemed disconnected from treatment, and her son seemed unresponsive to her attempts to perform the skills. The therapist investigated some way of providing her with counseling services to better support her progress in PCIT. Aiden few weeks later, one of the more experienced trauma therapists at the clinic began providing weekly adjunct services to the mother. Two weeks after beginning adjunct individual treatment, the mother regained full custody of both boys. Two weeks after this, in the 15th coaching session (three months after returning to PCIT), Aiden and his mother moved on to the second phase of treatment: The mother showed mastery of play therapy skills and her son was more consistently responsive to her.

The second phase of treatment, PDI, was conducted for 8 months. Altogether, the dyad received 14 PDI coaching sessions before the therapist was confident that the mother could manage her son's behavior, and that her son's behavior problems were sufficiently diminished. During this time, the mother received 15 of her own weekly individual services. For 4 months, Aiden and his mother's attendance was sporadic, receiving five coaching sessions. Then, Aiden's father filed an allegation of child physical abuse against the mother, which Aiden corroborated. Aiden's mother denied the allegation, stating that the father coached Aiden to corroborate it because of ongoing disputes about custody. She reported that the weekend before the abuse allegation was made, she sent Aiden's brother to his room for a time-out, and Aiden told her that if she didn't let the brother out of time-out, he would tell the social worker that she had hit him. Mother and son missed 3 weeks of PCIT during the investigation of the abuse allegation. Then the mother began to attend regularly, and the dyad made steady progress toward completion of the program and graduation. At PDI session 12, the family began to receive in-home services to help the mother generalize her skills to the home setting.

By the end of treatment, Aiden's mother reported significantly lower levels of disruptive (i.e., aggressive, destructive, defiant), anxious, and depressive behaviors on several standardized measures of children's behavior problems. She also rated Aiden as exhibiting fewer intrusive thoughts on a standardized measure of traumatic stress symptoms in young children. Behavior and symptoms ratings on all these scales fell from levels well above the clinical cutoff at pretreatment to well within the normal range of scores at posttreatment. In addition, the mother self-reported significantly fewer depressive symptoms posttreatment on a standardized measure of psychological symptoms. A comparison of pre- and posttreatment observational measures of relationship quality showed increases in the mother's sensitivity to her son's cues, increases in her engagement in the child's play, and less disruption when she needed the child to do something unpleasant such as cleaning up toys. Aiden was rated as more responsive to his mother and more likely to involve his mother in his play.

Description of Mother's Treatment

Knowing that the mother had a long history of domestic violence and a previous history of abuse and foster care, the therapist anticipated that he would be doing trauma-related therapy with the mother, uncovering triggers that made it difficult for her to implement the skills she was learning in PCIT. After initial clinical interviews, it was the therapist's opinion that the mother's long and unresolved history of trauma and maltreatment, manifest in elevated depressive symptoms, dependency needs, helplessness, and low self-efficacy, were the greatest barriers to progress in PCIT. Consequently, he implemented a two-pronged treatment approach: a cognitive-behavioral approach to help promote healthy cognitions and discourage depressive ones, and mindfulness training to help her control impulsivity and solve problems. Sessions were mostly devoted to disentangling problems she was having with her ex-husband and his girlfriend, the schools, the custody dispute, and how she could better use the skills she was learning in PCIT when dealing with her children's difficult behaviors. The parenting skills taught in PCIT supported her confidence in taking a responsive and authoritative role with Aiden, by planning ahead, considering his limitations, communicating clearly and directly, and being consistent in positively attending to Aiden's desirable behaviors and predictably following through with negative consequences. Practicing and eventually mastering these skills helped Aiden's mother to build self-efficacy as a parent, which may spill over into other life roles.

Conclusion

Much of the research and treatment on traumatized children has focused solely on the traumatized child's trauma symptoms—with much less attention to the disruptive behavior problems that are often exhibited by these young children. As is evident in this case, children who experience complex trauma often have both traumatic stress symptoms *and* disruptive behavioral problems. When examining the traumatized child through a broad lens encompassing functioning and social contexts, it becomes apparent that the parent–child relationship may be *both* a protective factor and a risk factor: It can both assist and hinder the child in his or her recovery from the traumatic event. For young children, this parent–child protection–risk balance suggests that any intervention for the child needs to incorporate the parent in the treatment process as well as to address the parent's capacity to provide a warm, positive, and protective relationship. In the same way that negative, coercive parent–child interactions can lead to a multitude of adverse outcomes, warm, nurturing, and supportive parent–child interactions can promote resilience. By targeting decreased negative interactions and increased positive interactions, PCIT is designed to enhance traumatized children's mental health by increasing the parent–child dyad's capacity to support resilience in both members.

Although we believe that the potential gain of strengthening the parent–child relationship is great, this case illustrates the complexity of people's lives and their ongoing vulnerability to risk. At several points in the course of treatment, this family could have terminated services. The mother was depressed and not really making positive changes; she was having trouble getting out of bed, much less getting to a therapy appointment. At one point, she lost custody of her children. It is a tribute to the treatment team, the social worker, therapists, and—most of all—the mother herself that the family continued to participate in treatment. In the face of seemingly overwhelming obstacles, the mother felt helped and supported, retaining her belief that the services make a difference for her future. By recognizing the mother's contributions *and* hindrances to her son's mental health, interventions could be put in place to support treatment of her son's problems.

This case also illustrates how services for the mother can be integrated with PCIT, and how each treatment modality can support progress in the other. Without antidepressants and her own counseling, it would have been difficult for this mother to overcome both the depression and the constant pressure of ongoing disputes (and retraumatization) in interactions with her ex-husband to learn to handle her children's very difficult behavior. It is more likely that the mother would have abandoned her parental rights, given her reaction to stress in the early weeks of PCIT. In summary, this case illustrates the way in which supporting and building a secure and nurturing parent–child relationship through PCIT is an approach to both reduce traumatic stress symptoms and build resilient parent–child relationships.

References

Abidin, R. R. (1995). *Parenting Stress Index: Professional manual.* Odessa, FL: Psychological Assessment Resources.

Achenbach, T. M., & Rescorla, L. (2000). *Manual for the ASEBA Preschool Forms and Profiles.* Burlington: University of Vermont, Research Center for Children, Youth & Families.

Biringen, Z. (2000) Emotional availability: Conceptualization and research findings. *American Journal of Orthopsychiatry, 70,* 104–111.

Briere, J., Johnson, K., Bissada, A., Damon, L., Crouch, J., Gil, E., et al. (2001). The Trauma Symptom Checklist for Young Children (TSCYC): Reliability and association with abuse exposure in a multi-site study. *Child Abuse and Neglect, 25,* 1001–1014.

Brown, E. J. (2005). Clinical characteristics and efficacious treatment of post-traumatic stress disorder in children and adolescents. *Pediatric Annals, 349*(2), 138–146.

Chu, A. T., & Lieberman, A. (2010). Clinical implications of traumatic stress from birth to age five. *Annual Review of Clinical Psychology, 6,* 469–494.

Cohen, J. (2003). Treating acute posttraumatic stress reactions in children and adolescents. *Biological Psychiatry, 53*(9), 827–833.

Derogatis, L. R. (1993). *Brief Symptom Inventory (BSI): Administration, scoring, and procedures manual.* Minneapolis, MN: NCS Pearson.

Eigsti, I. M., & Cicchetti, D. (2004). The impact of child maltreatment of expressive syntax at 60 months. *Developmental science, 7,* 88–102.

Eyberg, S. M. (2004). The PCIT story—part one: The conceptual foundation of PCIT. *Parent–Child Interaction Therapy Newsletter, 1*(1), 1–2.

Eyberg, S. M., Nelson, M., Duke, M., & Boggs, S. (2005). *Manual for the Dyadic Parent–Child Interaction coding system* (3rd ed.). Unpublished manuscript.

Eyberg, S. M., & Pincus, D. (1999). *ECBI and SESBI-R: Eyberg Child Behavior Inventory and Sutter–Eyberg Student Behavior Inventory—Revised: Professional manual.* Odessa, FL: Psychological Assessment Resources.

Fantuzzo, J. W., DePaola, L. M., Lambert, L., Martino, T., Anderson, T., & Sutton, B. (1991). Effects of interparental violence on the psychological adjustment and competencies of young children. *Journal of Consulting and Clinical Psychology, 59*(2), 258–265.

Fogel, A., Garvey, A., Hsu, H., & West-Stroming, D. (2006). *Change processes in relationships: A relational–historical research approach.* Cambridge, UK: Cambridge University Press.

Graham-Bermann, S. A., & Levendosky, A. A. (1998). The social functioning of preschool-age children whose mothers are emotionally and physically abused. *Journal of Emotional Abuse, 1,* 59–84.

Greenberg, M. T. (1999). Attachment and psychopathology in childhood. In J. Cassidy & P. R. Shaver (Eds.), *Handbook of attachment: Theory, research, and clinical applications* (pp. 469–496). New York: Guilford Press.

Guerney, L. (2000). Filial therapy into the 21st century. *International Journal of Play Therapy, 9*(2), 1–17.

Hood, K., & Eyberg, S. (2003). Outcomes of parent–child interaction therapy: Mothers' reports of maintenance three to six years after treatment. *Journal of Clinical Child and Adolescent Psychology, 32,* 412–429.

Hutton, D. (2004). Filial therapy: Shifting the balance. *Clinical Child Psychology and Psychiatry, 9*(2), 261–270.

Kaminski, J. W., Valle, L. A., Filene, J. H., & Boyle, C. L. (2008). A meta-analytic review of components associated with parent training program effectiveness. *Journal of Abnormal Psychology, 36,* 567–589.

Kazdin, A. E. (2000). Perceived barriers to treatment participation and treatment acceptability among antisocial children and their families. *Journal of Child and Family Studies, 9,* 157–174.

Kim, I. J., Ge, X., Brody, G. H., Conger, R., Gibbons, F. X., & Simons, R. I. (2003). Parenting behaviors and the occurrence and co-occurrence of depressive symptoms and conduct problems among African American children. *Depression, Marriage, and Families, 17,* 571–583.

Lovejoy, M. C., Graczyk, P. A., O'Hare, E., & Neuman, G. (2000). Maternal depression and parenting behavior: A meta-analytic review. *Clinical Psychology Review, 20,* 561–592.

Mannarino, A., Lieberman, A., Urquiza, A., & Cohen, J. (2010, August). *Evidence-based treatments for traumatized children.* Paper presented at the annual convention of the American Psychological Association, San Diego, CA.

Milner, J. S. (2000). Social information processing and child physical abuse: Theory and research. In D. J. Hansen (Ed.), *Nebraska symposium on motivation: Vol. 46. Motivation and child maltreatment* (pp. 39–84). Lincoln: University of Nebraska Press.

PCIT Training Center. (2012). *PCIT for traumatized children web course*. Retrieved from *www.pcit.tv*.

Reyno, S., & McGrath, P. (2006). Predictors of parent training efficacy for child externalizing behavior problems: A meta-analytic review. *Journal of Child Psychology and Psychiatry, 47*, 99–111.

Runyon, M. K., Deblinger, E., Ryan, E. E., & Thakkar-Kolar, R. (2004). An overview of child physical abuse: Developing an integrated parent–child cognitive-behavioral treatment approach. *Trauma, Violence, and Abuse, 5*(1), 65–85.

Scheeringa, M. S., & Zeanah, C. (2001). A relational perspective of PTSD in early childhood. *Journal of Traumatic Stress, 14*, 799–815.

Stevens, J., Ammerman, R., Putnam, F., & Van Ginkel, J. (2002) Depression and trauma history in first-time mothers receiving home visitation. *Journal of Community Psychology, 30*, 551–564.

Timmer, S., Ho, L., Urquiza, A., Zebell, N., Fernandez, Y., Garcia, E., et al. (2011). The effectiveness of parent–child interaction therapy with depressive mothers: The changing relationship as the agent of individual change. *Child Psychiatry and Human Development, 42*(4), 406–423.

Timmer, S., Urquiza, A., Zebell, N., & McGrath, J. (2005). Parent–child interaction therapy: Application to physically abusive and high-risk dyads. *Child Abuse and Neglect, 29*, 825–842

Timmer, S., Ware, L., Zebell, N., & Urquiza, A. (2008). The effectiveness of parent–child interaction therapy for victims of interparental violence. *Violence and Victims, 25*, 486–503.

Urquiza, A. J., Zebell, N. M., & Blacker, D. (2009). Innovation and integration: Parent–child interaction therapy as play therapy. In A. D. Drewes (Ed.), *Blending play therapy with cognitive behavioral therapy: Evidence-based and other effective treatments and techniques* (pp. 199–218). New York: Wiley.

Valentino, K., Berkowitz, S., & Stover, C. S. (2010). Parenting behaviors and posttraumatic symptoms in relation to children's symptomatology following a traumatic event. *Journal of Traumatic Stress, 23*(3), 403–407.

Werner, E. (1995). Resilience in development. *Current Directions in Psychological Science 4*(3), 81–85.

CHAPTER 18

Trauma Systems Therapy

Carryl P. Navalta
Adam D. Brown
Amanda Nisewaner
B. Heidi Ellis
Glenn N. Saxe

It's about a *trauma system*. This conceptual framework is what sets trauma systems therapy (TST) apart from other trauma models. The TST definition of a trauma system is: a traumatized youth who has difficulty regulating his or her emotions and behavior, and a social environment or system of care that is unable to help that youth regulate or to protect him or her from threats or reminders of threats (see Figure 18.1). TST addresses not only a traumatized youth's difficulty with emotional and behavioral regulation, but goes beyond this emphasis to focus equally on the role the social environment plays in triggering and maintaining this dysregulation. This interactive duality of dysregulation and the environment comprises the trauma system. TST is based on 10 treatment principles that guide teams in their approach to assessment, treatment, and the way they integrate their services and expertise (see Figure 18.2).

TST: Its Evolution, Clinical Rationale, and Evidence Base

Based in a large, urban general hospital, Glenn Saxe and his colleagues in the child inpatient unit had been providing interventions for children

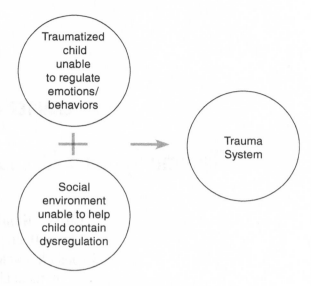

FIGURE 18.1. Trauma system.

with complex trauma histories in the "usual and customary" way—that is, in a clinic, in individual sessions, and with a primary focus on the child. Although our approach at the time was in line with evidence-based, individual child treatments (Wethington et al., 2008), we faced two major challenges. First, we had not recognized sufficiently that the children referred to us were coming from unstable home environments typically mired in poverty and affected by racism/discrimination, inadequate schools, and community violence. As such, these complex environmental and social factors were directly contributing to the children's presenting problems and suggested the need for intervention to reach beyond the individual. Second, we were uncertain about whether our work was having a positive impact on the children and their families. This uncertainty was reinforced when we realized that some of the children and families did not truly engage in treatment—a situation typically reflected by treatment dropout. Such attrition is especially prevalent in ethnic minority youth and with children and adolescents who have histories of child maltreatment (Lau & Weisz, 2003). As a team, we embarked on a mission to develop a different and better way to help the children and families we were treating.

As we set out to change the way we practiced, we followed four guiding principles: (1) treatment must be developmentally informed; (2) treatment must directly address the social environment/ecology; (3) treatment must be compatible with systems of care; and (4) treatment must be "disseminate-able." Affective (or emotional) dysregulation has been found to be one of the major problems experienced by children exposed to complex trauma

1. Fix a broken system.
2. Put safety first.
3. Create clear, focused plans that are based on facts.
4. Don't "go" before you are "ready."
5. Put scarce resources where they will work.
6. Insist on accountability, particularly your own.
7. Align with reality.
8. Take care of yourself and your team.
9. Build from strength.
10. Leave a better system.

FIGURE 18.2. 10 TST treatment principles. From Saxe, Ellis, and Kaplow (2007). Copyright 2007 by The Guilford Press. Reprinted by permission.

(Cicchetti & Toth, 1995). For such children, problems in emotion regulation (ER) can be understood as a core feature of traumatic stress associated with biological systems that help the individual survive in the face of threat (Frewen & Lanius, 2006; Hopper, Frewen, van der Kolk, & Lanius, 2007). When confronted with reminders of past trauma or actual threats, children who have been traumatized respond with hyper- or hypoarousal and other forms of emotional lability. We therefore chose to specify ER as a crucial focus of the treatment model, TST. This approach is consistent with other treatment approaches described in this book.

The seminal theorizing of Urie Bronfenbrenner (1979), with its emphasis on understanding the developing child in the context of his or her social ecology and the transactions that occur between that child and the various layers of his or her social environment, focused TST on the social ecology/environment of the traumatized child. Bronfenbrenner's framework is particularly appropriate to these children, due to the many threats and dangers that are in their environment and the absence of support or protection that may also be part of the environment. For instance, a child subjected to parental physical abuse who is also exposed to community violence may have difficulty recovering from symptoms due to the ongoing threat in the community. The treatment team decided to focus TST on addressing aspects of the social environment that directly relate to a child's emotion dysregulation. This focus is explained in detail below.

Although comprehensive approaches have been developed to coordinate and deliver an array of mental health services from multiple agencies (e.g., systems of care; Pumariega & Winters, 2003), our experience indicated that multiprovider approaches tend to be fragmented, uncoordinated, and thus not very effective. Consequently, we decided to devise an intervention approach that literally "brings to the table" each provider across all systems of care in a multispecialty clinical team. The TST team is typically comprised of home-based clinicians, a psychopharmacologist, psychotherapists, a legal advocate, and a supervising clinician with trauma treatment expertise. The intent was for TST to provide a team approach involving all systems of care with which a traumatized child is involved. These providers, in turn, were engaged with the various parts of the child's social environment (e.g., home, neighborhood/community, school). We thus decided that we needed to come up not only with an effective treatment model, but also one that could be successfully disseminated across a variety of "real world" settings.

One critical strategy that we used in the creation of TST was to create a model that is "disseminate-able" and that incorporates services that are available in most regions of the United States. TST is provided via a traditional multidisciplinary team that also possesses two unique members (i.e., home-based clinician and legal advocate). A second feature of TST that improves its successful adoption and implementation is that the model is fully operationalized in a published manual (Saxe, Ellis, & Kaplow, 2007), which is in line with other empirically supported, manualized, social–ecological models (e.g., multisystemic therapy; Henggeler, Schoenwald, Rowland, & Cunningham, 2002). Another feature of the TST model is the development of a treatment adherence approach to help ensure that treatment is delivered with sufficient fidelity. Specifically, fidelity is guided by adherence to the 10 identified TST principles and is consistent with the notion of "flexibility within fidelity" to lead to a child-centered, individualized treatment approach (Kendall, Gosch, Furr, & Sood, 2008).

The first study that initially demonstrated TST's efficacy was an open trial conducted at two sites: a child psychiatry outpatient clinic of a large, urban general hospital and a joint program of countywide departments of mental health and social services in rural upstate New York (Saxe, Ellis, Fogler, Hansen, & Sorkin, 2005). Each site had a team trained in TST, which was implemented prior to the study. One-hundred ten children ages 5–20 years old (mean age = 11.2, SD = 3.6) and their families were enrolled in treatment. The Child and Adolescent Needs and Strengths—Trauma Exposure and Adaptation (CANS-TEA; Kisiel, Blaustein, Fogler, Ellis, & Saxe, 2009) version was used as the primary treatment outcome measure after TST had been delivered for 3 months. For those children who remained in treatment (82; 72% of the enrolled sample), improvement was found in PTSD symptoms, emotion regulation, behavior regulation, caregiver's physical and mental health, caregiver psychosocial support and stability, and stability of the social environment. Positive changes in children's functioning were also strongly and positively correlated with changes in those dimensions that are specifically targeted by TST (e.g., ER and stability of the social environment). Moreover, 58% of the children transitioned from more- to less-intensive phases of treatment during the 3 months of the study.

The aforementioned joint program in upstate New York was the end result of the first successful TST dissemination effort (Hansen, Saxe, & Drewes, 2009). The adoption and implementation of TST came to fruition after the program's realization that (1) the primary reason for referral was "environmental–family dysregulation" as opposed to more isolated psychiatric disorders in the child being referred for services (e.g., oppositional defiant disorder, conduct disorder, posttraumatic stress disorder [PTSD]); (2) the majority of referred cases had histories of trauma, including abuse, neglect, and extreme poverty; (3) the clinical model used at the time had proven to be ineffective at providing services to these families, which presented as stressed, unable to organize themselves, and unable to keep members safe; and (4) resource barriers for the families (e.g., lack of child care and/or transportation) and a general mistrust of the system that resulted in poor engagement in therapy. As a consequence, the program decided to incorporate TST into its overall treatment framework, which also includes aspects of play therapy and cognitive-behavioral therapy.

Recent evaluation data provide empirical support for the program's clinical as well as cost effectiveness (Ellis et al., 2011). Across a 15-month period, 124 children between 3 and 20 years old who had experienced three to nine potentially traumatic events received TST. Measures of clinical course (hospitalization, need for intensive vs. office-based services), children's psychiatric and psychosocial functioning, and the stability of the social environment were taken at intake, at 4–6 months (early treatment), and at 12–15 months (late treatment). Cost savings were evaluated through a comparison of pre- and postimplementation hospitalization rates and lengths of stay for all children under the care of the county mental health department. Emotion regulation, stability of the social environment, and child functioning/strengths improved significantly over the course of treatment. Early treatment improvement in child functioning/strengths and social environment stability were associated with overall improvement in emotion regulation across the duration of the intervention. Children who were able to transition from crisis stabilization to office-based services during early treatment tended to stay in treatment and improve through late treatment. For the 72% of youth who completed treatment, the need for crisis stabilization services at 15 months was reduced by over 50%. Compared to children served prior to the implementation of TST, hospitalization rates were 36% lower and the average length of stay was 23% lower.

Such short- and long-term gains cannot be attained unless children and families are actively engaged early in treatment. Initial findings indicate that *Ready-Set-Go!*—the engagement approach used in TST—is associated with high levels of treatment retention (Saxe, Ellis, Fogler, & Navalta, 2011). In a small, randomized controlled trial of traumatized youth (*N* = 20), 90% of TST participants were still in treatment, whereas only 10% of "treatment as usual" participants remained at the 3-month assessment.

Dissemination: Real-World Settings

At the time of this writing, TST has been disseminated and implemented in 26 programs within 17 agencies across 10 states. Such programs include community-based outpatient programs, child welfare–mental health collaborations, foster care–mental health collaborations, shelters for unaccompanied undocumented minors, school-based mental health programs, residential programs, pediatric hospital-based programs, and substance abuse–mental health collaborations. Adaptations of TST have been developed for use in specialized settings, such as substance abuse programs, residential treatment, and foster care. Each adaptation adheres to key features of TST, while making crucial changes necessary to meet the individualized needs of the setting, demonstrating the concept of "flexibility within fidelity" (Kendall & Beidas, 2007).

The two major adaptations of TST are for child welfare and for refugee trauma. TST is uniquely suited for use in these types of programs in that, although the program placements are presumably more stable than the environment from which the youth was removed, triggers and reminders of interpersonal trauma are often highly prevalent. For example, a foster parent who may be well meaning but who adheres strictly to house rules may not understand that sleeping in the dark triggers the youth to become dysregulated. Similarly, staff in residential treatment programs may inadvertently contribute to signals of danger or fear by using loud voices or punitive limit setting. Also, residential programs that do not have systems in place to facilitate effective communication among team members may contribute to distress in the environment as well.

Key Practical Clinical Features

Assessment

In TST, each youth is assessed as being in one of three categories: regulated, emotionally dysregulated, or behaviorally dysregulated. Similarly, the social environment has three categories as well: stable, distressed, or threatening. By determining the relationship between these two ratings, the youth is assessed as being in one of five phases of treatment: surviving, stabilizing, enduring, understanding, or transcending. The TST assessment grid (Figure 18.3) is used to determine the phase of treatment, each of which is associated with a defined set of recommended treatment interventions.

Four key factors are considered when assessing whether a child is experiencing emotion dysregulation, behavior dysregulation, or neither. First, an episode of dysregulation is defined as changes in awareness (or consciousness), affect (or emotion), and action (or behavior) when the child is exposed to a stressor or triggering stimulus (these indicators are the tbree A's). If these three changes do not occur, the child is not considered to be dysregulated. Second, the rate or frequency of dysregulation episodes is taken into consideration. Typically, the number of weekly or monthly episodes is documented to help ascertain the degree to which dysregulation is present. Third, some evidence must exist that the dysregulation episode caused a problem with the child's school, family, peer relationships, or self.

		Stability of social environment		
		Stable	Distressed	Threatening
Emotion Regulation	Regulated	*Transcending*	*Understanding*	*Enduring*
	Emotionally Dysregulated	*Understanding*	*Enduring*	*Stabilizing*
	Behaviorally Dysregulated	*Enduring*	*Stabilizing*	*Surviving*

FIGURE 18.3. TST assessment grid. Adapted from Saxe, Ellis, and Kaplow (2007). Copyright 2007 by The Guilford Press. Adapted by permission.

This problem can either be related to the dysregulation episode itself or to feelings or behaviors related to the anticipation of a dysregulation episode (i.e., an impairment or distress criterion). Fourth, when a child engages in risky or potentially dangerous behaviors during an episode (e.g., aggressive, suicidal, self-mutilatory, or otherwise impulsive behaviors), he or she is considered to be behaviorally dysregulated. This distinction is the most severe emotion regulation tier in the TST assessment grid (Figure 18.3). In contrast, a child is categorized as emotionally dysregulated when changes in the three A's occur but with *no* risky or potentially dangerous behaviors (i.e., middle tier).

Within the framework of TST, a traumatized child who experiences a dysregulation episode transitions, timewise, across four emotional states: regulating, revving, reexperiencing, and reconstituting (the four R's). The development of the TST treatment plan is dependent on the designation of the child as regulated, emotionally dysregulated, or behaviorally dysregulated.

TST conceptualizes the social environment/system of care along a three-tier continuum of stability as well (i.e., stable, distressed, and threatening). The constructs of *help* and *protect* are critical in distinguishing among these three levels of stability. *Help* refers to the capacity of the social environment or system of care to help the child manage emotion and emotionally motivated behavior. *Protect* pertains to the capacity of the social environment or system of care to protect the child from stressors that may lead to dysregulated emotional states as described above. Collectively, the degree to which these capacities are present helps practitioners precisely ascertain the stability of the social environment/system of care.

A child's social environment/system of care is considered stable when the following three conditions are met: (1) the child's immediate caregivers are able to help him or her regulate emotion and to protect him or her from stressors; (2) the child's extended family, peer group, or neighbors are able to support the child such that any limitations of the immediate caregivers to help or protect are mitigated; and (3) the child's system of care has been accessed successfully to provide needed functions that the immediate caregivers and extended family are not able to provide. In contrast, a child's social environment/system of care is considered distressed when neither the child's primary caregivers, extended family, nor system of care is able to help the child regulate emotional states and/or protect him or her from environmental stressors.

Lastly, a child's social environment/system of care is considered threatening when one or both of the following scenarios exists: (1) The child's caregivers pose a true threat of harm to the child, and the child's extended family, peer group, or neighbors cannot adequately protect the child from this threat. Furthermore, the child's system of care has either not been accessed or has not adequately protected the child from this threat. And/or (2) a threat of harm to the child from outside the immediate caregivers exists, and the child is not adequately protected from this outside threat. In summary, the use of these three constructs (*stable, distressed,* and *threatening*) will determine the extent of stability/instability of a child's social environment and/or system of care and will help practitioners complete the TST assessment grid (Figure 18.3).

Treatment Planning

Rather than including nine disparate treatment phases that correspond to each of the nine areas in the assessment grid, TST has only five phases of treatment that align with unique foci and themes: *surviving, stabilizing, enduring, understanding,* and *transcending,* rank-ordered from most intensive (surviving) to least intensive (transcending) in terms of the acuity of service needs. Depending on the treatment phase, one or more of the TST service modules is clinically indicated (i.e., home- and community-based care, skills-based outpatient treatment, psychopharmacology, and services advocacy).

SURVIVING

The main theme of this phase of treatment is to protect the child from threatening environments and dangerous impulses and to set the stage for interventions in other phases of TST. A child in this phase is behaviorally dysregulated, and the social environment/system of care is threatening. Therefore, home- and community-based interventions are intensively used during this phase to acquire a comprehensive picture of the child's home environment and to assess the degree of threat and danger. During this treatment phase, a need to work closely with social service agencies, inpatient psychiatric units, and medication-prescribing clinicians is often present. Emotion regulation skills training and services advocacy can also be implemented in this phase when appropriate.

STABILIZING

The main theme of this phase is the creation of a safe social environment. Families who start in this phase usually have significant problems that will not be helped without home-based interventions. Typically, problems relate to family disorganization and/or to the child's school, peer group, and neighborhood, where stressors occur that routinely trigger the child. Interventions are delivered on site, usually in the home or school, and are designed to help stabilize the factors in the environment that are contributing to the youth's dysregulation. Interventions in this phase often include advocating for needed services. Many children in this phase will require pharmacotherapy and advocacy for additional help and support.

ENDURING

The main theme of this phase is the development of skills necessary to manage emotion and respond to the establishment of a safe social environment. The child and family must be taught skills that help them endure the impact of trauma so that extreme behavior can be minimized. In order for skill-based psychotherapy to be effective, the youth's environment must be safe and not triggering the youth to dysregulate. The primary mode of psychotherapy in this phase of treatment is emotion regulation skills training. If treatment has started prior to this phase, home- and community-based interventions should be mostly complete. For children who start in this phase, home- and community-based interventions may be required at some point.

UNDERSTANDING

The main theme of this phase is the establishment of therapeutic communication about the traumatic experience(s) so that the child and family are no longer consumed by the events. Techniques of cognitive-behavioral therapy are primarily used during this phase of intervention. Emotion regulation skills training should be completed before this treatment phase so that the child has sufficient skills to manage the processing of trauma-related cognitions and memories. Occasionally, medications will be necessary during this phase.

TRANSCENDING

The main theme of this phase is the creation of lasting meaning and perspective out of traumatic experiences once the trauma is over. The focus is to learn how to live in a way that is less defined by the past and more so by the future. This learning includes helping the child and family say goodbye to the therapist and moving beyond treatment. During this treatment phase, the child, family, and clinician work toward identifying and constructing culturally sanctioned activities that may create lasting meaning out of the child's traumatic experiences.

TST Intervention Modules

Interventions within TST are delivered according to a series of seven modules that are used in various combinations depending on the phase of treatment in which a child and family are assessed (see Figure 18.4). The seven treatment modules are briefly summarized here. For more detailed information on each module, refer to our treatment manual (Saxe et al., 2007).

1. *Ready-Set-Go.* This module is used with all families at the beginning of TST as a way of introducing our treatment approach, assessing families' capacities to engage, building a treatment alliance, and working to surmount barriers to engagement.

2. *Stabilization on Site (SOS).* This module involves intensive home-based and school-based services that focus on directly diminishing the sources of acute stress and traumatic reminders within the child's day-to-day environment.

3. *Services Advocacy.* This module involves explicit work with service systems that can offer needed resources to help with emotion regulation and, particularly, social environmental stability; such services may include housing, financial assistance, or domestic violence advocacy.

4. *Psychopharmacology.* This module applies psychopharmacology through the psychiatric consultant's role on a TST treatment team.

5. *Emotion Regulation (ER).* The emotion regulation (ER) module is a semistructured, office-based therapeutic approach that helps both parents and children gain greater awareness of emotions and specific skills and strategies for regulation;

6. *Cognitive Processing (CP).* The CP module is about learning cognitive-behavioral techniques of trauma processing so that the child will not become dysregulated when faced with stressors or reminders.

7. *Meaning Making (MM).* This module is about finding activities that the child, family, and therapist can do that will create lasting meaning about the traumatic event(s). These activities might include a ritual to "mark" that the child is beyond the trauma, art projects, or activities that involve helping others and are often syntonic with the cultural and religious background of the family.

	Surviving	Stabilizing	Enduring	Understanding	Transcending
Stabilization on site (SOS)	***	***	–	–	–
Services advocacy	***	**	*	*	*
Psychopharmacology	**	**	**	*	*
Emotional regulation	*	**	***	–	–
Cognitive processing	–	–	–	***	–
Meaning making	–	–	–	–	***

Note. *** = essential; ** = often helpful; * = occasionally helpful; – = not used or contraindicated

FIGURE 18.4. TST treatment intervention grid. From Saxe, Ellis, and Kaplow (2007). Copyright 2007 by The Guilford Press. Reprinted by permission.

The Moment by Moment Assessment

Gathering a clear, specific understanding of the environmental factors that trigger dysregulation is vitally important within TST. The Moment by Moment Assessment (MMA) is the tool used to identify these triggers in the environment that lead to changes in the three A's and the four R's. To identify and accurately define areas for intervention, the TST clinical team is expected to document episodes of emotion or behavior dysregulation and the stimuli that provoke them via the MMA. The following steps are used to conduct this assessment:

1. Inquire about episodes of dysregulation.
2. Understand how the three A's shift during these episodes.
3. Ascertain the precipitants to these episodes.
4. Understand how family members (or other members of the social environment) helped or made things worse.
5. Determine the cost to the child and family of these episodes.

Via this process, the team gathers exquisitely detailed information about what the youth was thinking, feeling, and doing immediately prior to, during, and after a specified instance of dysregulation. In addition, the team also gathers specific information about precise environmental conditions immediately prior to the episode. This information is gathered by interviewing the youth (only when he or she is back to a regulated state), interviewing other youth who may have witnessed the event, and interviewing other adults who were present as well.

TST Priority Problems

In usual care/treatment, the clinical targets for interventions parallel the diagnostic formulation. For a child diagnosed with major depressive disorder, for example, depressive symptoms such as sad/unhappy mood, social withdrawal/isolation, and neurovegetative symptoms are the foci whereby significant symptom reduction is the primary goal of treatment. Within TST, however, the trauma system is the focal point of all interventions—in particular, the TST *priority problems*, which precisely define the trauma system for a given child. The TST priority problems are based on the interface between the child's emotion regulation problems and stressful stimuli in the environment.

Once the information from the MMA is gathered, the TST team then establishes (1) links or patterns of links between emotion/behavior dysregulation and the stimuli that elicit them; (2) role of members of the child's social environment in helping or hindering regulation during these patterns of links; and (3) functional implications for these patterns of links. Then these patterns are assigned priorities, via clinical judgment, regarding the amount of dysfunction that they cause. Such dysfunction includes, but is not limited to, problems that jeopardize physical safety; engagement in treatment, home placement, school placement, or healthy development; problems that cause significant distress to the child or family members; and problems that can be solved relatively easily and are highly meaningful to the child or family members. The TST priority problems are thus those patterns that are assigned the highest priorities (typically one to four problems in total). Finally, the TST *priority solutions*, to address the corresponding priority problems, are formulated via the clinically indicated treatment modules, and the individuals who are responsible for carrying out these solutions are identified as well (e.g., child, parent, outpatient clinician, home-based therapist, advocate).

The TST priority problem is constructed utilizing the following sentence: Signals of _____, such as _____, lead to feelings of _____, which lead to emotional and/ or behavioral dysregulation, as evidenced by _____. In this sentence, which is designed to assist the team in the identification of the problem, the first blank space refers to the traumatic event(s), the second refers to the specific reminders of the traumatic event(s) within the social environment, and the remaining two spaces refer to the impact of these traumatic reminders on the youth's emotional and behavioral functioning.

Child Welfare Case Vignette

Identifying Information

Clara is a 12-year-old girl who was removed from her mother's home after she came to school and reported that she had been raped by her mother's boyfriend while her mother was in the home. School staff called child protective services (CPS), which investigated and arrested the mother's boyfriend, who was ultimately charged and sentenced. CPS determined that Clara was at imminent risk due to the mother's own mental health needs and consequently placed her in an emergency foster home.

Presenting Problem

Although Clara was referred to a community mental health clinic, she was very depressed and withdrawn in the foster home, where she made suicidal threats and gestures. The foster care agency brought her to an emergency room where she was admitted to a pediatric psychiatric inpatient unit.

Assessment and Treatment Planning

Staff at the hospital determined that she needed a higher level of care than a foster home could provide and facilitated a referral to a residential treatment program that used TST.

Trauma System and Priority Problem

Clara initially appeared quite anxious and withdrawn, with weekly incidents in which she would hide and, when found, would appear dissociated and have superficial self-inflicted scratches on her arms. The TST team conducted a MMA of this behavior by interviewing Clara (when she was not dissociated) and her mother. They found that these episodes occurred when a particular male staff member was on shift and that, though he treated Clara no differently than he did the other residents, she responded with great fear. Notably, his appearance was similar to the man who had raped her. With this crucial information, the team was able to create the following priority problem for Clara: "Signals of danger and victimization, such as being around someone who reminds her of the person who raped her, lead to feelings of fear and despair, which lead to emotion and behavior dysregulation as evidenced by dissociation, hiding, and self-harmful gestures." Clara was assessed as being in the stabilizing phase. The team thus needed to address Clara's behavior dysregulation while attempting to stabilize the environment.

Emotion Regulation Skills Training

In regard to helping Clara become better regulated, her primary therapist provided education about the impact of trauma and helped her understand her responses when reminded of traumatic events in some way. Clara's therapist also helped her develop skills to recognize when she was becoming dysregulated and to manage these distressing feelings by utilizing self-soothing skills and letting others know when she needed help. In regard to stabilizing the social environment, the residential leadership determined that Clara needed help to see that this staff member, although having a physical resemblance to her attacker, was in fact different, and that she was not actually in danger. With this staff member's agreement, he was temporarily assigned to another cottage so that the team could work with Clara while she was in a regulated state. Part of the plan involved looking at pictures of this staff member to help her learn to perceive him as a safe rather than an abusive man. The team helped Clara and the staff member to write letters to each other and eventually to have visits with her therapist present. The staff member was able to return to his cottage within 2 weeks. Not only did Clara come to experience the environment as stable, but she developed a very positive relationship with the staff member.

After 5 months of residential placement, the team determined that Clara had improved her behavior regulation sufficiently to be ready for a less intensive level of care. Clara's mother, however, did not follow through with recommendations from CPS. Although she visited with Clara, she did not attend all required parenting classes and did not regularly keep therapy appointments. Thus, although Clara's perpetrator was in jail, her mother was not ready to provide for her needs. The treatment team recommended referral to a therapeutic foster home within the same agency, which also utilized the TST model. The foster care TST team, having access to the residential team's assessment, first ascertained whether anyone in the foster home or immediate vicinity reminded Clara of the perpetrator. This possibility did not appear to be the case. Clara was placed in a home with two parents and one other foster child. The parents were caring and supportive and reported that Clara, though quiet, did well with them most of the time, but would become isolated and withdrawn at times and would lock herself in her room. The team then performed an MMA and determined that episodes of withdrawal usually occurred a day after Clara returned to her foster home from supervised visits with her mother. The visits appeared to be going well, but returning to the foster home after a positive visit with her mother was confusing and overwhelming to Clara. The foster care TST team worked with the foster parents to create a plan to anticipate and prepare for this reaction. One of the foster parents would meet her outside the apartment building when she came home from a visit and take her for a walk in the park to help her with the transition back to the foster home. Clara's outpatient therapist helped her identify, understand, and tolerate her feelings about not being able to live at home and to accept the support of her foster parents. In the meantime, Clara's mother became consistently involved in her own treatment and began family therapy sessions with Clara through the foster care agency. After approximately 1 year in foster care, Clara was able to return home to her mother with many supports in place.

Refugee Trauma Case Vignette

Project SHIFA (Supporting the Health of Immigrant Families and Adolescents) was developed to provide culturally appropriate mental health care for Somali youth and their families. Although many Somali youth have mental health problems related to varied adverse experiences (e.g., war and violence prior to resettlement, ongoing acculturative and resettlement stress), cultural and practical barriers have led to very few of them receiving mental health services. Project SHIFA thus grew out of a partnership among the Somali community, local education authority, and the mental health system in the Boston area in response to this high level of unmet need.

Identifying Information

A 12-year-old Somali male, Abdi, was referred to Project SHIFA by his school social worker. Abdi was born in Somalia but lived as a refugee in a camp in Kenya for the majority of his early childhood. When Abdi was 10 years old, he arrived and settled with his family in greater Boston,

Massachusetts. Upon their arrival, Abdi and his family moved around from shelter to shelter before being placed in permanent public housing.

Presenting Problem

Abdi had been suspended for fighting with his peers, and his teacher reported that he gets easily distracted, appears angry, and frequently talks back. She also expressed concern over his academic performance. At the time of the intake, he had a limited ability to regulate his emotions, which resulted in poorly modulated affect and impulse control. He exhibited signs of distress regarding his walks home from school and had begun to fear not only his safety but also his family's well-being.

Assessment and Treatment Planning

Once the initial referral was made, several conversations were conducted with Abdi's family and with the aid of a Somali cultural broker (someone who not only can speak the language [i.e., an interpreter], but also knows the person's cultural values, attitudes, and ways of life) about trauma and the services that comprise TST-Refugee (TST-R). Consistent with the overall Somali culture, stigma associated with emotion and behavior dysfunction was identified early on as a potential barrier to treatment engagement, as individuals who seek help may be seen as bringing shame to the family and consequently can be viewed as "the crazy one" in their community. However, Abdi's education became an entry point to developing a treatment alliance with the family, in that Abdi's success as a student was a primary goal for his mother. Thus, all interventions were framed with that goal in mind.

Trauma System and Priority Problems

Based on the presence of a threatening social environment (i.e., threats of physical harm while Abdi walked home from school) together with Abdi's behavior dysregulation (i.e., emotionally driven physical aggression), Abdi's trauma system was identified in the *surviving* phase. Implementation of several MMAs helped to elucidate a consistent pattern in which Abdi is triggered and becomes aggressive whenever he or his mother is made fun of or put down, such as being called a pirate. As outlined for the *surviving* phase, stabilization on site (SOS), services advocacy, and skill-based psychotherapy (emotion regulation skills training) were subsequently initiated. These intervention modules directly addressed the following two priority problems that were formulated, based on the TST assessment grid and the MMAs.

- *Priority problem 1:* Signals of danger and victimization, such as being harassed when walking home from school, lead to feelings of anxiety and distress in anticipation of the walk home, which lead to emotional dysregulation as evidenced by irritability and lack of focus in the classroom environment.

- *Priority problem 2:* Signals of rejection and alienation, such as peers making fun of him, lead to feelings of anger, which lead to behavioral dysregulation as evidenced by impulse dyscontrol, conflicts with peers, and physical aggression.

Services Advocacy

Priority problem 1 was immediately addressed by encouraging Abdi's family to file a proper police report. In tandem, school personnel were notified about the harassment incidents and the school consequently provided a bus pass for Abdi, which mitigated his anxiety regarding his own safety.

Emotion Regulation Skills Training

The school-based TST clinician began seeing Abdi on a weekly basis and focused on Abdi's emotion identification and relaxation skills. Abdi consequently had a much easier time describing his regulated emotional state and identifying the changes in his body when he gets triggered and feels out of control. Overall, Abdi's newfound skills in identifying what angers him and in calming himself down made a huge impact on his progress in treatment.

Another critical aspect of treatment was Abdi's and the school staff's enhanced understanding of how Abdi's Somali background and early experiences influence his present emotions and related behaviors. In Somali culture, males are raised to defend themselves and their families against insults or attacks of any kind by striking back, which is not acceptable behavior in a school setting. To address this issue, the clinician worked with Abdi to identify alternative ways to uphold his family's honor, which was fully supported by Abdi's mother when she communicated to Abdi that she would be even prouder of him if he were able to walk away from conflicts.

Toward the end of treatment, Abdi was beginning to smile and his affect was positively changing. He was also able to identify many things in his present life that make him feel happy, such as his family, playing basketball and soccer, and doing well in school. He reported that his primary goal for the rest of the school year was to not get into any more fights and, more importantly, to not have his mother come to his school for any type of meetings—a major "source of pain" that his mother articulated when treatment first began.

Conclusion

TST was created as a comprehensive treatment model for traumatized children, adolescents, and their families. TST also exemplifies the "broad-based treatments" advocated by Kazdin (1997) that "can be conceived in a modular fashion where there are separate components (modules) woven into an overall treatment plan" (p. 123). Although the primary treatment modules within TST are not new, a key innovation of TST is that the clinical model is embedded in an organizational model. That is, TST describes not only what is done clinically, but also how to integrate and orchestrate different clinical interventions so that children receive the right level of care, at the right moment in time, and in a tightly coordinated manner. In other words, TST provides both an organizing framework for identifying and coordinating the different service elements as well as a clinical model that describes exactly what providers do once they are brought together.

The major clinical innovations of TST are a focus on engagement, a phase-based treatment strategy, and an uncompromising focus on the intersection of emotion regulation and the social environment (i.e., trauma system). In addition, TST is a phase-based model in which services assembled in the treatment plan for any given child are more intensive for children with higher levels of need, but diminish in intensity as a child progresses through treatment. In contrast to other intervention models that specify a set number of sessions, a child moves from one TST treatment phase to the next based on his or her progress. Such an approach allows treatment to be tailored to the unique needs of an individual child and helps agencies strategically place their resources so that the children who need the most services actually receive them. Lastly, TST is all about the trauma system—addressing both the social environment and a child's emotion regulation capacity in a genuinely collaborative manner is the defining signature of TST. Fidelity to the model, while allowing for flexibility, is seen as critical, so that TST can be adapted for use in various settings. Fidelity is based on adherence to the 10 TST principles, (Figure 18.2) as a heuristic guide. These principles are based on the foundations that are succinctly highlighted above and fully described in the TST manual (Saxe, Ellis, & Kaplow, 2007). Sufficient fidelity to TST is anchored by these principles, and agencies that implement TST do so with training and technical support from the TST development team.

References

Bronfenbrenner, U. (1979). *The ecology of human development.* Cambrindge, MA: Harvard University Press.

Cicchetti, D., & Toth, S. L. (1995). A developmental psychopathology perspective on child abuse and neglect. *Journal of the American Academy of Child and Adolescent Psychiatry, 34*(5), 541–565.

Ellis, B. H., Fogler, J., Hansen, S., Beckman, M., Forbes, P., Navalta, C. P., et al. (2011). Trauma systems therapy: 15-month outcomes and the importance of effecting environmental change. *Psychological Trauma: Theory, Research, Practice, and Policy, 46*(6), 624–630.

Frewen, P. A., & Lanius, R. A. (2006). Toward a psychobiology of posttraumatic self-dysregulation: Reexperiencing, hyperarousal, dissociation, and emotional numbing. In R. Yehuda & R. Yehuda (Eds.), *Psychobiology of posttraumatic stress disorders: A decade of progress* (Vol. 1071, pp. 110–124). Malden, MA: Blackwell.

Hansen, S., Saxe, G., & Drewes, A. A. (2009). Trauma systems therapy: A replication of the model, integrating cognitive behavioral play therapy into child and family treatment. In A. A. Drewes (Ed.), *Blending play therapy with cognitive behavioral therapy: Evidence-based and other effective treatments and techniques* (pp. 139–164). Hoboken, NJ: Wiley.

Henggeler, S. W., Schoenwald, S. K., Rowland, M. D., & Cunningham, P. B. (2002). *Serious emotional disturbance in children and adolescents: Multisystemic therapy.* New York: Guilford Press.

Hopper, J. W., Frewen, P. A., van der Kolk, B. A., & Lanius, R. A. (2007). Neural correlates of reexperiencing, avoidance, and dissociation in PTSD: Symptom dimensions and emotion dysregulation in responses to script-driven trauma imagery. *Journal of Traumatic Stress, 20,* 713–725.

Kazdin, A. E. (1997). A model for developing effective treatments: Progression and interplay of theory, research, and practice. *Journal of Clinical Child Psychology, 26*(2), 114–129.

Kendall, P. C., & Beidas, R. S. (2007). Smoothing the trail for dissemination of evidence-based practices for youth: Flexibility within fidelity. *Professional Psychology: Research and Practice, 38*(1), 13–20.

Kendall, P. C., Gosch, E., Furr, J. M., & Sood, E. (2008). Flexibility within fidelity. *Journal of the American Academy of Child and Adolescent Psychiatry, 47*(9), 987–993.

Kisiel, C., Blaustein, M. E., Fogler, J., Ellis, B. H., & Saxe, G. N. (2009). Treating children with traumatic experiences: Understanding and assessing needs and strengths. *Report on Emotional and Behavioral Disorders in Youth, 9*(1), 13–19(7).

Lau, A., & Weisz, J. (2003). Reported maltreatment among clinic-referred children: Implications for presenting problems, treatment attrition, and long-term outcomes. *Journal of the American Academy of Child and Adolescent Psychiatry, 42,* 1327–1334.

Pumariega, A. J., & Winters, N. C. (2003). *Handbook of child and adolescent systems of care: The new community psychiatry.* San Francisco: Jossey-Bass.

Saxe, G. N., Ellis, B. H., Fogler, J., Hansen, S., & Sorkin, B. (2005). Comprehensive care for traumatized children. *Psychiatric Annals, 35*(5), 443–448.

Saxe, G. N., Ellis, B. H., Fogler, J., & Navalta, C. P. (2011). Preliminary evidence for effective family engagement in treatment for child traumatic stress: Trauma systems therapy approach to preventing dropout. *Child and Adolescent Mental Health, 17*(1), 58–61.

Saxe, G. N., Ellis, B. H., & Kaplow, J. B. (2007). *Collaborative treatment of traumatized children and teens: The trauma systems therapy approach.* New York: Guilford Press.

Wethington, H. R., Hahn, R. A., Fuqua-Whitley, D. S., Sipe, T. A., Crosby, A. E., Johnson, R. L., et al. (2008). The effectiveness of interventions to reduce psychological harm from traumatic events among children and adolescents: A systematic review. *American Journal of Preventive Medicine, 35,* 287–313.

CHAPTER 19

Conclusion

Julian D. Ford
Christine A. Courtois

The chapters in this book amply illustrate the remarkable progress that has taken place in recent years in the identification of complex trauma early in life and in the development, evaluation, and dissemination of treatments to help children and adolescents recover from its various aftereffects. These interventions are crucially important because they have the potential to keep these children from experiencing a lifetime of recurrent trauma-related adaptations, reactions, and symptoms. Deriving essential points from the material in these chapters, we leave you with a baker's dozen take-home points which we hope enrich your understanding and clinical work as much as they have ours.

1. Interpersonal traumatic stressors in early life have a biological impact that can fundamentally alter the structure and functioning of areas in the brain that are essential to a child's development of nonverbal and emotional forms of intelligence and an integrated sense of self (see Chapters 1 and 2), and how both the past and future are understood (see Chapter 2). It is important to think of psychiatric disorders as *neuro*psychiatric disorders that are influenced by and also alter child development.

2. When the shock and threat of traumatic stressors are compounded by the obviation, disruption, or loss of fundamental attachment bonds,

brain development is particularly vulnerable to impairment (see Chapters 1 and 2), and the corresponding development of a sense of self (see Chapter 3) and capacity to trust and engage in healthy relationships (see Chapters 3 and 4) often are profoundly impaired. Relational trauma is more than an event; it is a process that extends over time and that has significant compounding elements, such as betrayal of primary responsibilities and roles. Children are especially vulnerable due to their immaturity, physical size, lack of power, accessibility and dependency, and the fact that they are in the process of development, both physically and psychically.

3. Although a majority of children experience some form of psychological trauma before or during adolescence, there is a subgroup that can be identified in every community (in health care, school, and legal as well as mental health and child welfare systems) that experience multiple forms of trauma often involving adversity or victimization, such as abuse, neglect, and shattered families or family, community, or peer violence from an early age. These polyvictims suffer from the impact of cumulative trauma exposure, and as a result they are highly susceptible to extremely complex problems in physical, emotional, cognitive, and behavioral development and health (see Chapter 5).

4. Providing effective treatment for children and adolescents who are survivors of complex trauma (i.e., polyvictims) requires therapy models that have been tested scientifically and found to be effective (i.e., evidence-based treatments or practices), but also "clinical creativity, guided by sound clinical theory, evidence-based assessment, wise clinical judgment, and an evolving evidence base" (Chapter 6).

5. Formulating an understanding of the problems, needs, and strengths of a polyvictim child or youth is the essential first step in developing a plan and approach to therapy. The distinct but interrelated domains of self-regulation—including physiological, affective, cognitive, behavioral, relational, and identity—provide a conceptual framework and a link to validated assessment tools for the clinician (see Chapter 7).

6. No clinician can master all, or even most, of the available interventions and practices that have shown evidence of effectiveness in helping polyvictimized children and adolescents recover from the biopsychosocial impairments in self-regulation. Still, there is a core set of treatment practices and principles that can be taught (see Chapter 6) and systematically utilized (see Chapter 8) in order to take full advantage of the scientific and clinical innovations that have occurred in the traumatic stress field. These have also been addressed in a chapter devoted to the best practices in the treatment of children and adolescents in our previous book on the treatment of complex trauma (Ford & Cloitre, 2009).

7. Dissociation is a particularly challenging manifestation of trauma-related impaired self-regulation, and its manifestations in children's attentional, physical (conversion), information-processing, identity, and

behavioral and relational problems are crucial for therapists to recognize. Specifically: "Regardless of the therapist's approach to treatment, attention to the dissociated feelings, sensations, cognitions, experiences and/or self-states of the child is essential for the child to reconnect to all aspects of the self" (Chapter 9).

8. Many of the most refractory psychological problems in childhood or adolescence are exacerbated by the all-too-often undetected dilemma of persistent, intrusive reexperiencing of trauma memories and trauma-related physical and emotional states. With adaptations to address potential barriers and pitfalls that may interfere with safe and effective treatment, the two most widely used approaches to helping children and adolescents process trauma memories and create coherent personal narratives—trauma-focused cognitive-behavioral therapy (TF-CBT; see Chapter 10) and eye movement desensitization and reprocessing (EMDR; see Chapter 11)—have shown promise with polyvictimized children and adolescents.

9. A widely used therapy originally developed for other severe psychiatric disorders and dangerous behaviors, dialectical behavior therapy (DBT; see Chapter 12), and an innovative biopsychosocial "neurosequential" model (see Chapter 13) are potentially valuable additions to the clinician's toolkit for treating complex traumatic stress disorders.

10. The translational research approach to bringing the insights of science into clinical practice and the longstanding tradition of deriving innovations in psychotherapy from the creative clinical insights of experienced therapists (see Chapter 6) have resulted in a flowering of evidence-informed and clinically savvy intervention models for child and adolescent survivors of complex trauma and their families. Several complementary complex trauma-focused therapies have been explicitly designed to enhance trauma-impaired self-regulation and relational capacities (see Chapter 14).

11. Therapists working with children who are survivors of complex trauma can expand their perspective and their resource base by drawing on models of organizational change based on creating environments that provide a sanctuary from trauma (see Chapter 15) and systems of care that intentionally provide resources to restore self-regulation by children, adolescents, and their families and communities (see Chapter 18).

12. Families that have suffered generations of victimization, including historical trauma (see Chapter 16 on child–parent psychotherapy) or the severe strain of prolonged conflict and maltreatment (see Chapter 17 on parent–child interaction therapy and Chapter 18 on trauma systems therapy) may have to deal not only with posttraumatic dysregulation in their children but also with dysregulation in the adult caregivers, who have their own complex trauma histories and impairments. Helping caregivers and children to build (or regain) their capacities for self-regulation simultaneously is a key step toward ending what otherwise has become the tragedy of intergenerational cycles of complex trauma and breakdown of the family.

13. Even with all these inspiring advances in the understanding and treatment of children's and adolescents' complex traumatic stress disorders, every client with a complex trauma history remains a unique challenge for the clinician. Additionally, the client's ethnocultural influences must be assessed and treatment tailored to his or her particular needs and contexts (Brown, 2009). Each new case provides the opportunity not just to repeat the successful approaches of the past but to go a step or two further in building a scaffold from the current evidence or knowledge base to as yet undiscovered or unimagined innovations. As Tolstoy (p. 1) noted in telling the tale of a complex trauma survivor, Anna Karenina, "Happy families are all alike, and every unhappy family is unhappy in its own way" (p. 1). Understanding the "unhappiness" (i.e., trauma-related dysregulation) that is uniquely the case for each polyvictimized child and his or her family remains the core challenge, despite the wealth of knowledge and tools that innovative researchers and clinicians have provided us.

Beyond these key summary points, we would like to focus readers' attention on several thematic issues that run through this book and that point to the future of the field.

Evidence-Based Practice

In the predecessor volume to this book, we noted that, for children and adolescents (Ford & Cloitre, 2009) as well as for adults (Courtois, Ford, & Cloitre, 2009), empirically supported therapies are essential but not the complete answer to the effective treatment of clients with complex trauma histories and equally complex biopsychosocial developmental problems (see also Cohen, Berliner, & Mannarino, 2010; Lang, Ford, & Fitzgerald, 2011). The American Psychological Association (2006) Presidential Task Force on Evidence Based Practice recommended that the experience of skilled clinicians and the values and preferences of ethnoculturally diverse clients (in this case, children and families) should be included in any treatment plan and in related determination that a psychotherapy practice is "evidence based." Dissemination scientist-practitioners in the child and adolescent psychotherapy field similarly recommend that intervention models and their real-world implementation should be informed by the professional observations of clinicians and the lived experience of clients and their families (Chapter 6; Godley, Garner, Smith, Meyers, & Godley, 2011; Weisz et al., 2011). Thus, the empirically supported and informed therapy models described in this book must be applied in flexible ways that are responsive to the needs of the individual child and family and his or her particular ethnocultural and other contexts.

We also want to emphasize that the models described in this book are exemplary in two ways. They represent some of the best and most current thinking and the meticulous clinical and research efforts of leaders in the field. But they also are examples and not an exhaustive portfolio. In addition to the intervention models we noted in the "baker's dozen" conclusions above, and which were highlighted individually in earlier chapters, we refer readers to other innovative treatment models that have emerged from clinicians' careful observation and attunement to the experience and worldview of clients with complex trauma histories. These include four models briefly described in Chapter 14 (Trauma Affect Regulation: Guide for Education and Therapy [TARGET], Affect/Regulation/Competence [ARC], Structured Psychotherapy for Adolescents Responding to Chronic Stress [SPARCS], and Real Life Heroes [RLH]). Also important to acknowledge are therapy models that have been developed to address the need for integrating emotion and interpersonal regulation skills training with trauma memory processing (Skills Training in Affect and Intepersonal Regulation [STAIR]; Cloitre, Cohen, & Koenen, 2006; Trauma and Grief Components Therapy [TGCT]; Layne et al., 2008), treat co-occurring traumatic stress and substance use disorders (Seeking Safety; Najavits, Gallop, & Weiss, 2006), systematic early intervention (Child and Family Traumatic Stress Intervention [CFTSI]; Berkowitz, Stover, & Marans, 2011), and help victimized children in school settings (Cognitive Behavioral Intervention for Trauma in the Schools [CBITS]; Stein et al., 2003).

This remarkable array of therapeutic models and other approaches for children and adolescents with complex trauma histories (most of which have been developed or adapted in the past decade) demonstrate the extent and rapidity of innovation in treatment models that has been spurred by translation of developmental trauma science into therapeutic principles and practices.

Clinical Conceptualization and Diagnosis

We have followed the lead of several groundbreaking clinical research programs in emphasizing that the clinical challenge posed in understanding and effectively treating children and adolescents with complex trauma histories is complicated by the combination of traumatic victimization and by the loss of, or abandonment by, primary caregivers who are impaired (e.g., by mental health or substance use problems), neglectful, or victims themselves of past or current traumatic maltreatment or violence that interferes with their ability to parent successfully (Charuvastra & Cloitre, 2008; D'Andrea, Ford, Stolbach, Spinazzola, & van der Kolk, 2012; see also Chapters 1 and 3). As pointed out in Chapter 14, these kinds of "developmentally adverse interpersonal traumas" (Ford, 2005, p. 410) increase children's risk not only for anxiety or affective disorders (e.g., posttraumatic stress disorder [PTSD]) but also for a wide range of lifelong externalizing and physical health disorders due to deficits in core self-regulatory capacities (e.g., emotion dysregulation, dissociation, physical illness, social withdrawal or aggression; Cloitre, Stovall-McClough, Zorbas, & Charuvastra, 2008; D'Andrea et al., 2012; Felitti et al., 1998; Koenen, 2006).

Neurobiologically, this combination of threat/violation and loss/lack of protection seems to engender a shift in the brain (and body) from self-regulation via exploration and learning to hypervigilant dysregulation in service of threat detection and escape/avoidance or reactive aggression (Ford, 2009; Lanius et al., 2010; see also Chapters 1, 2, and 13). Hypervigilance and self-protective adaptations designed to promote survival involve very different patterns of brain activation that facilitate rapid automatic adjustments to avert harm and mobilize or diminish arousal (Neumeister, Henry, & Krystal, 2007), instead of neural connections necessary for the development of self-regulation (Lanius et al., 2010; Rauch, Shin, & Phelps, 2006). Survival-based dysregulation not only overutilizes bodily systems essential to preventing exhaustion, injury, or illness ("allostasis"; Friedman & McEwen, 2004), but in childhood it fundamentally alters ways of perceiving, feeling, thinking, interacting, and defining self or identity in ways that are extremely difficult to alter later in life and that can have lifelong negative impact (see Chapters 1 and 13). These dysregulated children tend to carry a large basket of internalizing (e.g., depression, bipolar disorder, anxiety disorders, eating disorders, reactive attachment disorder) and externalizing reactions and symptoms (e.g., intermittent explosive disorder, attention-deficit/hyperactivity disorder [ADHD], oppositional defiant disorder, substance use disorders) (D'Andrea et al., 2012). They often have severe PTSD symptoms (Ayer et al., 2009) but frequently are not diagnosed with PTSD (Cloitre et al., 2009). With all this baggage, it is tragic but not surprising that they are at risk for severe problems with psychosocial self-regulation in adulthood (Althoff, Verhulst, Rettew, & Hudziak, & van der Ende, 2010).

As noted in Chapter 14, a new psychiatric diagnosis has been proposed for dysregulated traumatized children, developmental trauma disorder (DTD; van der Kolk, 2005), but ultimately was not included in DSM-5. Although the danger of further burdening children who have emotional and behavioral problems with yet another diagnosis is always present, a principal purpose of diagnosis is to guide not only the delivery but also the design of treatment interventions. When children and adolescents receive multiple diagnoses and treatments for problems that may have a unique final common pathway—biopsychosocial dysregulation due to persistent survival-based hypervigilance—targeting that singular problem in adaptation could reduce the polytherapy and polypharmacy now deployed. And targeting specific symptoms or symptom dimensions may be no more direct or efficient than a diagnosis-based approach, and possibly less, because that too can lead to a menu of therapies rather than an integrated therapeutic strategy. The development of alternative approaches to diagnosing polyvictimized children that are not limited to the symptoms of PTSD and that do not impose the burden and risks of complex collections of comorbid psychiatric disorders, is not only consistent with the scientific evidence of complex sequelae of childhood victimization (see Chapter 14), but could spur the development and application of more efficient and safer treatments such as those described in this volume. Consistent with this view, developers of the best validated psychotherapy for traumatized children, TF-CBT, have proposed that treatment must address impairments in self-regulation when children present with severe behavioral or emotional dysregulation as a result of past or ongoing victimization (Cohen et al., 2010; Cohen, Mannarino, Kliethermes, & Murray, 2011).

Nevertheless, before undertaking the massive changes in mental health systems that are required when a new (or modified) diagnosis is established, it is important to determine whether the costs and effort are justified by the incremental clinical utility of a proposed diagnosis (First, 2005). One of the best tests—although by no means the only one—of clinical utility is whether a diagnosis both spurs the development of effective treatments and is shown to be ameliorated by therapies that address its core sources of pathology or maladjustment. Although the therapies described in this volume were not, with the partial exception of those in Chapter 14, developed purposefully to address DTD, the framework from which DTD evolved has been an inspiration for many of the key elements and features in those therapies (e.g., emotion regulation, restoring secure attachment working models). Results from an international field trial testing the DTD syndrome are providing a first indication of its potential clinical utility (Ford et al., in press). Meanwhile, clinicians who employ the therapy models that are described in this book will have the opportunity to use the structured interview for DTD (available from *jford@uchc.edu*) in their practices and evaluate clinically whether DTD provides a useful framework for conceptualizing and tracking progress in changing the posttraumatic self-regulation problems experienced by their clients.

Closing Words: Walking the (Self-Regulation and Attachment Security) Walk

The caveat that most commonly ends clinical texts and presentations is a call to therapists not to lose sight of their own professional and personal self-care in the midst of the excitement and turmoil of providing treatment to clients with complex trauma histories and severe self-regulation difficulties. The fascination with the "case" and with the "evidence-based treatment" can distract even the most experienced and savvy therapist from the impact of vicarious trauma and compassion fatigue. This can be a comforting distraction when the poignancy of clients' suffering, and the frustration and despair engendered by the inertia and setbacks that are endemic in their treatment (and in the systems that offer the treatment), weigh heavily on caring and diligent professionals. Yet, there are serious countertransference responses awaiting any of us when we choose avoidance over awareness (Brown, 2009; Kinsler, Courtois, & Frankel, 2009; Pearlman & Caringi, 2009).

Treating children and adolescents with complex trauma histories and complex forms of biopsychosocial dysregulation provides learning moments for therapists that don't arise in treating adult clients. Children tend to be much more transparent than adults in communicating (albeit often unconsciously or, at most, with a limited focal awareness) when they don't feel safe and secure or don't know how to handle what's happening or how the therapist is interacting with them. They react symptomatically, at times with some defensive disguise, but also quite often without guile or concealment. Adolescents tend to be less transparent but much more direct than either children or adults when they feel unsafe, unheard, or invalidated. And both children and adolescents gravitate away from adults who are dysregulated and toward adults who are aware of their own emotional states and able to regulate and to accurately respond rather than react.

Thus, regardless of one's theoretical orientation or technical approach to diagnosis and treatment, there is no hiding from the obligation to consciously self-regulate when treating children or adolescents with complex trauma histories. On a positive note, the therapies that are available to guide practice with these youths and their families offer a treasure trove of ways for therapists not only to teach but moreover to role model how to self-regulate under stress. "Walking the walk," therefore, is an opportunity to apply the best features of these therapies to our own biopsychosocial adaptation, and in so doing, to make therapy genuinely collaborative and a process of respectful co-learning and co-development. Our clients have the chance to resume, or finally begin, their personal development, and we as therapists have the opportunity to facilitate that essential recovery by applying what we teach to ourselves. In so doing, we can enhance the effectiveness of treatment by demonstrating directly that what we teach we also practice.

References

Althoff, R. R., Verhulst, F. C., Rettew, D. C., Hudziak, J. J., & van der Ende, J. (2010). Adult outcomes of childhood dysregulation: A 14-year follow-up study. *Journal of the American Academy of Child and Adolescent Psychiatry, 49*(11), 1105–1116.

American Psychological Association. (2006). Evidence-based practice in psychology. *American Psychologist, 61*, 271–285.

Ayer, L., Althoff, R., Ivanova, M., Rettew, D., Waxler, E., Sulman, J., et al. (2009). Child Behavior Checklist Juvenile Bipolar Disorder (CBCL-JBD) and CBCL Post-traumatic Stress Problems (CBCL-PTSP) scales are measures of a single dysregulatory syndrome. *Journal of Child Psychology and Psychiatry, 50*, 1291–1300.

Berkowitz, S. J., Stover, C. S., & Marans, S. R. (2011). The Child and Family Traumatic Stress Intervention: Secondary prevention for youth at risk of developing PTSD. *Journal of Child Psychology and Psychiatry, 52*(6), 676–685.

Brown, L. S. (2009). Cultural competence. In C. Courtois & J. D. Ford (Eds.), *Treating complex traumatic stress disorders: An evidence-based guide* (pp. 102–123). New York: Guilford Press.

Charuvastra, A., & Cloitre, M. (2008). Social bonds and posttraumatic stress disorder. *Annual Review of Psychology, 59,* 301–328.

Cloitre, M.,, Cohen, L., & Koenen, K. (2006). *Treating survivors of childhood abuse: Psychotherapy for the interrupted life.* New York: Guilford Press.

Cloitre, M., Stolbach, B. C., Herman, J. L., Kolk, B. V., Pynoos, R., Wang, J., et al. (2009). A developmental approach to complex PTSD: Childhood and adult cumulative trauma as predictors of symptom complexity. *Journal of Traumatic Stress, 22,* 399–408.

Cloitre, M., Stovall-McClough, C., Zorbas, P., & Charuvastra, A. (2008). Attachment organization, emotion regulation, and expectations of support in a clinical sample of women with childhood abuse histories. *Journal of Traumatic Stress, 21*(3), 282–289.

Cohen, J., Berliner, L., & Mannarino, A. (2010). Trauma focused CBT for children with co-occurring trauma and behavior problems. *Child Abuse and Neglect, 34,* 215–224.

Cohen, J. A., Mannarino, A. P., Kliethermes, M., & Murray, L. A. (2012). Trauma-focused CBT for youth with complex trauma. *Child Abuse and Neglect, 36*(6), 528–541.

Courtois, C., Ford, J. D., & Cloitre, M. (2009). Best practices in psychotherapy for adults. In C. Courtois & J. D. Ford (Eds.), *Treating complex traumatic stress disorders: An evidence-based guide* (pp. 82–103). New York: Guilford Press.

D'Andrea, W., Ford, J. D., Stolbach, B., Spinazzola, J., & van der Kolk, B. A. (2012). Understanding interpersonal trauma in children: Why we need a developmentally appropriate trauma diagnosis. *American Journal of Orthopsychiatry, 82,* 187–200.

Felitti, V. J., Anda, R. F., Nordenberg, D., Williamson, D. F., Spitz, A. M., Edwards, V., et al. (1998). Relationship of childhood abuse and household dysfunction to many of the leading causes of death in adults: The Adverse Childhood Experiences (ACE) study. *American Journal of Preventive Medicine, 14*(4), 245–258.

First, M. B. (2005). Clinical utility: A prerequisite for the adoption of a dimensional approach in DSM. *Journal of Abnormal Psychology, 114*(4), 560–564.

Ford, J. D. (2005). Treatment implications of altered neurobiology, affect regulation and information processing following child maltreatment. *Psychiatric Annals, 35,* 410–419.

Ford, J. D. (2009). Neurobiological and developmental research: Clinical implications. In C. Courtois & J. D. Ford (Eds.), *Treating complex traumatic stress disorders: An evidence-based guide* (pp. 31–58). New York: Guilford Press.

Ford, J. D., & Cloitre, M. (2009). Best practices in psychotherapy for children and adolescents. In C. Courtois & J. D. Ford (Eds.), *Treating complex traumatic stress disorders: An evidence-based guide* (pp. 59–81). New York: Guilford Press.

Ford, J. D., Grasso, D., Greene, C., Levine, J., Spinazzola, J., & van der Kolk, B. (in press). Clinical significance of developmental trauma exposure and symptoms: Results of an International Survey of Clinicians. *Journal of Clinical Psychiatry.*

Friedman, M. J., & McEwen, B. (2004). Posttraumatic stress disorder, allostatic load, and medical illness. In P. Schnurr & B. L. Green (Eds.), *Physical health consequences of exposure to extreme stress* (pp. 157–188). Washington, DC: American Psychological Association.

Godley, S. H., Garner, B. R., Smith, J. E., Meyers, R. J., & Godley, M. D. (2011). A large-scale dissemination and implementation model for evidence-based treatment and continuing care. *Clinical Psychology: Science and Practice, 18*(1), 67–83.

Kinsler, P. J., Courtois, C. A., & Frankel, A. S. (2009). Therapeutic alliance and risk management. In C. A. Courtois & J. D. Ford (Eds.), *Treating complex traumatic stress disorders: An evidence-based guide* (pp. 183–201). New York: Guilford Press.

Koenen, K. (2006). Developmental epidemiology of PTSD: Self-regulation as a core mechanism. *Annals of the New York Academy of Sciences, 1071,* 255–266.

Lang, J. M., Ford, J. D., & Fitzgerald, M. M. (2011). An algorithm for determining use of trauma-focused cognitive-behavioral therapy. *Psychotherapy, 47*(4), 554–569.

Lanius, R. A., Bluhm, R. L., Coupland, N. J., Hegadoren, K. M., Rowe, B., Theberge, J., et al. (2010). Default mode network connectivity as a predictor of post-traumatic stress disorder symptom severity in acutely traumatized subjects. *Acta Psychiatrica Scandinavica, 121,* 33–40.

Layne, C. M., Saltzman, W. R., Poppleton, L., Burlingame, G. M., Pašalić, A., Duraković-Belko, E., et al. (2008). Effectiveness of a school-based group psychotherapy program for war-exposed adolescents: A randomized controlled trial. *Journal of the American Academy of Child and Adolescent Psychiatry, 47*(9), 1048–1062.

Najavits, L. M., Gallop, R. J., & Weiss, R. D. (2006). Seeking Safety therapy for adolescent girls with PTSD and substance use disorder: A randomized trial. *Journal of Behavioral Health Services and Research, 33,* 453–463.

Neumeister, A., Henry, S., & Krystal, J. (2007). Neurocircuitry and neuroplasticity in PTSD. In M. J. Friedman, T. M. Keane, & P. Resick (Eds.), *Handbook of PTSD* (pp. 151–165). New York: Guilford Press.

Pearlman, L. A., & Caringi, J. (2009). Living and working self-reflectively to address vicarious trauma. In C. A. Courtois & J. D. Ford (Eds.), *Treating complex traumatic stress disorders: An evidence-based guide* (pp. 202–222). New York: Guilford Press.

Rauch, S., Shin, L., & Phelps, E. (2006). Neurocircuitry models of posttraumatic stress disorder and extinction: Human neuroimaging research—past, present, and future. *Biological Psychiatry, 60,* 376–382.

Stein, B., Jaycox, L., Kataoka, S., Wong, M., Tu, W., Elliott, M., et al. (2003). A mental health intervention for schoolchildren exposed to violence: A randomized controlled trial. *Journal of the American Medical Association, 290,* 603–611.

Tolstoy, L. (1877/2000). *Anna Karenina* (R. Pevear & L. Volokhonsky, Trans.). London: Penguin.

van der Kolk, B. (2005). Developmental trauma disorder. *Psychiatric Annals, 35,* 439–448.

Weisz, J. R., Chorpita, B. F., Frye, A., Ng, M. Y., Lau, N., Bearman, S. K., et al. (2011). Youth top problems: Using idiographic, consumer-guided assessment to identify treatment needs and to track change during psychotherapy. *Journal of Consulting and Clinical Psychology, 79*(3), 369–380.

Index

An *f* following a page number indicates a figure; a *t* following a page number indicates a table.